GREAT JOYS, GREAT SORROWS

AN IMMIGRANT'S JOURNEY THROUGH SURGICAL RESIDENCY

A SURGEON'S TALE
BOOK 4

MICHAEL M MEGUID MD

This story was written using the ancient method of typing with two fingers, using antique references called diaries, letters, and occasionally photos, and drawing on the prehistoric ingenuity of the human brain.

ISBN: 978-0-9992988-6-2

M3 Scientific Media Publications, LLC
Marco Island, Florida 34145, USA
michaelmeguid.com

1970S SURGICAL RESIDENTS' SURVIVAL GUIDE WHO WORK 110 HOURS PER WEEK

- Eat when you can.
- Sleep when you can.
- Read when you can.
- Crap when you can.
- Go home when you can.
- Have sex when you can.
- Don't stand when you can sit.
- Don't sit when you can lie down.
- Don't stay awake when you can sleep.
- Don't fix it if it's not broken.
- Don't mess with the pancreas.
- A good operation is better than good sex.
- A bad operation is worse than a cold pizza.
- A wound heals from side to side regardless of the incision's length.
- During an operation, the enemy of good is better.
- Shit flows downhill.
- When there is a question between a resident and a nurse, the nurse always wins.
- Residents can be replaced. Nurses cannot.

- When in doubt about a patient, call your senior staff to keep them informed.
- Always ask for help if you don't know how to do something surgically.
- When called by the nurse, see the patient and the nurse to assess a problem.
- Answer your pages promptly.
- Learn to prioritize the many tasks that you have.
- Tell it like it is! Don't lie! Get the correct information.
- Engage in damage control when making a mistake. Accept liability for actions.
- Be courteous to others. Remember that respect breeds respect.
- Be a team player. What goes around comes around.
- Own your education. Invest time and effort in surgical practice.
- Be punctual; others depend on you. Respect their time.
- Document for the record often, wholly and accurately.
- Be helpful to fellow residents who become your colleagues and friends for life.
- Develop the skills to be efficient, dependable, and trustworthy.
- Sign in and sign out to avoid errors in management.
- Write a summary note to ensure continuity of patient care upon leaving the service.

CONTENTS

A SURGEON'S TALE

A HISTORICAL AUTOBIOGRAPHICAL EPIC MEDICAL SERIES

Spanning nearly a century—from the tumultuous 1930s to the early 21st century—the ongoing six-part story of *A Surgeon's Tale* is a sweeping historical biographical medical series that chronicles not only the life of Michael Meguid but also the intricate, often harrowing tapestry of the times in which the author lived. Set against an extraordinary backdrop of global upheaval and transformation, this profound human narrative of surgery explores the profound intersections of surgery, identity, multiculturalism, and personal destiny.

At its core, *A Surgeon's Tale* transcends the boundaries of memoir. It is a rich and multifaceted journey that explores the realm of medical discovery, ethical dilemmas, and the relentless demands of surgical life. It examines the broader social, political, and psychological forces that influenced him. Throughout its pages, a narrative unfolds of child neglect, intrigue, scientific deceit, and the revelatory process of discovery within the medical field. Illicit passions and heartbreaking betrayals emerge alongside stories of unyielding ambition and even family murder.

Meguid's journey—from his birth on the Giza Plain next to

the mighty pyramids, Cairo surrounded by opulence of grandparent's love with markets brimming with fresh fruit to food scarcity in a devastated post-war childhood in Hamburg, Prussian corporal punishment, maternal abandonment and neglect leading to childhood complex-PTSD (*Roots & Branches**), and through demanding competitive medical school in London (*Mastering the Knife**), with the distraction of illicit love (*Surgeon & Lovers**), followed by intense surgical training working 110 hours per week at Harvard hospitals (*Great Joys, Great Sorrows**)—*A Surgeon's Tale* is filled with both noble and nefarious characters—mentors, rivals, and liars—each revealing something essential about the human condition. The series exposes the rituals, hierarchies, language, and codes of surgery while navigating the raw emotional landscapes of childhood abandonment, love, betrayal, loss, alienation, and belonging.

A Surgeon's Tale is a human story that reveals a radiant thread of resilience. It serves as a testament to the endurance of the human spirit, the passion that propels us forward, and the triumph that can emerge even from the darkest corners of a life dedicated to the pursuit of meaning, truth, the seeking of love, and healing.

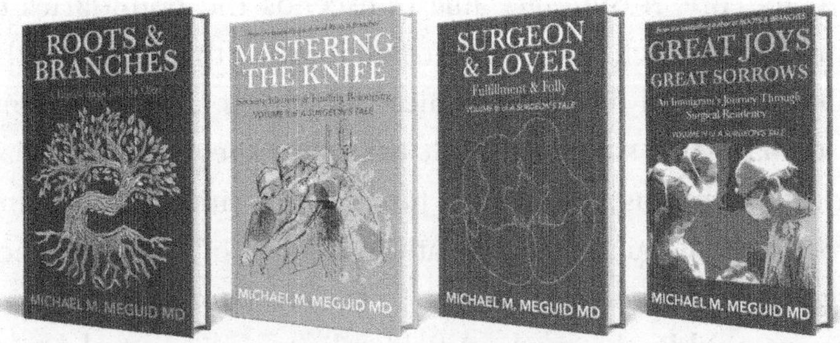

*Books are available on Amazon, Audible, and Kindle.

DEDICATION

To my surgical teachers, mentors, nurses, and fellow residents—many of whom ultimately became my esteemed colleagues—who taught, shaped, and nurtured my growth into a skilled surgeon.

I also dedicate this volume to all my patients, whom I have served with humility, and who continue to be a part of my memory.

Most medical students are attracted to surgery . . .
The bloody drama of the operation fascinates them.
The dramatic force of some great operator stirs their admiration.
They hear little of failures and know nothing of the haunting anxieties, the keen disappointments,
The baffling perplexities, the dread responsibilities,
And the numerous self-reproaches of one who spends his life as an operating surgeon.
—John Chalmers DaCosta, MD LLD

FOREWORD

Availability, Affability, and Ability
—Surgical Aphorism

In *Great Joys, Great Sorrows, An Immigrant's Journey Through Surgical Residency,* Michael Meguid continues to share with the reader the ins and outs of his life's voyage through time. In this book, the fourth in the series, *A Surgeon's Tale,* we learn of the relentless demands, emotional tolls, family sacrifices, and triumphs—the pleasures and pains of operating and caring for patients. We discover how surgical residents were molded in the 1970s—how Dr. Meguid was transformed from a naïve London intern into a skilled, independently operating Chief Surgical Resident and budding scientist through the forces imposed by a rigorous Harvard and Boston medical education. It was a historic time when residents worked 110 hours weekly to learn their skills and had no unions to give them a voice.

Meguid's book contains arresting details about the pressures of early general surgical residency, where some residents got divorced, others developed depression and burnout, and most worked for giants of surgery—all for a pittance! This occurred only a few decades ago in the same hospitals that are still pillars of our society.

With great humor and a prose style as exacting as a surgeon's scalpel, Meguid paints portraits of his fellow residents and professors, the titans and superheroes who taught, sculpted, and mentored his growth into a mature, competent surgeon.

Arriving in New York as an immigrant with a young wife and $48 in his pocket, he entered the American medical hierarchy. Fresh from an internship in London, England, he began as a lowly immigrant resident at The Peter Bent Brigham Hospital, Harvard Medical School. In this account of his journey, Meguid writes at times like a memoirist and at other times like an anthropologist or ethnographer.

I met this extraordinary, dedicated man in July 1971, shortly after I had graduated from medical school at Cornell University Medical College in New York City. I arrived in Boston to begin my surgical training at Harvard, at the Beth Israel Hospital under the direction of the preeminent (and my future lifelong mentor) Dr. William Silen. My first rotation was across the street on Longwood Avenue at the prestigious Boston Children's Hospital of Harvard Medical School. I was a surgical intern in the pediatric surgical service. One year above me, the second-year junior resident, who traditionally came from the Harvard sister teaching hospital, was Michael Meguid, from the famous Francis D. Moore's surgical residency at the Peter Bent Brigham.

We had the luxury and privilege of sharing some of our most precious and memorable surgical experiences while working together. We spent every waking hour operating, handling all the necessary chores, caring for very sick children every other night when we were on call, and sleeping, when possible, in the hospital (36-hour work on the weekends!) This was years before the mandatory "80-hour work week" or the recent introduction of the Residents' Union.

From the beginning, I recognized in Michael an intelligent, caring, and empathetic man with an insatiable curiosity—someone I genuinely enjoyed being around. Despite his seniority, he had an inclusive and humble manner when caring for his colleagues and surgical patients. The Children's Hospital was the pinnacle of pediatric surgery in the country, surrounded by true icons in the field. To say that it was somewhat intimidating would be an understatement!

Life is remarkable. Little did we know that some 50 years later, our paths would cross. Yet, it was a chance to relive the minute-by-minute drama I experienced at the beginning of my surgical training. This book recounts our shared experiences at Boston Children's Hospital, and it is just one part of this remarkable story.

Volume IV of *A Surgeon's Tale*, a unique and captivating series, is now available. This riveting life story, which began in Cairo and traversed war-torn Germany before reaching present-day Boston, is a must-read for those who appreciate a distinctive narrative style in medical literature.

For those of you who enjoy books, plays, television dramas, and movies about medicine, *Great Joys, Great Sorrows* will be a delight. Since colorful lives, careers, and relationships are intriguing and captivating, Meguid's fourth memoir is all that and more. I venture that its singular content and his responses to the challenges in his life would provide interest and fascination to any reader. I encourage you to enjoy a wonderful escapade. I would not miss it, as I couldn't put down each book in the series *A Surgeon's Tale*.

Richard A. Lynn, MD, FACS, RPVI
Past 2nd Vice-President of the
American College of Surgeons

AUTHOR'S NOTE

Life can only be understood backward, but it must be lived forwards.
—Søren Kierkegaard

Great Joys, Great Sorrows: An Immigrant's Journey through Surgical Residency continues the saga of *A Surgeon's Tale*. In this chapter of my life story, I share the intensity of my surgical journey as I learn the craft of surgery at Peter Bent Brigham Hospital and Boston Children's Hospital. This life intertwines with my role as a husband to Victoria and, after she completed a three-year pediatric residency, as a father to our young daughter, born out of love. I never imagined we would also bear the responsibilities of the "sandwich generation." Thus, the characters that readers met in previous volumes—Victoria's mother, Shirley, and particularly my biological mother (Mother), who has managed to elbow her way into this story with her unrealistic demands—remain relevant. In the second part of my residency training, found in Volume V of *A Surgeon's Tale*, space is generously dedicated to my cherished Oma—my surrogate mother of adoration and emotional support, for no story would be complete without her. Interwoven with my residency tale, I included memories of my childhood upbringing, including how growing up in different cultures at various ages has impacted current events in my life.

I've strived to be as authentic as possible in retelling the events of my surgical training in Boston during the 1970s, drawing on my personal archives, letters, photo albums, a log of operations performed, and copies of correspondence. Letters written over fifty years ago, once deemed private, are now included to enhance the narrative and contribute to a more subtle depiction of events and personalities. Certain characters and scenes are composites, and specific experiences have been rearranged to create a cohesive narrative. Names and identifying characteristics of individuals and patients have been omitted to protect their privacy. In some cases, I used names based on historical facts and records. As unique individuals, they may still find themselves represented in these pages. This account does not aim to provide the entire story. Others may recall the events differently or have their interpretations of what transpired.

To illustrate certain surgical conditions and complement the text, I have included drawings depicting aspects of an operation, created in collaboration with a young artist, Trent Muller. Poetry and music were my therapy for decompressing from the intense burnout I experienced, particularly while working at the Boston Children's Hospital. This volume features poetry and music that soothed my soul during those days and offered comfort throughout the lengthy process of solitary writing.

Furthermore, I found inner peace through the insightful and poignant writings of Maria Popova in *Brain Pickings*, which eventually became *The Marginalian*. I also listened to the Poet-a-Day streaming from the Academy of American Poets because, for me, poetry provides a sense of silence—"that quiet space," quoting Ada Limon, US Poet Laureate. I appreciate the sentiments expressed by the writer and poet Ursula K. Le Guin, who penned those lines with great clarity.

Science describes accurately from outside,
Poetry describes accurately from inside.
Science explicates; Poetry implicates.
Both celebrate what they describe.
—Ursula K. Le Guin

My account of the techniques used to train surgical residents toward the end of the last century reflects the forces that shaped present-day surgeons, who are now wise older men on whom we rely to maintain our health. I fully recognize that the structure and time limits of surgical residency have changed, and the institutions where I trained now have resident unions to advocate for better working conditions. I applaud them.

A Surgeon's Tale is an autobiographical series that represents a profound personal journey I began writing for my children and grandchildren, who were born in the land of the free. They know their grandparents were immigrants, like millions of others who came motivated by the desire for a better life and to contribute to this society, quoting Alfred, Lord Tennyson: "*To strive, to seek, to find, and not to yield.*" However, my offspring only have a vague understanding of the details; I don't burden them with the past when we are together. Instead, we focus on their budding launch into the society we helped create. If they are interested in my life—all its strivings and failures—they need look no further than the first three volumes and future installments, including this one of *A Surgeon's Tale.*

This book continues *A Surgeon's Tale*, exploring an immigrant's adaptation to American culture while learning the discipline and art of surgery during my two-year intensive surgical residency at Harvard.

The second part of my six-year residency, *The Enemy of*

Good . . . is Better, Volume V of *A Surgeon's Tale*, will continue the story of my surgical training as I complete my research commitment in Dr. Moore's Laboratory for Surgical Research, followed by my training at the renowned Boston City Hospital.

Michael M Meguid, MD, PhD, FACS, MFA
Marco Island
July 2025

PART I

1970-1971

Peter Bent Brigham Hospital, Harvard University

Assistant Junior Surgical Resident
PG-2

Life is short, and the Art is long.
The occasion is fleeting.
Experience is fallacious, and judgment is difficult.
—First Aphorism of Hippocrates

PROLOGUE

Oaths are but words, and words but wind . . .
—Samuel Butler

"The Chief is dead!" A voice came over the crackling landline.

"Who? Dr. Moore?"

I was a guest lecturer on surgical nutrition at the Surgeons' Nutrition Congress in Pretoria, South Africa, when his son, Chip, called to share the devastating news. My surgical role model's life ended on November 24, 2001, about 27 years after I physically left the Brigham, although my emotional connection lingered on.

"Would you be coming to his memorial service at the Harvard University Chapel on Friday, December 21?" Chip, the young Francis D. Moore, asked.

What a measured question! Would I attend?

1

THE CHIEF OF CHIEFS

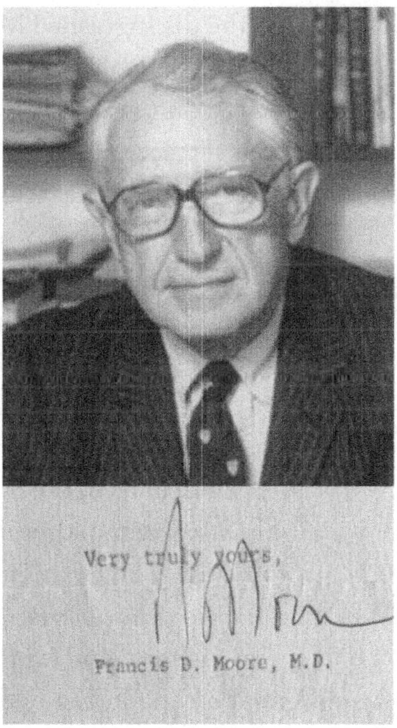

In caring for patients, don't trip over a blade of grass.
—Francis D. Moore, MD

Considered the most influential force in American surgery during the second half of the twentieth century, Dr. Moore was larger than life—an inspiring, stimulating, yet demanding figure at the pinnacle of the surgical world. I respected him as a surgeon-scientist par excellence and sought the opportunity to work with him. His philosophy of assuming complete responsibility for the patient's welfare appealed to me. Furthermore, I endorsed his views that surgeons should be obligated to participate in approved clinical studies involving patients to apply the lessons we learn to the next patient.

The true seduction of Michael Meguid began some three years previously, on December 13, 1967, when I first met Dr. Moore. The esteemed man was the Surgeon-in-Chief at Peter Bent Brigham Hospital and the distinguished Mosely Professor of Surgery at Harvard Medical School in Boston. The iconic surgeon-scientist had appeared on the cover of Time Magazine for his groundbreaking surgical research.

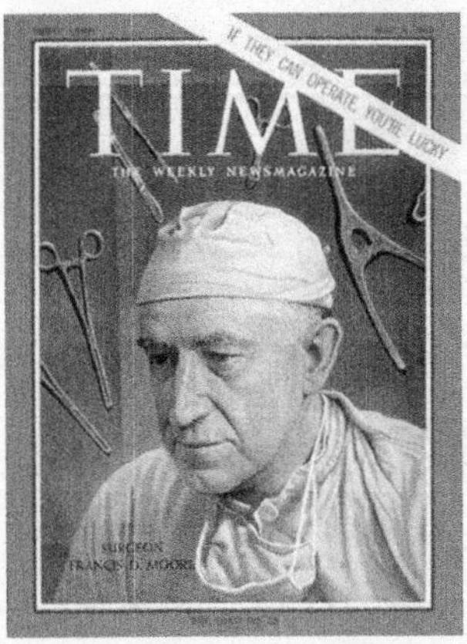

These characteristics drew me to my idol, who once said, "The surgical investigator must be a bridge tender, channeling knowledge from biological science to the patient's bedside and back again. He traces his origins from both ends of the bridge; he is thus a bastard, and everyone calls him this. Those at one end of the bridge say he is not a very good scientist, and those at the other say he does not spend enough time in the operating room." I profoundly believed in and trusted his philosophy.

I became an apostle, an emissary of his belief, practicing according to "St. Francis of the Brigham." I imagined him embodying my father's features; like any admirer, I wanted to be like him.

Before my first meeting with him, I completed a six-week elective at Mass General Hospital from November to December 1967 at the invitation of Dr. Gerald Austin. He was another surgical giant I met in Boston while fulfilling my elective requirement in general surgery for the University College Hospital Medical School curriculum. The American concept of structured residency training in surgery over five years appealed to me, as this model had not been widely implemented in Britain at that time.

"If you want to do some research as well," my senior resident at Mass General, Dr. Sugarbaker, had said, "then the place to go is the Peter Bent Brigham Hospital, where the chief of surgery is a surgeon-scientist." Given that it was already December and late in the selection process for new residents, he encouraged me to call Dr. Moore's office and apply for an interview immediately.

Two days later, on the same day Victoria flew in from London for our wedding in Boston, I had an eleven o'clock interview with Dr. Moore. While we waited outside his office, the door suddenly opened, and an imposing figure in a white coat greeted us. We stood up. He appeared intensely curious, scholarly, and professorial, with horn-rimmed glasses and graying temples. His charismatic presence absorbed all the oxygen in the anteroom, for such was the quality of his company. He embodied charm and grace, congratulating us on our marriage and shaking Victoria's hand. She looked glamorous in her mother's luxurious mink coat over a red suit and stayed outside during my interview.

Sitting across from me at his neatly organized, paper-covered desk, he leaned forward, holding a pad and pen, jotting down notes as we spoke. Serious, probing, and compassionate, he matter-of-factly asked a series of questions—who was my father, what had he done, what did I want to do in life, and what were my research interests?

"I am interested in physiology and metabolism and in how the body functions or reacts to the stress and injury of a surgical operation, with particular emphasis on body fluids and electrolytes."

He sat back in his chair, pensive, and eyed me. Further questions followed. Finally, he asked me the names of the individuals I had worked with during my time on the surgical service at Mass General. After reflection, he said, "There may be an opportunity as a second-year resident for two years starting next July 1968, followed by research for one or two years in my lab." He nodded at the end of the sentence as if painting a full stop, signaling the interview's conclusion.

I smiled joyfully at his optimistic tone and heard the cautionary, "I'll write to you shortly." With that, he stood up. The interview lasted barely ten minutes—quite formal, albeit constructive. I liked the man and his decisive thought process, despite being amazed by the abrupt change in demeanor when greeting and interviewing me—one congenial and social, the other entirely businesslike. As I got to know him professionally while working at the Brigham, and then personally over five years of my many Friday morning visits when he was retired and writing his memoir, *A Miracle & A Privilege*, I unearthed the various pieces of the puzzle that defined Dr. Moore's complex persona. He gradually opened up to me, yet I felt he never quite revealed himself.

Perhaps others, too, felt the same.

Captivated by his dynamic character during our brief interview, I overlooked some critical facts. First, I would graduate from University College Hospital Medical School in London in July 1968. After that, I needed to complete a one-year house job/internship, a mandatory requirement to finish my medical training in England and become a fully registered physician in the UK, which I would need if America didn't work out.

The second, equally important point was that Victoria, who was a year behind me academically, would graduate in July 1969. She, too, would need to complete her year of house jobs to become a qualified physician—a security I wanted for my wife. Therefore, we could not go to Boston until July 1970, which was later than Dr. Moore had initially understood and planned. Lastly, the possibility of a pediatric residency for my wife had not yet been explored.

Weeks later, through a series of letter exchanges, I realized he couldn't recall much from our interview. I sensed the precariousness of my job offer. Amid the ensuing confusion, he requested several letters of recommendation.

I requested letters from Mr. Hart, a senior surgeon for whom I had done a locum while I was a student, who quaintly described me as "my surgical dresser"; from Mr. Kingdom, with whom I completed my six months as a house surgeon at the Royal Ear Hospital; from Dr. Gilliland, my chief at Bethnal Green Hospital during my medical house job and the man who taught me to publish or perish; from Dr. Stern, the neurology consultant who first taught me clinical medicine; and from Nobel Laureate Professor Huxley, my professor of physiology and the president of the medical school's Physiology Society, for whom I served as chairman. All of them kindly vouched for my competence and integrity.

Afterward, I received a charming letter of appointment, along with academic student non-immigrant visas issued by Harvard at his request, which allows Victoria and me to stay in the USA for five years. After that, we would have to return to England.

ORIGINAL COPY.

HARVARD MEDICAL SCHOOL
DEPARTMENT OF SURGERY

FRANCIS D. MOORE, M.D.
Moseley Professor of Surgery

Peter Bent Brigham Hospital
721 Huntington Avenue
Boston, Massachusetts 02115
Telephone 617 - 566-6226

17 June 1969

Dr. Michael Marwan Meguid
15 Albany Street
Regent's Park
London, N.W. 1
ENGLAND

Dear Dr. Meguid:

I have received fine recommendations about your work. We will therefore plan to have you join our residency staff in July, 1970, for two years of junior residency.

One of these years can be spent in the laboratory, if you so wish, but it is my understanding that you would like to have primarily clinical training.

Do let me know if this fits in with your wishes and plans.

Thank you very much.

Very truly yours,

Francis D. Moore, M. D.

FDM:scr

2

TRANSATLANTIC DREAM

We were strangers once, too.
—Barack Obama

I embarked on a lifelong dream of Victoria and me becoming doctors in Boston, Massachusetts, which began in 1967 when Victoria and I married in the city. In June 1970, we departed England on a scheduled transatlantic crossing aboard Cunard's iconic QE2 from Southampton to New York, bringing along two large steamer trunks on a late-summer day.

I passed the Royal College of Surgeons Primary Fellowship exam in London the previous week. This grueling written and oral exam tested my knowledge beyond the medical school level in applied anatomy, clinical physiology, and surgical pathology. Passing it, along with 20% of the other candidates, indicated that I was ready to begin surgical training and ascend the British surgical ladder. However, the thrill of success didn't bring joy. Instead, after two years of studying, I was overwhelmed by a tiredness and a fatigue that seeped deep into my bones, draining me physically, mentally, and emotionally.

Three years earlier, in November 1967, I interviewed with Dr. Francis D. Moore while completing my surgical elective at Mass General Hospital. In a letter I received after returning to London, he offered me two years of surgical training as a *provisional* resident, starting in July 1970, at the postgraduate (PG) levels PG-2 and PG-3. Following this, I had the option of pursuing one or two years of research, which I desired if the opportunity was available.

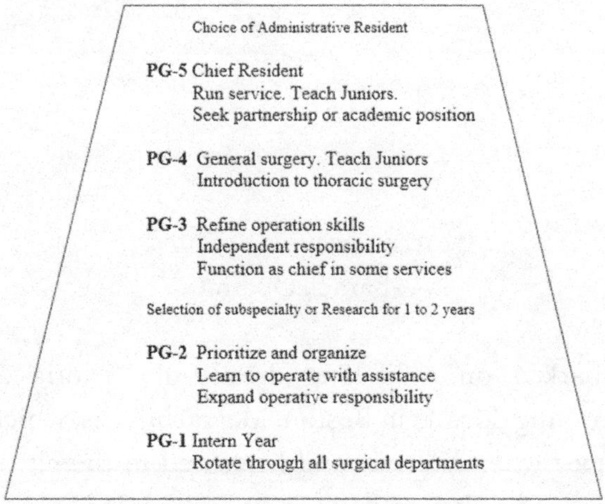

Ideally, I would have liked to be offered the chance to complete two additional clinical years as a PG-4 and PG-5, achieving five years of surgical training in this prestigious program under the aegis of Dr. Moore. I planned to sit for the American Board of Surgery certification examination and then return to London to take the final Royal College of Surgeons certification exam, thereby qualifying in both the United States and England, accommodating Victoria's potential wish to return to her country of birth. However, the PG-4 and PG-5 years were reserved for the *categorical* residents who had started their internships at Brigham. The term provisional resident inherently suggested that I could be weaned out if I didn't meet the standards of my categorical colleagues. Upon completing the PG-5 year, there was an option to become an Administrative Resident to assist Dr. Moore, commonly referred to by his acronym—"FDM"—in managing the residency. At the same time, he was also busy traveling and engaged in non-administrative work.

How could I have expected Dr. Moore to offer me more than his generous proposition? He didn't know me, my academic track record at London University, my drive and determination to succeed, or my willingness to work endless hours. If I pursued a second year of research in Dr. Moore's lab, waiting for a potential opening for a PG-4 and PG-5, that second year in the lab would be counted by the Accreditation Council for Graduate Medical Education as part of a five-year general surgical training to graduate as a fully qualified surgeon after passing the certification examination.

Victoria and I felt exhausted as we boarded the QE2 in Southampton, bound for New York, a result of ten years of relentless study. My journey included three years as a student at a grammar school in Manchester after arriving from Cairo, followed by three years studying clinical medicine at University College Hospital, and two years focusing on basic medical science at University College London. While wandering through the anatomy dissection hall, I met the love of my life, Victoria Perfect. After completing the basic sciences, she pursued her clinical training at Westminster Hospital. We concluded our years of study with a six-month medical and surgical internship to apply everything we had learned. This mandatory internship in the distinguished British National Health Service (NHS), required by the General Medical Council, ensured our registration in the United Kingdom as bona fide physicians, granting us the right to practice general medicine in the community. It took me another two years to prepare for and pass the Primary Fellowship of the Royal College of

Surgeons. In the meantime, I completed a clinical elective in surgery at Mass General in Boston, where Victoria and I got married.

Victoria had completed nine years of stressful, continuous study, culminating in the mandatory internship. We had undertaken most of it as individuals at two medical institutions, with me a year ahead of her schedule. As a result, we faced different clinical training, vacation, and examination schedules, which put a strain on our marriage.

During this trip across the pond to Boston, we planned to relax, recuperate, and recapture the intimacy of love that stress and work had displaced while preparing ourselves for our new adventure in America. Given our considerable fatigue, achieving this was a significant challenge in just five stormy Atlantic days.

We boarded the QE2, the pride of the Cunard Line, in Southampton. Standing at the railing, we waved goodbye to our mothers on the quay while comforting each other and reflecting on the strain in our marriage caused by our disconnected schedules. Exhaustion affected us both since we hadn't had regular meals and had only managed fragmented sleep for months. We had endured intense periods of concentrated study, examinations, and a lack of consistent emotional or physical closeness. This trip was our chance to escape from our books and endless studying, allowing us to reconnect with one another.

The ship steamed into the English Channel to cross the pond. Our routine on board the QE2 was to sleep as long as possible and have breakfast in our cabin around 10 a.m., followed by lunch at an assigned table with an elderly American couple who had just returned from a much-cherished trip to their former Yugoslavia. They managed a gas station in Ohio, and when they learned we were new doctors, they told us we would become wealthy. We didn't grasp their meaning because we had become doctors in our idealistic youth with the lofty goal of serving mankind.

After lunch, we hurried to catch the 2 p.m. movie in the theater. At 4 p.m., we savored a traditional English tea that was hardly affordable for medical students—Kenyan black brew with milk, thinly sliced cucumber sandwiches, warm scones served with clotted cream and strawberry jam—luxuries we couldn't indulge in on our modest NHS doctors' incomes.

After a much-needed late afternoon nap, we dined again at our table with our new travel companions. After dinner, we escaped into a fantasy world by attending the 8 p.m. movie.

Depending on the nightly weather, we strolled the deck, gazing at the shimmering Atlantic when the sea was relatively calm, huddled together against the Atlantic gusts in our warmest clothes, or bobbed up and down in the ship's pool to avoid post-dinner seasickness during the roughest weather before crawling into bed at the early hour of 10:30 p.m.

Four days of this leisurely and luxurious routine at sea helped me get in touch with my beloved Victoria again. Love budded once more. Battling headwinds and choppy waves, the QE2 took five days to cross the Atlantic, reaching the shores of America on July 5, 1970.

We arrived in New York as academic students with non-immigrant visas. Although we didn't see ourselves as immigrants, we had brought all our earthly possessions to America, along with our emotional past and personal histories. I thought landing in America with $100 in my pocket would be sufficient. For a brief moment, we felt quite wealthy. The car we rented for $52 through the ship's radio, which was waiting for us at the dock while we were at sea, left us with $48, the only cash we had.

The Pontiac Executive four-door sedan resembled a behemoth shimmering in the dockside sun. At nearly nineteen feet long, it was twice the length of the average car on London's streets. Until then, I had only driven my mother's stick-shift Volkswagen and my mother-in-law Shirley's Ford sedan. Neither Victoria nor I was sure we could handle this steel beast.

The vehicle was large enough to hold our sea trunks. We placed one in the back seat, causing the car's rear to sag, while the other filled the trunk, making the back droop even more. The Pontiac's hood pointed upward, resembling a rocket more than a car. Unfamiliar with the automatic three-speed V-8 engine, I inadvertently shot off the docks into traffic, nearly sending us through the windshield when I slammed on the brakes to avoid a collision.

Before our departure, we almost canceled our trip to Boston after watching the movie Easy Rider. It left us feeling uneasy, anxious, and fearful. The film revealed a side of America we were unaware of—drugs, racial bigotry, sinister bikers, and long-haired hippies who rode through the American South with an indifferent attitude toward America's Black community. Our fear stemmed from our limited view of America portrayed in the movie and its reviews. However, we rationalized that Harvard was as safe as the institution where we had trained in London. We had a commitment, a booked passage, and the determination to go to America. I would gain insight into America's many contradictions and paradoxes in the years to come. The various contrasts between England and America struck us vividly. I could not understand how I had failed to notice these differences when I was a surgical student at Mass General three years ago.

America was at war, yet it pulsed with vitality and smiling faces. It was strikingly different from the effects of the two wars I experienced in 1948 and 1956 between Egypt, where I lived, and Israel. The wailing air raid sirens inflicted panic, fear, and anxiety on my sister and me as we rushed into the cellar upon hearing jets fly overhead, punctuated by the repeated cracks and booms of antiaircraft guns and the bombing in downtown

Cairo. The distant destruction of military installations and the reverberating explosions that shook the house instilled a feeling of terror. During the 1956 war, the toxic mix of unending propaganda echoed resounding victories from Cairo radio, while conflicting reports about the destruction of our air force and the defeat of our army heard on the BBC left us in a chronic state of mistrust and apprehension. We endured shortages of national consumer goods and commodities while fear, terror, and uncertainty prevailed daily among friends, family, and the nation. Here in America, the war was thousands of miles away from New York, but it wasn't always on everyone's mind.

The Vietnam War made headlines, as did the peace talks in Paris. Despite the Kent State massacre just two months earlier, everyday life continued at its privileged, leisurely pace. To celebrate the birth of American independence that July, Arthur Fiedler conducted rousing patriotic music with the Boston Pops for a festive crowd at the Hatch Memorial Shell. The Red Sox were playing at Fenway Park in their 70th season of Major League Baseball, finishing third in the American League East with 87 wins. Baseball grew in interest for us, especially after the Brigham gave us complimentary tickets to Fenway Park. This was America, Victoria, and I arrived in 1970, one day after Independence Day.

I drove while Victoria navigated us out of New York City through slow-moving traffic, marveling at the skyscrapers that loomed over us. The car's powerful engine purred as we traveled about 200 miles north from Brooklyn along Route 95 to Boston. The car's tilt gave me the impression that we were driving uphill as we headed north, dragging our heavy treasures behind us. We listened nonstop to country music and endless advertisements because we were unfamiliar with the preset channel buttons; pressing them resulted in garbled stations and static. Finally, we found a pop music station with "Raindrops

Keep Falling on My Head" and the rowdy "American Woman," which replayed repeatedly, interspersed with Simon and Garfunkel's melodious "Bridge over Troubled Water" and The Beatles' "The Long and Winding Road"—songs with nostalgic lyrics that reminded me of the London we had just left behind.

Unlike the rainy weather in England, the sun felt pleasant, and a warm, welcoming breeze flowed through the open windows. After a few hours, we stopped at Howard Johnson's for our first American meal—a generous serving of fried clams and a gigantic ice cream cone.

There still wasn't a cloud in the sky or a drop of rain on the horizon when Victoria and I finally arrived at 45 Marion Street, in a quiet, leafy residential area of Brookline, a suburb of Boston.

My friend Sheila, Professor Huxley's assistant secretary in London, now works at Harvard. She found an unfurnished second-floor apartment—two rooms with a kitchenette. She wrote that the rental "was nice, a bit pricey, a new building, and within walking distance to the hospital." We discovered it to be twice as large as our flat at 15 Albany Street in London. But then, we knew everything in America was "bigger and better."

Victoria and I were trying to haul our first trunk up the stairs when our new neighbors, Karen and Neil Goodman, appeared. Tall, athletic, and friendly, Neil immediately introduced himself and his wife, reminding us that Americans shake hands and always smile. They did this not only out of cordiality but also because they had perfect teeth. This highlighted the differing state of public dentistry in Europe, where having perfect teeth is not a priority. I had noticed the smiles of the immigration agent, the young and cheerful server at Howard Johnson's, and now Neil and Karen—something to practice.

Karen, a clinical psychologist, was as bubbly as Neil was reserved. They had moved into the building a year ago when

Neil started his first-year residency in Internal Medicine at Beth Israel, another nearby Harvard hospital.

Walking through our two-room flat with white-painted walls and parquet floors, they noticed our two trunks next to a couple of suitcases in our larger-than-life, empty condo.

"Where are you guys going to sleep?" Karen pondered.

We wondered, too.

They chatted and watched as we partially unpacked and spread out our British bedding, my Egyptian grandfather's blanket, and my German grandmother's pillows on the floor beneath the bedroom window.

"Right there!" we pointed. "We'll eventually get a box spring and a mattress."

"We recommend a Sealy, don't we, Neil? Macy's has a white sale this weekend with big discounts. You should go," Karen said.

"What's a white sale?"

"Steeply discounted household linens, bedding, towels, and similar merchandise."

"And they deliver," Neil added. "Is that your car?" he asked, nodding toward the street.

"No. It's a rental. Do we need one?"

"Aren't you going to work?"

"Yes, I hope we'll both work. Victoria has an interview near the end of July at the Children's Hospital Medical Center, and I started at Brigham a few days ago."

"But you're late," he said pensively. "Do they know? You better go soon."

"Yes, they consented to my late arrival."

"The hospital is at the other end of Longwood Ave. You'll need a car."

"No bus?"

He shook his head, looking at us in bewilderment. By

British standards, it was within a customary walking distance. For an American, maybe not.

Seeing our empty refrigerator, Karen took us to Stop and Shop. Victoria and I strolled through the endless aisles, amazed by the abundance of goods and various brands for a single staple. Unlike in England, peaches were cheaper than eggs! This was incredible. We shopped wisely, knowing we had just under $50. Our first grocery bill was around $35, which we paid in cash. Karen's bill exceeded $80, which she paid with a credit card. On the way to the mall, she filled her car at twenty-eight cents a gallon. It's cheaper than milk!

At Macy's, we selected a double-sized Sealy Posturepedic mattress with a base that would be delivered C.O.D. in three days. By then, we would have set up a bank account and transferred the remaining money from London from Mr. Winterberry, my first surgical patient during medical school. He was a rectal cancer patient and a stockbroker by trade who had invested my £5, which was one week of my food allowance, into a speculative mining company in Australia. "You might lose it, young man. But your small investment will become a fortune if they strike uranium as it's rumored."

He was right!

Karen told us people place unwanted furniture along the curb for trash collection on Tuesdays. "If you see an item you need, just pick it up.

"Really?"

"Yeah . . . and it's often good quality. Just help yourself."

Going through other people's discarded items felt inappropriate. It reminded me of my childhood in post-war Hamburg in 1948, when my sister and I lived with our elderly German grandparents, who spoke no Arabic. Anything that survived the war was salvaged from the ruins or rubble piles and given a new purpose. It evoked a sense of poverty and destitution, feelings that young doctors couldn't understand, but it may have been necessary.

We were immensely grateful to Neil and Karen Goodman for their kindness and guidance in providing information that helped us begin the lengthy acclimatization process: how to obtain a Social Security number, where to go to the bank, how to apply for a credit card, where to buy fresh food, and how to order a landline with AT&T. Even though we were both physicians and needed the phone, the landline wouldn't be installed for three business days. However, the noteworthy aspect was the cost—significantly cheaper than in London. Life was looking up as we navigated the social intricacies of America.

We unpacked lethargically, drained by Boston's summer heat, humidity, and the time zone difference, as we continued to organize our lives in our unfurnished apartment, uplifted at midday by the sound of a distant church bell. The only tangible link to our past life was what emerged from the trunks. The personal items from my steamer, once meaningful in London, now seemed almost insignificant in the uncertain shape and vastness of our new life. I grew apprehensive and restless in this amorphous and unclear mood, worrying about starting my surgical training late and missing the crucial orientation programs. By mid-afternoon, we experienced overwhelming fatigue and a mindset aptly described as 'jet-lag psychoses,' a disorientation due to the time zone difference afflicting us. Our reactions and emotions responded sluggishly, as if through molasses, impairing and distorting coherent thought and action.

We drank plenty of water that afternoon to combat the effects of travel dehydration and the oppressive heat. Weary from the intense sunshine, we rested in the late afternoon on our simple beds. We lay apart, sweating.

I wanted to embrace my wife, feel protected, and experience her affection. I had intensely missed her over the past year while she took care of the house chores, and I felt desperately alone with the fear of abandonment I had faced as a child. Being with her eased my sense of insecurity and anxiety about the decision to come to Boston. We held hands as our afternoon rest transformed into a confusing kaleidoscope of sleep, disrupted by disorientation. I was thankful to have her beside me now, free to touch and caress the porcelain skin of her face and body and stroke the places I cherished. She appreciated my touch, even despite the sticky sweat.

We woke up around 4 a.m., our bodies still on English time, suffering from jet lag—a desynchronized sleep disorder. The early morning sun streamed through our curtainless windows, causing our flat's temperature to rise to nearly 80°F with high humidity. Unused to air conditioning, despite having a built-in unit, we kept the windows open, comforted by our British habit of enjoying fresh air.

3

THE MIGHTY BRIGHAM

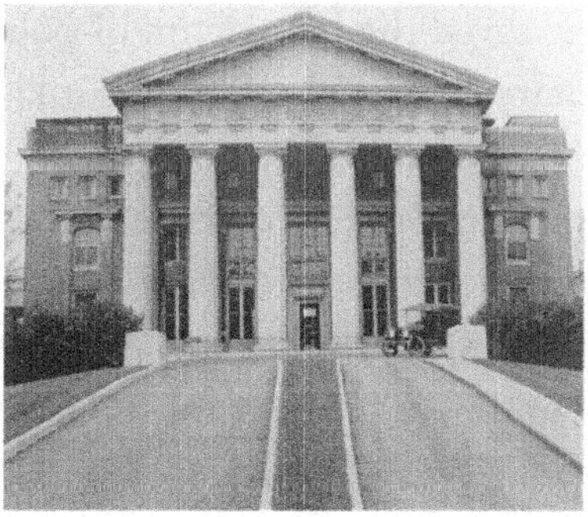

Assume complete responsibility for the welfare of the patient.
—Francis D. Moore

The day after we arrived, in late morning, I hurried under the warm sunshine to Peter Bent Brigham Hospital. Upon entering the remarkable rotunda, the milestones of the Brigham's legendary medical discoveries weighed heavily on my shoulders.

During the first decade of the twentieth century, a legacy from real estate baron Peter Bent Brigham and public funding established the hospital adjacent to Harvard Medical School. Opened to the public in 1913, its mission was "to provide for the care of sick persons of indigent circumstances." The hospital was designed with the lingering concept of contagion: the wards were spaced far apart and connected by a long corridor that spanned the entire length of the building, known as The Pike. Branching off to the south were four wards along Francis Street, while the administrative buildings extended opposite toward Shattock Street, the site of Harvard Medical School.

The institution's reputation was established through a series of distinguished surgeons and physicians. In 1923, Dr. Elliott Cutler conducted the world's first successful open-heart valve operation. Drs. Murphy, Whipple, and Minot received a Nobel Prize for curing pernicious anemia with vitamin B12. In 1929, the iron lung saved the first victim of polio, while Joseph Murray (Nobel Laureate) performed the first kidney transplant in 1954.

"The Department of Surgery office is in the basement," the clerk at the information booth told me. "Go down that main Pike," he said, pointing to a very long corridor that extended beyond the eye, "until you reach Ward D. Opposite it, take the stairs down one floor, and it'll take you into Dr. Moore's office suite."

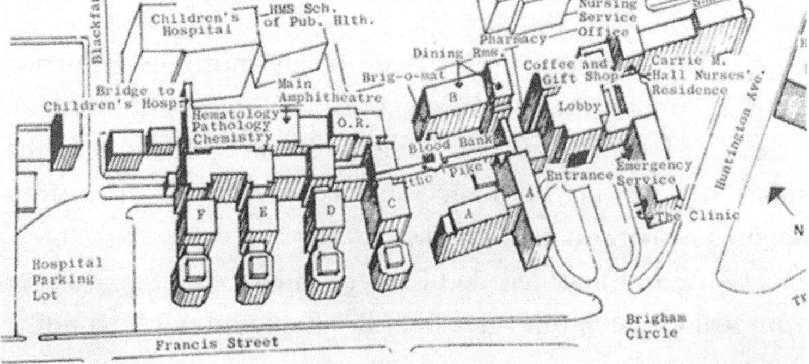

I walked into a hubbub of noise. Secretaries were typing or on the phone, some rushing about like a frantic bee colony. I stood at a counter in my gray suit, feeling very self-conscious. A woman paused her work and approached me with a welcoming, professional demeanor. When I announced myself, the young brunette with curious eyes and vibrant energy paged someone.

"I'm Gail," she added, "one of Dr. Moore's assistants." Then she walked away, only to return with a welcome package.

"Here is the key to your on-call room. When you return to the lobby, you'll notice narrow stairs leading up to the on-call rooms on the second floor."

"In that direction?" I questioned, pointing.

She nodded and resumed, "I'd show you, but women aren't allowed up there. You'll find six white uniforms and a leather Dopp kit on your bed." Seeing me question her statement, she added, "Toothbrush, comb, hairbrush, shaving kit, and face cloth—yours to keep. Dr. Moore wants the residents to look sharp." This was a different start to a job than in England.

"A staff dining room is open during the hours shown in this brochure. If you miss the assigned mealtimes, you can eat for free in the cafeteria when it closes to the public at eleven o'clock at night. You'll meet a lot of other residents there and . . ." As she spoke, a young man appeared, shot me a glance, and interrupted Gail's instructions.

"Are you the guy from England?"

"Yes?"

"You're late," he said to me. "I've been covering for you for days . . . at least six or eight fucking days and nights . . ." Before I could show him Dr. Moore's consenting letter, he continued in an angry voice tinged with venom, "Here." He shoved a pack of cards into my hands. "These are your orthopedic patients. This is your page receiver. You're on call today and this weekend."

"On call, now? Today? But I only arrived yesterday."

Still angry, he continued, "Yeah. Rounds with the team tomorrow at 7 a.m."

"But I'm a *general surgical resident*," I said emphatically. "I'm here for general surgery," I protested, "not orthopedics. Won't I be working with Dr. Moore?"

"You're assigned to start with ortho," and as if to emphasize facts, he added, "for the first rotation. And don't fuck it up."

"Where is this ortho team?"

"In the O.R. Don't ask me when they'll come out."

Dazed, I stood still, speechless. He abruptly took off. Gail's demeanor softened with a look of empathy; then she turned away and returned with a stack of books in her arms. "You'll need to read these to understand Dr. Moore's surgical philosophy, which dominates your training, the other residents tell me. It's the right way to do surgery."

While scanning the titles, I discovered that the first three contained material I would incorporate into my surgical identity—my philosophy as a surgeon and my interests: two on metabolism and one on breast disease, which greatly intrigued me.

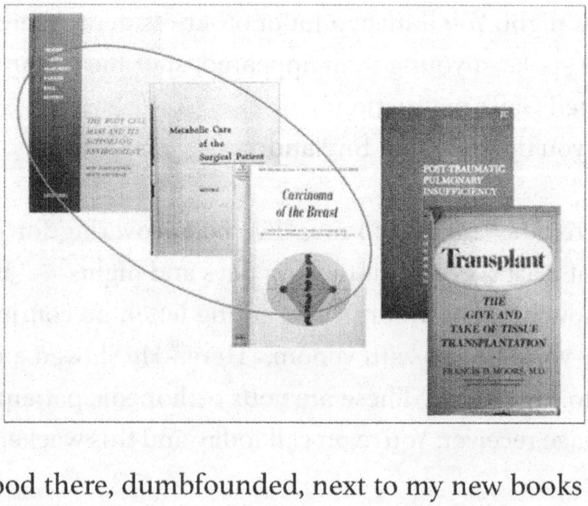

I stood there, dumbfounded, next to my new books stacked

on the counter in my gray suit, holding a bulky pager in one hand and a stack of 3x5 patient cards in the other.

Gail blushed at witnessing the handover. In medical school, I shied away from orthopedics, the field that focuses on the body's framework. I wanted to understand the body's function and physiology, and I didn't care much about its anatomical structure.

I asked Gail, "Can I see Dr Moore now to let him know I've arrived?"

"He's in Marion near the Cape on his summer vacation. He likes to sail. He pops in from time to time. I'll let him know you're here. There is a party for the residents on Labor Day weekend at his house in Marion. You'll meet him there." The prospect of meeting Dr. Moore at the party on Labor Day weekend filled me with excitement and curiosity.

"Labor Day weekend? When is that?"

"The weekend of September 7. You'll get a flyer in your mailbox."

"What happens at the party?"

"All the new residents are invited to a beach party and clam bake at the end of summer. You know, cooking lobsters, clams, corn on the cob, and things like that. He'll take you out on his sailboat if you want, and then there's singing around the piano in his home. He generally meets each resident one-on-one. I'm sure he'll talk to you then." She paused.

"Didn't you get a schedule of your rotations?"

"No. When do I rotate through Dr. Moore's service?"

"Well, he doesn't exactly have one, so to speak. When you're on the Ward Service, if he is free and in town, he'll do rounds with the residents, so you'll work with him then."

She must have detected my confusion.

"See here," she said, pulling out my schedule from the envelope of papers on the counter. I moved closer to view my scheduled assignments.

"You're assigned to start on the Ortho Service. We didn't know when you'd arrive, so that's a good place to start because you can assist the ortho residents."

"But I'm not interested in ortho; it's general surgery that I thought I'd be doing."

"Well, Dr. Megee... am I pronouncing it right?"

"The 'd is pronounced, like Megeed."

"OK. So, after ortho, you'll do general surgery next..." she said, pointing to the schedule before us. I nodded. "Every six weeks, you'll move from one surgical service to another, getting the chance to operate on a variety of illnesses. They say it rounds you out as a surgeon."

"He doesn't have a service?"

"He sees his established private patients in his office. Otherwise, he is overwhelmed with the Surgical Services for the United States project for the American College of Surgery—the SOSSUS project—which aims to determine how many surgeons should be trained for the population, often taking him out of town."

In a moment of panic, I lost myself in a sea of questions. Where was my senior registrar or resident? How do I reach him? Where is the orthopedic ward, and where are the patients? Where are the cafeteria and the restrooms? I have no American money. How do I tell Victoria I won't be home tonight or this weekend? Will she be all right alone in this strange new place? What about tomorrow? Where are the morning ward rounds? Are there rounds later today?

I attempted to organize my mental priorities while experiencing fleeting cognitive impairment, overwhelmed by the constant barrage of irritating messages from the overhead PA system. This relentless noise elevated my stress levels. The weight of the new responsibilities was palpable.

Gail inserted herself into my thoughts. "Why don't I keep the books until you've settled?"

"Yeah, that would be helpful. Thanks."

"Did you get a copy of this booklet and your contract in the mail?"

"In England?"

"No. In your internal mailbox."

I shook my head, unaware I had one. It consisted of ten mimeographed pages listing standard American medical abbreviations—most of which differed from those we used in England—and general phone numbers for wards and departments.

"Fancy having to re-learn medical terms."

She chuckled. "Sign your contract and return it to me. You'll also need a chest X-ray. Once cleared and you have no TB, we'll give you your Massachusetts license, narcotic license, and malpractice insurance papers."

"How much is my pay?"

"To start, $3,000. But don't worry, I understand it's going up to $6,000 soon."

Bewildered, I leaned against the counter and took stock. Gail brought me a paper cup of ice-cold water. "Here, this might help."

Walking back to Marion Street, I felt as if I had entered a different world, one of Zielschmerz—the dread of finally pursuing a lifelong dream. My fellow residents were older, more high-strung, goal-oriented, and demanding—unlike the surgical environment in London, where I felt comfortable and in control. This was the competitive world of residents, emblematic of American individualism.

Victoria was surprised to see me. While I explained the events, she made me a cup of tea and a sandwich. Throughout my time at home, the pager squawked endlessly, filled with numerous meaningless messages that were out of context, as well as others instructing me to call various nursing stations to discharge and admit patients, and so on. Unable to answer, since we had no phone, I was repeatedly paged with increasing urgency, which gradually raised my blood pressure.

Reassured by Victoria that she would lock the flat door and inform our new neighbors of her situation, I left with some cash and walked steadily down Longwood in my gray wool suit.

4

AN ETERNAL DAY

Health care is really health management.
Healing has *morphed into treating.*
Where is the care?
—Bernard Lown, MD

The on-call room was small, with a narrow window under an old wooden desk and a rickety metal chair. Against one wall stood a metal-framed bunk bed. The lower bunk showed signs of having been occupied. Next to the bunk bed, the telephone rested on the floor. I flung my stuff on the upper bunk, where I found a starched, short white coat and trousers. I slipped them on and saw *Terra incognito*—the orthopedics ward.

As far as I can remember, we had no orthopedic lectures or focused teachings in this field during medical school in London. We had only one off-the-cuff discussion, hardly meriting the tutorial title, given by two jovial young registrars who lounged on a gurney in an anteroom. Their chat was more of a formality than an education. There wasn't even an orthopedic question on my surgical qualifying finals in England.

One learned orthopedics as a specialty after passing the Primary Fellowship examination. I wanted to be a soft tissue cutter rather than a bone carpenter.

I recalled learning the basic treatment of long bone fractures: alignment, immobilization, traction, and elevation to avoid edema. I would prescribe pain medications as needed, and when the fracture had healed, days or weeks later, I would prescribe physical therapy. Concerning the issue of arthroplasty—joint replacement, I knew nothing except for having observed a couple of archaic procedures in Casualty's minor O.R. in London.

Before joint replacement, the common practice was to remove the head of the femur when it was fractured—an excision arthroplasty. The femur would form a pseudo joint with the articulating cup of the pelvis. A pseudo-arthritic joint eventually developed many adhesions that prevented the patient from walking and occasionally kept them bedridden.

A procedure to break up the pseudo-joint was first introduced in 1826 by John Barton, a surgeon in Philadelphia. As a medical student in 1969, I observed Mr. Hamilton-Evans, an elderly, heavy-set surgeon with a pronounced limp, bring patients who had undergone excision arthroplasty into the minor operating room in Casualty.

The scene was reminiscent of the early days of surgery when operations were done in a pit watched by an audience in their street clothes—this was theater! While the fully clothed patient lay down on the O.R. table, he'd place a mask over their nose and mouth and give them a whiff of gas to put them to sleep. Then, to my horror, he'd lay their leg on his thigh and forcefully break their stiffened, fused, ankylosed hip joint. I could hear the cracking and tearing of adhesions. I thought this was a barbaric procedure.

"This procedure," he casually said to the students, "helps the patient mobilize their frozen hip, allowing them to walk with a cane until it freezes again in about three to four months. Then they come back and see me again."

The entire practice had the quality of a biblical scene. The patient would awake from the whiff of gas, rise, and walk out of the O.R. with their cane, clutching a prescription for pain medication. I only attended his clinic twice because the cracking of bones upset me.

In Boston, the era of arthroplasty, or joint replacement, was in full swing, as each version of a joint was replaced by a more sophisticated version—progress for treating patients with large joint disease. My knowledge in this field was a big zero compared to the orthopedic residents I would now work with.

Unlike in England, I found my new patients mixed in with non-orthopedic patients scattered throughout the ends of Wards C and D. All the nurses on the wards wore white dresses, without pinafores, distinguishing nursing caps, or different-colored belts to indicate a hierarchy of responsibility.

Who was the head nurse?

Who was the nurse in charge?

Did all the nurses here have equal status?

I couldn't figure it out.

This was so different from the nursing setup in England. At the nursing station, the phones were manned by a secretary sitting in front of a screen next to a set of order books. She transcribed a physician's order into nursing actions—all very practical. It didn't take me long to grasp how the system worked, although I missed having a nurse accompany me on rounds who had a comprehensive knowledge of each patient's condition. A nurse spotted me. "Are you the new resident? We've been paging you like crazy. You must discharge a couple of patients. Their beds are needed." Discharging a patient wasn't simple. A nurse couldn't just take a verbal order from me.

Instead, I had to read through the patient's record to determine what was happening. Apart from a brief "op note" describing the name of the orthopedic procedure that the patient had undergone, I was struck by the paucity of the resident's notes. I wondered if these patients were ever formally rounded on in the traditional sense or had been physically examined by the ortho residents, and whether a comprehensive or meaningful note was ever written concerning the patient's hospital stay.

Per my British education, I wrote three prescriptions for each patient being discharged: one for pain, one to prevent constipation, and one for a sleeping pill. The head nurse, Joanne, amused by my unfamiliarity with the names of local medications, was happy to translate the British medication names to their American equivalents. When it came to patient vital signs—pulse, temperature, blood pressure—these data were surprisingly kept by a different nurse in a different location. The patient's nursing care seemed fragmented. It didn't seem like patient care but patient management.

While I wandered about the ward, I bumped into Joanne again. This time, she smiled. "What's your name?'

"Dr. Meguid."

Joanne was young, perhaps in her early to mid-twenties, pleasant, with fair hair, and helpful. I sensed a general air of despondency.

"Are you tired or sort of sad?" I said, trying to ingratiate myself.

She told me, to my dismay, that she was a widow. Today was the first anniversary of her husband's death. Joanne said that he was killed in Vietnam. I was stunned. She couldn't have been older than Victoria and was already a widow.

She hung around, sensing I was lost. As I tried to learn how to discharge a patient, she instructed me to tell them to call their surgeon's office for a follow-up appointment.

"And what about physical therapy?"

"Their surgeon's office will arrange that, too."

I began to see the differences between American-style private and British socialized medical practices. Both showed strengths and weaknesses.

Continuing my rounds, I reviewed the relatively thin charts of my orthopedic patients, most of whom were in their 50s to 70s. Each had a brief history and a physical exam that focused explicitly on their orthopedic problem—barely a page. I discovered that a more comprehensive record was often located in their physician's private office notes, frequently tucked away in the back of the chart. Most patients had numerous consultations with specialists, including cardiology, general internal medicine, and urology, among others, to ensure they were healthy enough to undergo an operation.

I wondered why the orthopedic resident couldn't do that. Had they not gone to medical school?

While I puzzled over this question aloud, Joanne told me it was to protect against litigation.

"You mean lawsuits? For what?"

"Anything that goes wrong, you know. An 'expert' had given the green light," she said. I was confused. Wasn't the orthopedic resident a qualified physician? Did the patient's doctor not carry any authority?

Where orthopedic notes existed, they were brief and focused mainly on the joint that was to be or had been replaced. There were endless—almost daily—notes of the patient's blood work and X-ray findings, duplicating the lab results in the chart. A few notes were concerned with the patient's complaint or well-being. My surgical teacher in London, Professor Robin Pilcher, suggested "Treat the patient, not the disease." I wondered if treating their symptoms instead of treating the whole patient led to more or less litigation.

On the Ortho service, the discussions, emphasis, and focus were primarily on the diseased joint, almost as if the patient was of secondary concern. This conflicted with Dr. Moore's philosophy about the practice of surgery—"assume complete responsibility for the welfare of the patient"—as I had learned and practiced in England. I felt uncomfortable with this approach to surgery. It reminded me of a car assembly line, where each worker was focused on doing one thing, only vaguely aware that they were assembling an entire vehicle.

I found the new admission. She shared a room with another patient who didn't have the same Attending. Pulling a curtain about her, I said, "Hello, Mrs. Norris. I'm Dr. Meguid. You're having surgery tomorrow, and I want to examine you." She looked startled as I put on the light above her bed. "Dr. Turner is my doctor," she said emphatically. "He's already examined me in his office. I saw him last night. A nurse had already taken my blood. Is everything all right?"

"I'm sure it is. I'm here to listen to your lungs and heart and check the hip we'll be operating on tomorrow."

"I had a chest X-ray early this morning and an EKG just now. Is there a need to recheck my heart? The specialist was here and has already done this. He said everything was OK."

"Mrs. Norris, please show me which hip you're being operated on." She reluctantly and slowly lowered her blanket.

"They both hurt. But this one," she pointed to her left side, "hurts more. I can hardly walk."

"May I examine you?"

"Are you a student?"

I flashed a smile and began to examine her hip.

"Who's doing the operation tomorrow?" she asked.

I continued my exam, eliciting a few "ouches" and "That's painful, and you are hurting me."

"Dr. Primo is your surgeon, so he'll operate on you. I'm a general surgical resident—part of his *team* who cares for his patients." Covering herself again, she asked me, "I filled out a menu for dinner, but I've not had a tray yet. Would you know when I'll get something to eat?"

"Let me ask your nurse."

"It's Jennifer," she said.

As the afternoon progressed, individual residents of the ortho team, accompanied by some medical students, came straggling out of the O.R. They looked weary, hungry, and tired. In response to my questioning, the residents became quite animated by their arthroplasty adventures—the new technological marvel and the frontier of orthopedics. Eventually, the acting chief orthopedic resident appeared shorter and pudgier than the rest, with curly hair and small, squinting eyes. The Chief Resident had been called up for Vietnam, and this one took his place.

"Are you this English guy, Mike McQuid?" he asked in a high-pitched voice without introducing himself.

"Hi. It's pronounced Meguid—like Megeeed."

"Great Irish name. You're on call tonight. Have you seen any patients yet?"

"I'm working my way through them." The rest of the ortho team, his PG-2 and PG-3 orthopedic residents, had gathered around, eyeing me as we stood in the corridor. His question made me wonder if he saw me in the capacity of an intern rather than the PG-2 resident that I was.

"So, how are they?"

"They're holding their own."

"Hey guys, did you hear that? They're holding their own!" He laughed, slapped his side, and gave me a crooked stare, which made me uncomfortable. The others pretended to chuckle, more out of apprehension. I wasn't sure what to make of it. I didn't get the joke, which was evident to me. I didn't like his mocking attitude or insistence on calling me McQuid. In my mind, this callow fellow couldn't be taken seriously. He was behaving like an idiot.

"OK, guys. It's time for rounds. Let's go," he said, and with that, I turned right toward the ward. They all turned left, heading to the X-ray Department. I turned around and trailed them.

We viewed X-rays displayed on a continuous, sizable white screen, a practical innovation compared to the series of light boxes used in London, which the acting chief raised and lowered as needed. The X-rays showed diseased heads of femurs, evidence of osteoarthritis, or old trauma of the acetabulum, the cup that made up the hip joint.

Ignoring the human patient, the acting chief focused only on the disease. He framed the world through the narrow window of doing joint surgery "because that's where the money is," instead of helping a suffering human. I thought his interest was limited to the operations he was excited to do. Had arthroplasty become the tip of the arrow that led to the market-driven delivery of surgical care that would erode the core values of the high ideals of American medicinal practice: research, teaching, clinical care, and doctor-patient interactions?

I agree with Dr. Moore that this could end conventional patient care. It would prove to be the underlying cause of my unhappiness with the Ortho service and maybe explain why the medical profession isn't viewed in such high regard.

As if with a vision of a giant neon green dollar sign on the horizon, he talked endlessly about how he wanted to handle all the big operations, while his curiosity about the patient's history—the story of the human being, their occupation, and life—was lacking. He relied too heavily on expert interpretation of X-rays, often getting the different patients mixed up as he whizzed up or down the mobile screens. This non-systematic approach to viewing X-rays was unfamiliar to me, irritating, and made me uncomfortable. That's how mistakes are made.

My orthopedic residency was long and hard. The residents had a reputation for being smart, as sharp as a tack, goal-oriented, and laser-focused on ortho at the expense of general surgical knowledge, despite some having completed a year or two of general surgery. They worked very hard to acquire specific technical skills. After four years of orthopedic residency, they'd sit for their specialty exams. In passing, they could start independently or join an orthopedic practice to enjoy the fruits of operating. I wondered if the financial reward was the motivation since I came to understand that orthopedic procedures were reimbursed favorably.

Nevertheless, I felt that hands-on examination, which allows for personal contact with a patient, was an essential part of treating a patient, showing empathy and respect to sick patients, particularly those dependent on the surgeon, who often felt vulnerable and helpless.

As young surgeons, we were confident that our actions were right for the patient. The less experienced, the greater the degree of hubris. The more skilled and knowledgeable a surgeon became, the more he knew that complete certainty was elusive.

As suddenly as the three residents and the medical students had appeared, they left the X-ray Department and melted away. There was no thought of going to do patient rounds. Standing alone in the hallway, I felt redundant.

I learned that the Ortho Department consisted of three or four full-time professors or associate professors making up the permanent faculty of the orthopedic service. Then, six or seven instructors, clinical assistants, or clinical associates were younger and affiliated with the department. They saw patients in their private offices and scheduled them for surgery at the Brigham or other community hospitals. Although I cared for their patients, I did not know how to contact them should a problem arise, which made me uneasy.

There was a large age difference among the orthopedic surgeons. The established ones had served in WWII or Korea, while the younger ones had recently returned from Vietnam.

Their approaches to common orthopedic problems differed, reflecting the influence of their respective war experiences.

I returned to the wards and worked my way through the new admissions. I listened to patients' complaints in the context of their lives, how their symptoms limited their jobs and affected their social lives, and addressed their concerns as best as I could. I hadn't yet joined the bold, enthusiastic era of arthroplasty joint replacement, not knowing the operation's limitations, complications, and longevity of these joints. Would they need replacing in a few years?

I was uncertain about what to put on the consent form because I hadn't done a hip replacement. The consent form is a complex document with legal consequences. It mostly fell to residents to get it signed. In a sense, it was an abrogation of the surgeon's responsibility. I felt uneasy filling it out and having the patient sign it. How informed is the patient to consent, and how can they understand what they are signing? I always thought it should be completed by the *patient's surgeon* rather than a third person. It should be signed after discussing the operation, the desired outcome, and possible complications with the patient and their family member. Had this been done during the private office visit? I had no way of knowing.

Around 5 p.m., a lull in the hustle and bustle descended onto the ward as if everyone had agreed they were tired and needed to rest, and visiting hours had begun. As I, too, slowed down, I suddenly realized my incredible fatigue, more so than hunger.

5

DESYNCHRONIZED SLEEP

"Sleep-psychosis"—a mental disorder in which thought and emotions are so impaired that contact is lost with external reality.
—Spalding Gray

To rest for a while, I dragged myself up to my bunk bed, feeling exhausted, dehydrated, and disoriented. Without undressing, I lay down to relieve my body and aching legs. That's all I wanted to do.

Abruptly, I was awoken by a blinding ceiling light.

A stocky man stood in the open doorway, swaying slightly as he steadied himself against the door frame, astonished as he stared at me. He turned off the overhead bare bulb just as a young, lithe, tanned woman pushed past him and threw herself onto the lower bunk, shaking the entire bed frame. The room went dark. The silhouette, backlit by the corridor light, swayed slightly while standing in the doorway.

He burped. "Who the hell are you?"

Disoriented, parched, and with a buzzing headache in the stuffy room, I tersely replied Michael Meguid, alert from the rude awakening.

"I'm Bertus. This is my room. You can't camp here." I remained silent, trying to grasp what was happening. He raised his voice, saying, "Hey kaffir . . . are you awake? Do you hear me? You need to find another room." I recognized his Afrikaans accent. Like me, he was likely a provisional resident, but originally from South Africa.

"Alright," I murmured as I turned to face the wall, still wearing my shoes. Every bone in my body ached. Exhausted, I was drawn back into the abyss of sleep. The door closed. He approached. He began rattling the metal frame of the bunk bed. "Hey, fokken kaffir. You heard me. You can't stay here. Go find another room."

The shaking continued. A whiff of alcohol penetrated the depths of my sleep-lag psychosis.

"Honey, come lie down. He's too far gone to trouble us. Leave him be," she said. And with that, Bert gave up. The metal frame shuddered again, absorbing his weight on the lower bunk. I heard murmurs, curses, and titters drifting up to me as I floated in an ambiguous state of consciousness between reality and sleep.

Sometime in the pitch darkness of the night, the phone rang. It rang for what felt like a long time. Finally, he picked it up. There was a pause. "Hey, kaffir. It's for you." He slammed the receiver against the metal frame of our bunk bed.

A faraway female voice asked, "You on call?"

I vaguely remembered the word "on call" from earlier in the day, which felt light-years ago.

"Yes."

The voice said, "Your patient is having some pain. No post-op orders . . . written . . ."

I couldn't figure out what she was saying in my foggy state. Her words lingered in my mind, but I couldn't make sense of them.

"What?"

"He's having . . ." something about pain, she repeated more firmly and loudly, adding, "Doctor, are you awake?"

"Yes, yes." I didn't understand the context of what she was saying. Pain where? What kind? Which patient? I couldn't focus or wake up. I felt lethargic and detached from the words being spoken.

"Pain!" she yelled.

"Oooh, pain! All right. Give him 100 mgs i.m. Pethidine."

"What's that?"

"Pethidine, you know, Pethidine?" I replied irritably, unsure about what there was not to understand about a simple order. "Pethidine . . ." but she'd hung up. I dropped the receiver onto the floor.

A voice soared up from below. "It's Demerol. Get up, you sod and see the patient. Nurses can't take narcotic orders. Don't you know that? Get up, see the patient, and write it in the order book," as the banging of the metal frame recurred.

Glancing at my luminescent wristwatch, I noticed it was around 2 a.m. I had almost slept for nine hours, yet I still felt groggy and thirsty. My body and brain weren't in sync. It was pitch dark. How can I get out of an upper bunk in complete darkness? Where are the toilets? As these questions swirled through my mind, I fell asleep again. In retrospect, it wasn't a brilliant idea to be responsible for caring for sick patients while jet lag disrupted the body's circadian rhythm. I made a significant medical judgment error that still embarrasses me to this day.

An alarm went off.

At 5:30 a.m. I was wide awake, as it was now 10 a.m. London time. Even with our four study-free days as we crossed the pond, my body hadn't fully adjusted to Boston time. I had to pee urgently.

The light flickered on, blinding me once more. The naked woman walked slowly toward the door, her bare feet silent on the floor. She had a white bottom and a narrow, tanned waist. Without any rush, she slipped on her gown and turned around, revealing pale, youthful breasts, a tanned torso, and a patch of darkness below. She looked up and saw me. Her short hair was tousled, yet she remained attractive.

"Hi, I'm Molly."

I waved as she left the room. I saw Bert's hairy legs swing out of bed. He looked up and said, "Hey, you. This isn't your room. Find another."

I dangled the key that had been given to me.

He failed to snatch it.

By mid-morning, I sensed that the entire hospital seemed to be aware of my appalling mistake. When the nurse called, I should have done exactly what I usually did in London: get out of bed, go to the ward, examine the patient, and write an order and a note in the patient's chart for the pain medication.

But in the dead of night, I had inadvertently fallen back asleep, which indicated that I was an unreliable resident. Already, I had a permanent stain on my reputation and record.

6

ORTHOPEDIC INFERNO

One of the essential qualities of the clinician is an interest in humanity,
The secret of patient care is in caring for the patient.
—Frances Weld Peabody

Going home meant that all the scheduled operations and ward rounds had finished. I'd walk home slowly, often in the dark, to decompress, breathe fresh air, and reconnect with life. During those times, I wished I could drink, as I would have stopped at a bar in Coolidge Corner to unwind from the stresses and irritations of the surgical day. Instead, Victoria made me a tea and chatted about her day while preparing dinner.

"I don't work with Dr. Moore," I said. She continued chatting. "I repeat, I don't work with Dr. Moore."

"Why not?" I told her what had transpired.

"Did you know that before we came?"

I shook my head. After a silence, she said, "Well, sounds like a rounded training. Don't you think?"

I raised one eyebrow, which she understood reflected my mixed feelings about the situation.

I arrived at the hospital by 6 a.m. and worked that day, that night, and the following day until the team could go home and the coverage was handed over to the second-year ortho resident. The general rule was that the resident in the operating room had to care for the post-operative patients and then write a note after examining them. He would then prepare the new admissions for the next day's surgery, dictate discharge summaries, and complete the countless patient and administrative chores on the scut list while collaborating with the nurses. Their shifts generally corresponded to those in England: 7 a.m. to 3 p.m., 3 p.m. to 11 p.m., and 11 p.m. to 7 a.m. He'd be lucky to get three to five hours of cumulative sleep during the night. The pattern repeated itself the next day.

The 30- to 36-hour shifts added up to a 110-hour workweek. Weekends and national holidays passed unnoticed by the on-call residents because, from the moment they entered the hospital, their minds were consumed by the welfare of the patients and the hospital routine. It was such a successful working model that it was applied to all the other services and rotations within the Harvard system.

We had a free evening every other night. When I got home, after a cup of tea and a shower, I wanted a meal and sleep. If I had to prepare for a conference or a patient presentation, I needed to get up at 4 a.m. to do my homework or read during those incredible morning hours, avoiding the sticky summer heat. We still hadn't figured out how to operate the air conditioner.

Victoria's interview with Dr. Janeway, conducted toward the end of July, was successful. Her arrival had helped him solve a problem. Dr. Laurie Harken, the daughter-in-law of the renowned cardiac surgeon Dr. Dwight Harken and the wife of Alden Harken, one of my esteemed senior residents, sought a flexible 50% part-time pediatric residency to accommodate her small children. Victoria became her partner, the other 50%.

I was still in the orthopedic service when Victoria started her residency in pediatrics at the Children's Hospital Medical Center, also known as Boston's Children's Hospital. Although her schedule was less stressful, she focused mainly on catching up on sleep upon her return home. Our evening meals together became irregular. Grocery shopping, dining out, or going to a movie were mainly saved for weekends. Lovemaking took a distant second.

When Victoria wasn't home during this time, I'd have dinner in the peaceful stillness, as we had no radio or TV. My lack of sleep and the quiet apartment heightened my old phobias related to childhood abandonment, the early loss of my father, insecurity from chronic stress, and the fear of loneliness—anxiety, depression, and codependency. My disinterest in orthopedics also contributed to these feelings. I'd collapse into bed exhausted, shutting out the world.

Apart from one another, as new immigrants, we had no support system—neither family nor friends. My beloved Oma wrote a few letters, but none came from my sister, Gulnar. Occasionally, a letter from Mother would arrive. Her whereabouts varied with each letter—London, Hamburg, Cairo, or with her friends in Landstuhl in the German Rhineland. I lost track of her location. Since Victoria's schedule differed from mine, Mother Teresa best described my loneliness at home: "The most terrible poverty is loneliness and the feeling of being unloved."

After a few days of Ortho service, the acting chief instructed me to scrub in for the following morning's case. Rose, the fierce, no-nonsense O.R. supervisor reputed to exhale fire through her nose, shuffled papers until she located my name. "You're the new resident," she said briefly. Her accent confirmed her Armenian origins. While I stood in front of her desk waiting to verify that I had a Massachusetts license and malpractice insurance, she caught a resident from another service trying to sneak into the O.R.

"Hey, you," she yelled. "Yes, you . . . you can't scrub. Go to the record room and dictate your outstanding op notes." He slunk away. Without an op-note, the hospital couldn't bill the insurance companies.

Turning to me, she said, "You're here for two years. Use locker 33. And scrub your hands for a good ten minutes, do you hear? An 8 a.m. case starts at 8 a.m. It doesn't mean you come here at 8 a.m. Don't lose this slip with the combination of your locker number."

I nodded and wrote the combination in Arabic with a Sharpie at the top of the locker door. Unfamiliar with combination locks, I was certain I would forget both the numbers and the next turn when I was in a hurry. After that, I changed into O.R. whites.

At 8:15 a.m., I stood next to a female patient lying on the O.R. table, anxiously looking around as the anesthesiologist and his two residents inserted various intravenous catheters into her hands and arms while administering oxygen through a face mask, waiting for her doctor before anesthetizing her. We observed. It was understood that placing the patient under general anesthesia was most perilous during both the induction and emergence phases.

Finally, Dr. Primo, the attending physician and professor, an elderly and experienced surgeon, entered the room. He spoke reassuringly to his patient while the anesthesiologist and his residents hovered nearby, preparing to begin. He then reviewed her chart.

"Who wrote the consent?" he asked.

"I did."

"Who are you?"

"He's the guy from England. Mike McQuid," said the acting chief resident.

"I'm Dr. Primo. You need to specify the type of operation and include all potential risks or complications on the consent form, including the post-operative ones . . . blood clots, infection, and death." The acting chief stared at me and hissed under his breath, "Can't you even do that?"

Addressing Dr. Primo, I said, "Sorry. I'm Michael Megeed. I'm accustomed to the legal practice in England where the patient's surgeon is responsible for obtaining the consent."

Dr. Primo nodded. "Where in England are you from?"

"University College Hospital, London."

His eyebrows raised, and he smiled—a smile of recognition.

The anesthesiologist lifted the sheet that separated the operative field from the anesthetic team, commonly referred to as the "blood-brain barrier," where the surgeons represented the blood and the anesthetic team was the brain. I disliked that concept because I viewed the anesthesia team as a vital part of the surgical team—not a separate, independent entity.

"Dr. Primo, your patient is now asleep, but she can still hear your conversation," the anesthesiologist said.

Dr. Primo crossed out what I had written and signed the consent form after writing something. "Hey, Mark, until Mike becomes familiar with our system, I expect you to get the consent forms." The acting chief shot me a deadly stare.

Dr. Primo looked around. "Where is Chris?" Chris walked in as Dr. Primo asked. I quickly realized he was a technician from the medical company that manufactured the joint implant.

"OK. Let's go."

The acting chief and I scrubbed and gowned while the scrub nurse assisted us in putting on gloves. A quiet shuffle surrounded the patient until it became clear that Dr. Primo, not the acting chief resident, would operate.

Dr. Primo positioned the patient with her right hip secured on a yellow beanbag on the O.R. table while the acting chief observed passively. Even with a mask on, it was clear that he was sulking. The circulating nurse evacuated air from the beanbag using a vacuum pump to stabilize the patient's position on the table. The acting chief cleaned the upward-facing left hip, then Dr. Primo applied a brownish Betadine antiseptic solution and covered the entire area with a transparent adhesive hypoallergenic film dressing—something I hadn't seen in London. The company technician, Chris, stood on a low stool behind Dr. Primo, looking over his shoulder.

After Dr. Primo made the incision in the skin and muscle, the technician muttered instructions about each step of the operation. There was a lot of hammering and what seemed to be carpentry as the technician guided Dr. Primo through the procedure to create a new hip joint, acting as an assistant. The acting chief showed no enthusiasm and stood there brooding and watching, leaving me to mop the floor dry of blood. As Dr. Primo operated, he requested each surgical instrument he needed. I noticed that all the instruments had different names here than the ones I had learned in England. I would have to relearn their American names.

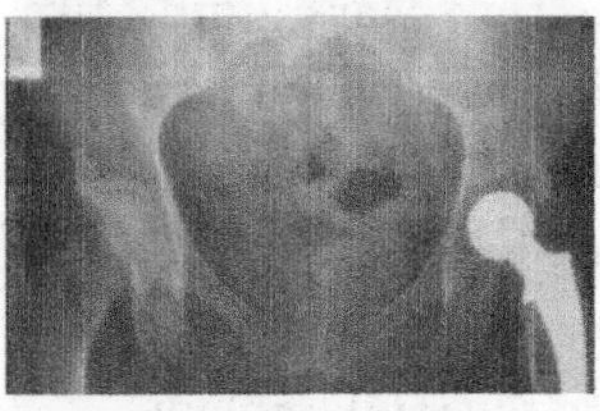

When Dr. Primo had completed the joint replacement and was satisfied with the X-rays of the new implant, he and Chris departed.

"Hey Mark, dictate the op note," came the order as he left. The acting chief cursed under his breath, "You did it, you should dictate it, asshole."

Eager to assist him, I said, "I can close for you if you like."

"Sure."

Turning to the scrub nurse, I requested a 2-0 cotton suture on a straight needle. The size of a suture indicates its diameter in millimeters, and the more zeros that follow the number, the smaller the diameter.

"Are you crazy?" the acting chief said in a raised voice. "Cotton? NEVER use cotton! Where did you learn that stupid stuff? We only use Chromic sutures." I nodded, realizing that the more rigid the dogma, the deeper the ignorance.

Healing depends not on the type of suture but on the inflammatory reaction in the tissue surrounding the suture and incision. Professor Pilcher in London taught me this and often added a chest surgeon's motto: "Wounds heal from side to side, no matter how long they are."

"You don't know how to close. Change sides. I'm closing," he told me sharply. I didn't argue. I saw no way to please him or soothe his insecurity.

Facing him, the scrub nurse announced firmly, "Before you go any further, we're missing a 3-x-3-inch sponge."

We checked the various layers of the wound. "It's not here. You probably counted wrong. Count the swabs again. Let's close."

The scrub nurse held a humongous Kelly clamp in midair as if she was about to crack his skull or knuckles and repeated emphatically, "*I said a sponge is missing.* We don't close in my O.R. until the sponge count is correct. Do you get it?"

There was no doubt that, like the scrub nurses in London, this one understood her authority over the residents and didn't take her responsibilities lightly. Years ago, I learned to view scrub nurses as a surgeon's ally and to respect them. I'd heard that scrub nurses were considered second wives to some surgeons. They were invaluable and made my life easier during operations. I revere them and always take them seriously.

We reexamined all the layers of the open wound and the drapes around it while the circulator nurse crawled eerily around us on the floor and under the drapes, searching. The 3-

x-3 sponges have a blue metallic stripe woven through them, allowing them to be detected by X-ray.

Professor Rodney Maingot, who guided me through my first appendectomy on my first private patient at St. George's Hospital in London about a year ago, had warned me not to use 3-x-3-inch sponges to avoid leaving one in the wound, as this could lead to an abscess and necessitate a second operation to retrieve it, potentially resulting in a lawsuit. At his insistence, I had always used the larger 9-inch x 9-inch lap sponges. His reasoning now made complete sense to me.

"Not here," came the muffled voice from under the drapes.

"God-damm-it," shouted the acting chief. "I bet that fucker took it with him just to make me get an X-ray of the wound. They told me he does it every time. I'll get even with him." At this stage, the acting chief was getting on my nerves.

The X-ray technician was called.

While waiting, I asked, "What do you mean you'll get even?"

"At Harvard, we don't get mad—we get even," he said, scathingly quoting Robert Kennedy.

"How?" I asked.

"You'll see." The acting chief spoke with venom and a scornful squint in his eyes.

The anesthesiologist, who had begun to lighten the patient's anesthesia, readjusted his gases to deepen the level of the patient's subconsciousness. We lingered nearby.

Twenty minutes later, an X-ray of the wound, including the surgical area, did not reveal a sponge.

"See, I told you. He took it with him. Count them again and file a goddamn report. I'm closing," the acting chief crowed in triumph. His foul mood led him to close the wound carelessly despite my best efforts to assist him. He wasn't a decent person, nor a good surgeon, as he ignored the fundamental principle of surgical technique: treating the patient's tissue with care. No doubt, this behavior and attitude would reach Dr. Primo's ears. Long ago, I learned that a bond existed between a scrub nurse and a surgeon. It was best to keep one's thoughts to oneself and one's mouth shut regarding an attending. He was beginning to inflict moral injury; if not on the scrub nurse, then on me, contributing to my feelings of distress and depression and diminishing my passion for surgery.

The circulating nurse reported a missing 3-x-3-inch sponge. The American College of Surgeons estimates that about one thousand sponges are left in patients' bodies daily in America. To avoid or minimize this error, the scrub and circulating nurses acted as our guardian angels; they kept the count. We closed and wheeled the patient into the recovery room. It was 12:45 p.m.

7

TRIUMPH OF AMPUTATIONS

Do not mistake the line of discoloration in gangrene for the line of demarcation. The former spreads, and the latter rarely moves.
—Augustus Charles Bernays

On this day, only a few minor operations were scheduled for the morning. The acting chief divided us into four groups, with each group seeing a quarter of the patients. He went to lunch, and twenty minutes later, we joined him at a nearby deli on Huntington Ave.

We squeezed into his booth and placed our orders. I was starving. The acting chief had already devoured half of a large pizza and didn't offer us any of the leftovers. I ordered an Italian sub—cold cuts I remembered from my childhood in Wedel, Germany, with my Oma. The others shared two enormous pizzas and drank Coca-Cola. My sub measured six inches long—a perfect size. The bread roll was sweet and soft, unlike the dense rolls typical of German bread. Still, it was delicious. Unused to large American portions, I could hardly finish it! Growing up in post-war Germany, we had to clean our plates. I couldn't leave food behind, so I always ate it all.

Between bites of pizza, the acting chief hinted that he was the top dog on the team, which he hardly needed to remind us —despite being a fourth-year resident instead of a fifth. "Marty Schultz has been interviewing for jobs," he said, leaning over to me. "His family comes from Wisconsin, so he's looking to join a practice there. That's great for me. I get to do most of the cases. I'm becoming good at it."

We ate; each engaged with their food and private thoughts.

"Mike how are your patients?"

"They are stable. Mrs. Lobos is running a low-grade fever."

"From what?"

"Not sure yet. Her wound looks benign."

"Do a fever work-up."

"What's that?"

"Where did you go to medical school? Mexico or some forsaken African country? You know, blood work, urine cultures, blood cultures, a chest X-ray," he whined.

I felt like shoving his pizza down his throat.

"Oh, you mean an FUO work-up."

"What the shit is *that*."

"Fever of Unknown Origin work-up—don't you know that? I've already got the blood work and urine, and she's having X-rays as we speak because her sputum looked greenish. That's why I was late."

He glared at me. "You probably just got saliva," he said offhandedly.

"No. I got sputum using a trans-tracheal cough tickler.'

"Yeah? What shit is that?"

"One injects 1 ml of sterile saline into the trachea through the cricopharyngeal membrane just below the thyroid cartilage. This makes them cough and expectorate sputum."

"That's dangerous! Who the hell does that?"

"The residents at Mass General."

He took a swig from his Coke. "Be sure to check the results."

"Of course. Why would I otherwise get them?"

"Let me know if anything funny. I don't want Primo to bite my ass off again after you fucked up with the consent form."

A quietness followed. "I'm sure glad to be leaving this shit behind when I go to Vietnam as my deferment finishes at the end of this residency. The women there are hot." I wanted to say I hope you step on a mine or get the clap, but I held my tongue.

We continued to eat in silence. Then he burped and asked, "So, what's this fancy exam you did that kept you from starting on time? One of the guys in the research lab covered for you, which created many problems."

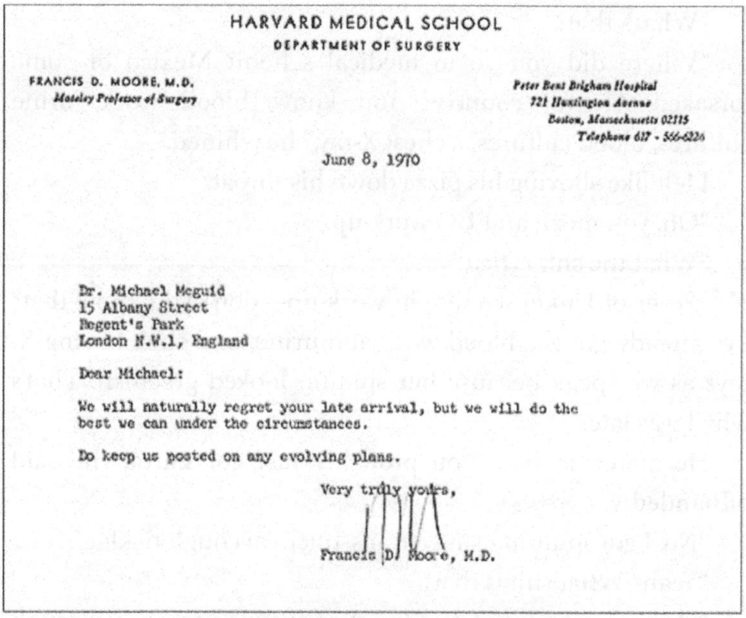

HARVARD MEDICAL SCHOOL
DEPARTMENT OF SURGERY

FRANCIS D. MOORE, M.D.
Moseley Professor of Surgery

Peter Bent Brigham Hospital
721 Huntington Avenue
Boston, Massachusetts 02115
Telephone 617 - 566-6226

June 8, 1970

Dr. Michael Meguid
15 Albany Street
Regent's Park
London N.W.1, England

Dear Michael:

We will naturally regret your late arrival, but we will do the best we can under the circumstances.

Do keep us posted on any evolving plans.

Very truly yours,

Francis D. Moore, M.D.

I wish I had Dr. Moore's letter to shove in his face. "I informed the chief of my late arrival."

"And what did he say?"

"Well, something to the effect that he looked forward to seeing me when I arrived."

"Yeah?"

I nodded, thinking what a jerk he was. Then, reluctantly, I explained the Primary Fellowship and its pass rate of 20% in the hope of impressing him. He wasn't impressed.

"Couldn't you have done this earlier?"

I stared at him, wanting to bash his face. I held him in the highest of low regard. "I think the operating surgeon should get the consent before a witness, just like we did in England. Legally, it's his responsibility, as I told him in the O.R." Facing him directly and looking him straight in the eyes, I firmly said while measuring each word, "To set the record straight in your mind, not only did I pass all my British medical exams, do internships in London, an elective at Mass General, and pass my advanced surgical exam, but I also passed the American Medical Boards just as you did, so don't you goad me with Mexico or some forsaken African country. Do you get it?" As if to cut him down to size, I added, "I'm way overqualified to do the scut work that you should be doing on your patients."

He appeared visibly pale and shaken. As he reclined in the cubicle, he dropped his piece of pizza, as if expecting me to punch him in the face. He picked up his pizza again, then dropped it again. "I'm not hungry." He remained silent. The others were silently glancing at me. He shifted his attention to the third-year resident sitting across from him.

"Yesterday's operation was a joke. I could have done it better and faster. Primo is an old guy." I cringed at his braggadocio. He continued, "He doesn't know what he's doing when it comes to hip arthroplasty. He should leave this kind of ops to us young guys. He should retire," he said, chuckling.

I was reminded of the saying, "Intelligent people talk about ideas, ordinary people talk about things, and small people talk about other people."

I was at the bottom of the totem pole, so the acting chief had already sent me to manually disimpact the hard, concrete stool from a constipated patient because of the opioids he had prescribed. This was a procedure where I put on gloves and, using plenty of K-jelly, removed the stool as far up the rectum as I could reach while a nurse held the wailing patient in the left lateral position. I would do anything to help a patient. However, assigning me this task reflected his attitude toward a kind of power play, and I understood the acting chief's message. I tried not to show my contempt for his personality.

To keep me busy, he designated me to assist with what he called "minor procedures,"—such as helping junior attendings with amputations. These ranged from cutting off a single necrotic toe or an entire foot, leaving the heel as the stump to fit a prosthesis, or creating a stump after amputating above or below a knee for an artificial limb.

In my view, there is no such thing as a minor operation. Every procedure is a significant operation for the patient, with both physical and emotional repercussions.

The acting chief resident was either unaware of, or more likely indifferent to, the historical and cultural significance of amputations. I believed that lacking even an inkling of the historical background of an operation did not contribute to being a good surgeon. It reduced one to a surgical gigolo, performing a job merely for money—worse than an itinerant technician. I approached amputations with a deep sense of sorrow for the patient, who was facing the consequences of vascular insufficiency, diabetes, chronic infections, or gangrene. I showed the acting chief no satisfaction with my outward reluctance to perform such operations, honoring the immense history of this age-old procedure.

Many military surgeons shared their experiences performing amputations during the eighteenth-century wars, at a time when anesthesia had not yet been discovered.

Among them were Napoleon's surgeon, Dominique Jean Larrey, and the father of British surgery, John Hunter, who eloquently recounted amputating a leg in seven seconds. Additionally, Walt Whitman depicted numerous amputations of limbs during the American Civil War of the nineteenth century. The advances in surgery stemming from battlefield amputations include the use of hot tar pitch to stem wound bleeding. These vivid accounts pay tribute to the sophisticated art of surgery. Surgeons, including Abu al-Qasim al-Zahrawi al-Ansari, born in 936 CE, recognized the profound consequences of limb removal. Thus, amputation is one of the most thoughtful and philosophical procedures, requiring meticulous attention to serve the patient's best interests. To restore a patient's sense of humanity and self-worth, it was essential to provide them with the best available prosthesis. In those historical times, amputation was as revolutionary as modern-day arthroplasties for restoring a victim's mobility. Having never performed an amputation in England, I viewed this opportunity as a chance to become an expert and deliver the best care for my patients.

I had a sense of history catching up with me. During my anatomy class in medical school, we were required to complete the dissection of our cadaver, Fred. By the last term, all that was left of him was the lower limb—the thigh, knee, leg, ankle, and foot. Terrified of failing the epic 2nd M.B. in 1965, Bachelor of Medicine examination, I made a strategic decision. Instead of studying the muscles, arteries, veins, and nerves of Fred's leg, I'd focus on revising and re-learning all the basic sciences I had learned during the previous 18 months. My rationale was that man could live without legs. I left the dissection to my dear colleague Jonathan Marrow, a consummate dissector. The gamble worked. There wasn't a single exam question in anatomy on the leg, nor in the advanced courses and exams of the Royal College of Surgery a couple of years later. I passed the dreaded 2nd M.B. and moved on to study clinical medicine without learning this crucial knowledge.

I needed to fill my knowledge gap with a nightly crash course in reading about leg anatomy in R. J. Last's book on *Applied Anatomy* and *Gray's Anatomy*, which are two of the most influential works. After that, I borrowed Richard Warren's book *Procedures in Vascular Surgery*, a surgical atlas focused on lower limb vascular procedures and amputations.

In Dr. Warren's atlas, each amputation was elegantly illustrated with step-by-step diagrams showcasing the procedure, from the skin incision to the operation's steps and skin closure. Instructions were provided for patient care before, during, and after the operation. I enjoyed reading his book, which made a procedure I didn't aesthetically prefer more palatable due to its impact on the body and the patient's functionality. Dr. Warren's atlas detailing the operative procedure and my studies on prostheses to restore mobility made the operation more acceptable to me. Throughout my surgical career, whenever such an operation was needed, I felt confident performing it because I had learned the anatomy and considered myself an expert in amputations.

The young attendings who returned from Vietnam taught me a great deal. The blood supply to the lower limbs in an infected leg was a critical determinant of the level of amputation and, consequently, the success or failure of the procedure, including the prevention of stump infection and the maturation and healing of the weight-bearing stump. I learned to handle the tissue with care, using fine-toothed forceps to address the bleeders and avoid tying a suture around nerves, which could lead to stump and phantom pain. Instead, I retrieved the artery that retracted alongside the nerve bundle and tied it off separately from the nerve, allowing the nerve to retract into the tissue.

My first procedure involved performing a below-knee

amputation on a patient with gangrene in the foot, assisted by an amiable junior attending who had recently returned from Vietnam.

"How many have you done?" he asked me.

"This is my first, and I'd appreciate it if you could walk me through the operation step by step."

He nodded.

After the patient was anesthetized, a blood pressure cuff was applied to the thigh and inflated to a pressure above the patient's normal blood pressure to minimize bleeding. After washing and draping the leg, he marked the incision on the calf with a purple medical skin marker that resembled Victoria's eyeliner. "That will be the incision."

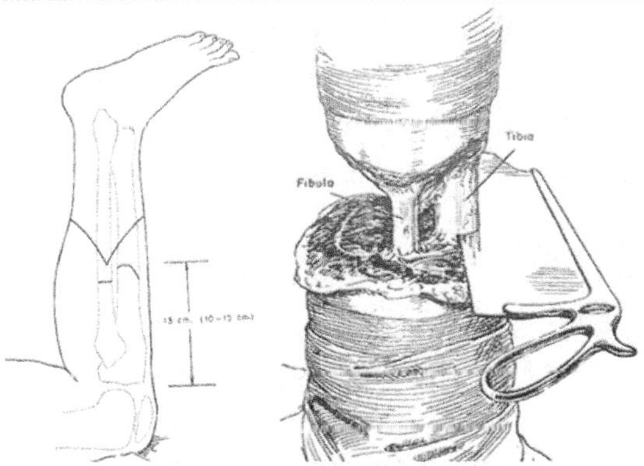

Diagram on the left shows the fish mouth incision about 13 cm below the knee is made. Muscles, vessels, and nerves are divided. On the right, the tibia and fibula are sawed through.

The scrub nurse handed me the scalpel. I beveled the skin incisions so that the upper flap of tissue would come together easily with the lower tissue flap and amply cover the bone to form a firm stump. I carried the cut through the muscles to the bone and tied off the arteries. The attending scraped back the periosteum towards the knee at a preselected level. The periosteum is a fascia-like tissue around the bone. There was minimal bleeding from the bone despite the cuff occluding the main blood supply, which surprised me. He then passed me the handsaw and instructed me to saw the tibia, the main bone of the leg, and the fibula, the thinner bone, while he held the foot. Sawing was tougher than I thought it would be, and my effort at dividing the bone resulted in smoke lingering in my nostrils. After I finished, he removed the gangrenous foot and lower leg from the operative field.

"Now cut the fibula about an inch and a half lower than the tibia."

I did.

The nurse deflated the cuff. The remaining tissue oozed some blood, indicating it was healthy. He removed the extra fibula piece and rasped, beveled, and smoothed the sharp edges of each bone. I controlled the bleeding from the bone edges with sterile beeswax, pressing it into the pores of the bone. Then, I covered them with the remaining muscles, subcutaneous tissues, and skin to form a firm stump.

He handed me the needle holder. I closed the deep fascia and placed the skin sutures apart to allow any blood to ooze out. The attending physician wrapped the stump and applied a posterior splint to prevent knee contracture.

Opinions between older and younger generations of surgeons regarding post-operative care were controversial. The attending physicians from Vietnam dressed the stump immediately, just as we had done. By day three, when the stump showed signs of healing, we called Livingstone, a knowledgeable African American orthopedic technician, to create a mold of the socket to place over the stump. He attached a metal pipe that ended with a foot rocker, allowing the patient to stand, bear weight, and walk several times a day. The patient stood tall. Each step was a significant achievement toward a new life.

The older generation of surgeons who had experience from World War II or the Korean War waited six to ten days before creating a prosthesis socket. During this time, the patient remained in bed and was largely inactive.

I operated, with the assistance of an older surgeon, on a patient who required an above-knee amputation. On the fourth day of his bed rest, my patient developed a thrombus in the femoral vein above the knee stump. A massive embolus, a blood clot, broke free and traveled to his lungs, resulting in his death. In those days, using low-molecular-weight anticoagulants or aspirin wasn't routine.

I was devastated and mourned his loss. I became depressed as I remembered my father, who died from a pulmonary embolism caused by a thrombus in his left polio-stricken leg after ten days of bed rest for heart failure. His death occurred when I was nearly twelve. I thought I had processed the anger and grief of losing him, but the loss of my patient reawakened deep feelings of guilt and sorrow.

The death of Mr. Brynmor was my first post-operative death in Boston. The French surgeon, René Leriche, contemplated in his 1951 essay on La philosophie de la Chirurgie—The Philosophy of Surgery—that "Every surgeon carries within himself a small cemetery, where from time to time he goes to pray—a place of bitterness and regret, where he must look for an explanation for his failures." With the loss of Mr. Brynmor, I began my cemetery of regret and grief.

There wasn't anyone I could go to discuss my struggles with the emotional turmoil of self-doubt, guilt, and a degree of failure because I had operated. During Thursday morning's ortho discussions, his death was mentioned and merely glossed over. Like others in the room, I had to become more detached so I could continue functioning as a surgeon and a human. Nevertheless, his death left a scar.

Using standardized, repeatable surgical techniques helped me perfect the operative procedure of amputations and the patient's pre-operative and post-operative care. My preference became to mold the socket to place over the stump and affix a metal pipe with a foot rocker to get the patient out of bed very soon after an operation, minimizing pneumonia, loss of thigh muscles, thrombosis of the vein, and the potential of death from a preventable pulmonary embolism. I began to appreciate that the higher up the leg I amputated, the more difficult it was for a patient to get out of bed, since the legs were a counter-weight to the torso. As my competence grew, I gained a sense of accomplishment, satisfaction, and a sense of learning and improving my surgical skills. It brought me much personal joy and pride, which somewhat compensated for the angry scut boy I had become. The pleasure of these leg procedures was entirely mine. I marveled at my detailed knowledge of the leg's anatomy—a joy of surgery not shared with the acting chief to prevent his interference in these operations.

I also learned a valuable lesson about coping with grief after an amputation. Before I performed one, I sat down with the patient and asked some straightforward questions. Often, these questions compel the patient to confront reality. How would they manage both physically and emotionally with a change in their body image? They needed to reflect on the role and significance of their leg. How would an amputation—the loss of a limb—impact their mobility? Emotionally? How would it affect their partner, children, or friends?

Every day, I did rounds in the ward and documented each patient's status. My notes reflected my conversation and examination. Each note wasn't cluttered with blood or X-ray results. These reports were in the back of the chart. I noticed Dr. Primo would trail me, writing a note below my note. This puzzled me, especially when his notes were a modification of mine. He would sign them and stamp his name below his note.

Worried my note wasn't sufficient, I approached him. "Dr. Primo, do you not like my notes? Am I doing it correctly, or not? Am I doing it inadequately?" My questions startled him. He rose from his chair, looked at me, and said, "Oh no. The problem is that if I don't write a daily note on my patients' charts and stamp my signature, Medicare won't pay me for each day the patient is hospitalized."

Okay. That information will be helpful if our future is in the United States.

Attitude

by Charles R. Swindoll

The longer I live, the more I realize the impact of attitude on life.
Attitude is more important than the past, education, money, circumstances, failures, successes, than what people think, say or do.
It is more important than appearance, giftedness, or skill.
It will make or break a company, a church, a home.

The remarkable thing is we have a choice every day regarding the attitude we will embrace for that day.
We cannot change our past,
We cannot change the fact that people will act in a certain way.
We cannot change the inevitable.

The only thing we can do is play on the one string we have, And that is our attitude...
I am convinced that life is 10% what happens to me,
And 90% how I react to it.
And so, it is with you...
We are in charge of our attitudes.

8

RECKLESS & INDIFFERENT

People can be divided into three groups:
Those who make things happen,
Those who watch things happen,
And those who wonder what happened.
—John Newbern's Law

At 7 p.m. one night, the ward nurse informed me that the E.R. had admitted a male patient with a closed fracture of the right leg. The lower limb seemed as if someone had kinked it backward at mid-calf. The E.R. doctor had neglected to perform the most basic procedures to stabilize the leg. I examined the patient, and the pulses in his foot were strong—the leg was pink and viable. Following surgical protocol, I called the acting chief, my senior backup. I described the situation and let him know that it was beyond my capacity to manage and that the emergency required surgery tonight.

"Does he have good pulses beyond the fracture and in his feet?"

"Within five seconds, even though his foot is cold, I can feel strong anterior and posterior tibial pulses, the peroneal artery, capillary refill, and venous drainage."

"Doesn't sound like an emergency to me. I'm having dinner with my wife. It can wait until the morning." He hung up.

I wanted to scream down the phone that he was a selfish, lazy, arrogant son-of-a-bitch. He needed to come in and mobilize a surgical team. I sensed deep within me when a case was an emergency, and I'd tackle it as best I could. But in this situation, I was out of my depth. My senior should have come into the hospital and backed me up. It's always safer to look and see than to wait and see. The acting chief was negligent in his duties.

I found the orthopedic technician, Livingstone, in the ortho supply room. He examined the patient's leg and agreed that we could create a plaster splint to stabilize the leg from the knee down to the ankle, across the fracture site, and to the toes, thereby minimizing his pain and preventing his foot from drooping. I communicated my thought process to the patient and provided him with some morphine for sedation while Livingstone prepared his cart. Soon, he arrived at the bedside with his trolley, plaster bandages, and buckets of warm water to construct a posterior splint. I worried throughout the night and checked the patient's leg and foot pulse hourly. All hell broke loose in the morning when Dr. Primo saw our back slab. To him, it was an emergency that should have been plated and screwed in the O.R. after the accident the previous night. The blame for the stabilizing treatment was placed on me. I explained to Dr. Primo that I had done what I could without help.

I understood and could predict who participated in the downward flow of negativity. It's human nature. The blame and responsibility typically fall on the person disseminating problems down the totem pole to the individual with the least authority or ability to stop it from happening. If those purveyors of negativity were to analyze the cause of the adverse event, they would recognize that shifting the blame downward only exposes their lack of moral integrity, maturity, and leadership. During my training, I met residents and attendings who embodied moral righteousness and honesty—those I admired.

Perhaps the acting chief's inaction has caused another blemish on my record. He approached being an egocentric psychopath—a man devoid of guilt or compassion—a dangerous physician, a less-than-mediocre surgeon.

He and the ortho rotation brought me down. The Brigham wasn't what it was cracked up to be. It was not a place for training general surgeons. Why not return to London instead of staying and feeling like a failure every day? I loathed my situation in Boston.

In my depressed state, quitting crossed my mind several times. At the Co-op, which I passed while walking home, I saw a poster of a poem entitled "You Mustn't Quit." I bought it and hung it up at home. Whenever I entertained the thought of quitting, the line "Success is failure turned inside out" kept staring back at me. No! I wasn't going to let that bastard define me or my life.

The thought of quitting when things didn't seem right wasn't new. Had I not considered quitting when I lived alone in Manchester at sixteen and failed the first year of grammar school? Packing my bags and flying back to Cairo would have been easy. Instead, I repeated the year and overcame my social and academic challenges.

No, I had to push through this horrible rotation. My coming rotations were in general surgery.

On Thursday mornings, there were no scheduled operations. The service gathered in the Roman-style auditorium—the attendings sat in the front rows, while the residents occupied the back, emphasizing the surgical top-down authoritarian structure. One morning, as I stood before the assembled crowd, I presented the history and physical findings of a challenging new patient with an unusual bone-related problem. After I finished, I sat down. A wide-ranging discussion followed among the senior staff regarding how to manage the patient surgically.

Dr. Primo stood at the podium and detailed his experience. I noticed that the acting chief had left, and Dr. Primo's pager repeatedly went off with a loud, garbled message that interrupted his discussion. He paused to listen to the squawking dispatch. The audience fidgeted when he resumed his talk. His pager squawked again.

It had to be the childish behavior of the acting chief.

"Why do you do that?" I asked him one day.

"He operates on all the cases I should be doing," he replied. "It's not fair."

"Fair? Or just? They are *his private* patients. There isn't anything fair about this system."

"Then don't have a training program."

"C'mon. Residency is mutual abuse or exploitation: you operate on his patients, and he teaches you. He expects you to care for them day and night for a few years. Seems reasonable to me," I said, trying to put some perspective on the situation. "After all, when you graduate, you become a competitor in this medical marketplace."

He looked at me. "What do you know, McQuaid? Wait till I evaluate him. I have that power."

"You evaluate your bosses?" I asked in consternation—no such thing in England. In Dr. Primo's defense, I said, "Occasionally, he must get up to speed with new operations to remain certified. He's learning new techniques for joint-replacement implants to teach you."

He made a dismissive jerk of his head, consistent with his character. I was reminded of the saying, "Perhaps no sin so easily besets us as a sense of self-satisfied superiority to others," especially when he stated that he would evaluate me, too, when the orthopedic rotation ended. I sensed that his evaluation would threaten my reputation at the Brigham. It never occurred to me that I, too, would assess him. I reckoned the Almighty would see to that—indeed, the Army had his number by sending him to Vietnam!

My feelings of dejection and unhappiness deepened. This training wasn't what I wanted. Where was the cutting I had expected? I felt trapped, as if I were in prison with no way out. Among the three groups of people defined by John Newbern's Law, I was not the individual who made things happen, as I had in England. Was my move to America a big blunder? I didn't feel inclined to climb or participate for the first time, hoping to minimize my contact with the acting chief. I preferred to stay on the wards to examine the patients, handle the paperwork, and chat with the nurses.

You Mustn't Quit

by Edgar Albert Guest

When things go wrong, as they sometimes will,
When the road you're trudging seems all uphill,
When the funds are low and the debts are high,
And you want to smile but you have to sigh,
When care is pressing you down a bit—
Rest if you must, but don't you quit.

Life is queer with its twists and turns.
As everyone of us sometimes learns.
And many a fellow turns about when he
Might have won had he stuck it out.
Don't give up though the pace seems slow—
You may succeed with another blow.

Often the goal is nearer than it seems
To a faint and faltering man;
Often the struggler has given up when he
Might have captured the victor's cup;
And he learned too late when the night came down,
How close he was to the golden crown.

Success is failure turned inside out—
The silver tint of the clouds of doubt,
And when you never can tell how close you are,
It may be near when it seems afar;
So stick to the fight when you're hardest hit—
It's when things seem worst,
You must not quit.

9

BLESS THE IRISH

When life gives you lemons, make lemonade.
—Elbert Hubbard

I dictated discharge summaries in the basement medical records room. The clerks who managed the filing room were mainly middle-aged women originally from Ireland. The staff befriended me. I welcomed their friendship and often took refuge in the records room to rest and recuperate from the hustle and bustle, the commotion on the ward, particularly when the burden of caring for a disorganized service became too much—when I felt, as the aphorism stated, "I was fed shit and expected to grow surgically." I shared this saying with them, and they found it hilarious.

They'd often make me a cup of tea to console me when I dictated the orthopedic discharge summaries on blue round plastic sleeves. They showed me an entire shelf of undictated "derelict" medical records. "The hospital can't collect from the insurance companies if they don't get a final discharge summary."

"Whose records are these?"

"They were ignored by residents who left and didn't do their summaries. The hospital will pay anyone $5 for each dictation. There are plenty of skinny records that you could do. It would help us clear some of these shelves."

What a deal! I browsed through the shelves of the filing cabinets and selected the slimmest charts, especially those related to abdominal operations, subjects with which I was familiar. The art of dictating a discharge summary involved asking,

"What information did the next person need about this patient's treatment and status?" This often led to several short paragraphs totaling half a page—clear, concise, organized, and accurate! It took only ten minutes. No one wanted to read a summary of War and Peace. The report would be typed and placed into my pigeonhole. The next time I was down there, I'd read it, make corrections, review the re-typed version, and sign it. It was an easy $5.

Over the months, long after I'd left the ortho service, I dictated records on non-busy nights when I was on call at the Brigham and later at the Children's Hospital across the street. I continuously received extra checks, eventually covering our first summer vacation.

Early on, my new Irish friends discovered that we had just arrived from London and were trying to set up a home.

"Did you get any furniture from the departing chief residents?"

"No, we arrived late. Looks like we missed that chance."

"There is overflow furniture, odds and ends in the storage garage. Have you had access to that, you know, for your pickings?"

"No."

Their surplus furniture—bookshelves, a desk, kitchen chairs, and extra lamps—overwhelmed us. They dropped these off on weekends, and Victoria, who was amazed by the variety of kitchen chairs, particularly the old, well-crafted wooden ones we cleaned and repainted, met them. With the furniture I picked up from the side of the road, our flat gradually transformed into a home. We still have some solid wood pieces to this day.

The emotional meaning of home was a place where Victoria and I felt safe, secure, loved, and accepted; a place where I didn't have to define my strengths or explain myself. It was where I could be myself 24/7, be the champion, be insecure, and still be cherished by my wife. It served as a refuge, a joyful space where I could also feel sad, laugh, sing, and whistle to my heart's content—although she insisted that my whistling was too shrill for her.

Home represents more than just four walls and a place to eat and sleep; it's where our deepest relationships flourish and many of our most significant life events unfold. It also enhances my connection to my roots and society. My home is a sanctuary of music, books, and even more books—bathed in plenty of sunshine and natural light.

While waiting for her interview with Dr. Janeway, Victoria borrowed Karen's sewing machine and made curtains. During an off weekend, I painted a wall red and the unused metal medical record shelves white. Gradually, with the help of our Irish friends, we transformed our space into a comfortable home, hanging some artwork we had brought. Paychecks were typically received at the end of each month. We lived off blood money during the first few months of our stay. Victoria and I became monthly donors at the Children's Hospital, where platelets were needed for children undergoing chemotherapy. In return, they paid us $50. At the end of the month, I received my stipend, followed by Victoria's after she became a resident at the Children's Hospital. In the meantime, the $5 and $50 payments sustained us.

As the orthopedic service was concluding, Dr. Primo

observed me repeatedly on the ward performing the duties of an intern instead of being allowed to operate at the level of a second-year resident. He decided to guide me through the hip replacement procedure. He had learned the lateral approach from a technician. He was now passing on his knowledge using the "learn one, do one, teach one" method attributed to William Stewart Halsted at Johns Hopkins University. This concept suggests that by actively teaching others, learners solidify their knowledge and demonstrate mastery of the subject.

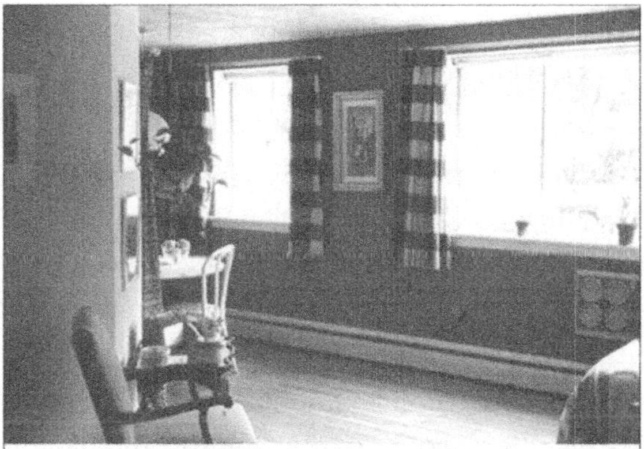

Livingroom Showing Acquired Secondhand Furniture.

The night before the operation, I met with the patient. She was in her sixties and suffered from pain in her left hip, which resulted in back pain. Over time, her hip pain and mobility had not improved despite pain medications, physical therapy, and cortisone injections; therefore, hip replacement promised pain relief and an extension of her physical activity— "returning my youth," as she described it. I marveled at the scientific ingenuity behind the design of the artificial hip.

I made the skin incision and followed Dr. Primo's instructions for separating the hip flexors. He excised the old joint, and we replaced it with a shiny new hip ball. Then, I closed the wound layer by layer while the acting chief observed from behind his mask, his beady eyes revealing a passive-aggressive expression. The sponge count was correct, and I was expected to dictate the operation, which I did.

When the operation was completed, Dr. Primo said, "Well done." This was one of the few pieces of positive feedback I received during my early residency. The overall philosophy was that a resident did well until they made an egregious mistake or worse. Then, you'd hear about it from the top.

I disliked this viewpoint. There are countless ways to encourage a trainee. Fostering confidence and well-being didn't cost anything, and I decided to adopt a positive approach when I had juniors working with me.

This operation was the only joint replacement I performed. I understood its necessity in an aging population; yet, strangely enough, I didn't feel the same elation or satisfaction I had previously experienced in the field of general surgery, and there didn't seem to be an intellectual challenge in this bony field. Despite it being Sunday, I, in my gray suit, decided to make quick rounds on the patients. Walking down The Pike, I heard, "Help. He's bleeding," coming from a non-ortho patient room. I backtracked.

Upon entering a two-bedroom, I noticed the first patient bleeding profusely from the site where a long-standing central venous catheter had just been removed. I attributed the bleeding to a venous-cutaneous fistula and sat on the patient's blood-soaked bed, applying significant pressure with several 4x4-inch sponges over the fistula's skin opening. I instructed the patient in the other bed to call the operator and shouted across the room to inform them that we had a code blue.

"We have a bleeding patient who needs to go to the O.R. immediately," I shouted. Following the alarm, a team of physicians gathered around the bed. They quickly assessed the situation and determined that I needed to stay on the bed while continuing to apply pressure. Within minutes, the bed was rolled out of the room and down The Pike to an operating room. The bed carrying the bleeding patient and a street-clothed Michael Meguid was wheeled into the O.R., where the nurses and an anesthesiologist were prepared to receive the patient. A surgeon took my place, holding back the dam to prevent further massive blood loss from the pale and light-headed patient. I calmly walked out of the sterile operating room in my gray suit, much to the astonishment of the operating room desk nurses. I received no accolades for saving a patient's life; I was foolish to have expected any.

Throughout this rotation, my unhappiness grew, compounded by the disjointed nature of patient care, my inability to perform at the level I was accustomed to as a surgical resident in England, and my struggle to connect with the other ortho residents. There was no support from the acting chief resident or the senior resident, who were isolated; there wasn't a team where I could flourish. There were no formal rounds and, consequently, no bedside teaching. I didn't experience camaraderie, cohesion, or collaboration among the residents as I had at Mass General some years earlier. Here, they all seemed apprehensive or even threatened by this "fill-in" acting chief resident.

"You're going to the Fig-Leaf service next and then the Ward Service, where the residents will eat you alive," said the Acting Chief with a chuckle.

"Fig-Leaf service?"

"Yeah. You know, it covers the private parts," he said, irritated that I didn't find his flippant comments amusing.

As the rotation concluded, I realized I had developed an aversion to orthopedics as a specialty, likely influenced by the acting chief's general attitude, especially toward me. I felt relieved when it ended.

10

SURGICAL CULTURE

God found some of the strongest people and made them nurses
—Anonymous

I continued to question my decision to come to Boston. I came close to quitting on several occasions. With a non-immigrant visa, I felt at the mercy of Dr. Moore and the residency system. No matter how hard I tried to escape the treadmill, it would have irreversible repercussions. I felt trapped. I hadn't yet met Dr. Moore, and Victoria had started her pediatric residency. I didn't dare admit my feelings of personal failure to her. In the absence of feedback from the chief, which I believed was related to my performance in ortho, I surmised that despite the poor fit between myself and orthopedics—and my profound unhappiness—I might have performed better than I thought. Nevertheless, I longed to return to London and work for Professor Wilkinson at The Hospital for Sick Children to do general surgery—to operate on the hallowed, beloved abdomen.

Considering the advantages and disadvantages, I reflected on pursuing a mandatory internship in London to become a licensed physician in the UK. After successfully passing the Primary Fellowship examination, I would need to take on various surgical registrar positions, moving from one post to another on my journey to becoming a surgeon. After passing the final Surgical Fellowship examination, I became a Fellow of the Royal College of Surgeons.

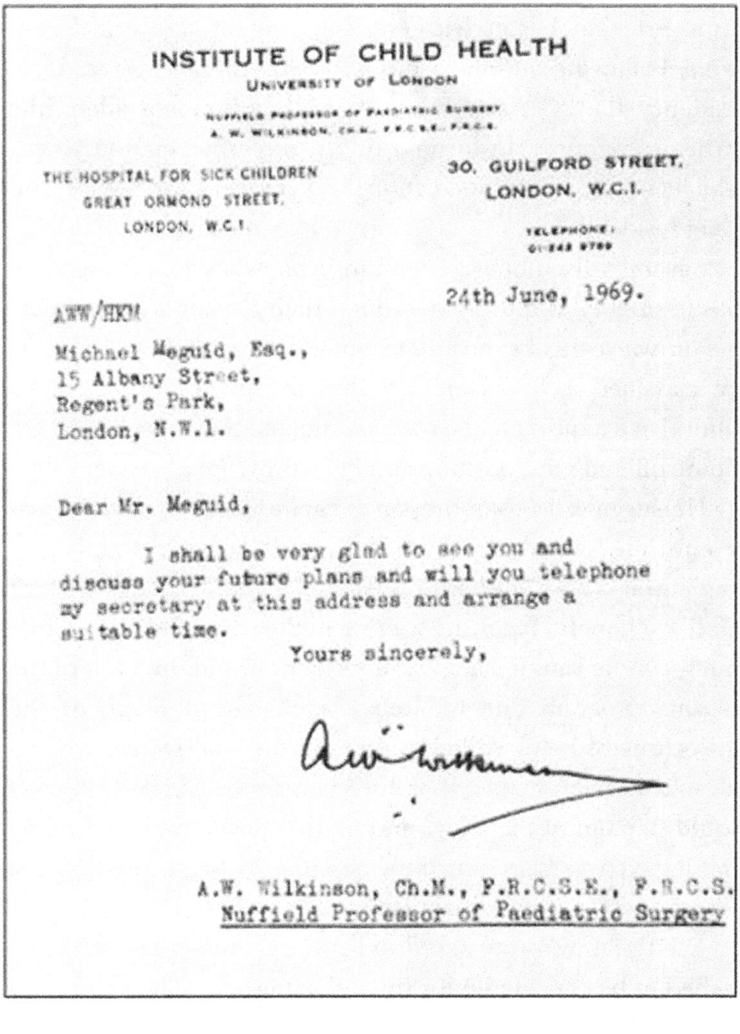

INSTITUTE OF CHILD HEALTH

UNIVERSITY OF LONDON

NUFFIELD PROFESSOR OF PAEDIATRIC SURGERY

A. W. WILKINSON, CH.M., F.R.C.S.E., F.R.C.S.

THE HOSPITAL FOR SICK CHILDREN
GREAT ORMOND STREET,
LONDON, W.C.1

30, GUILFORD STREET,
LONDON, W.C.1.

TELEPHONE:

24th June, 1969.

AWW/HKM

Michael Meguid, Esq.,
15 Albany Street,
Regent's Park,
London, N.W.1.

Dear Mr. Meguid,

I shall be very glad to see you and discuss your future plans and will you telephone my secretary at this address and arrange a suitable time.

Yours sincerely,

A.W. Wilkinson, Ch.M., F.R.C.S.E., F.R.C.S.
Nuffield Professor of Paediatric Surgery

In contrast, I would need to complete five years of training in an accredited general surgery program in the U.S. After that, I would be eligible to take the written and oral examinations of the American Board of Surgery. If I passed, I would become a Fellow of the American College of Surgeons.

After completing my training, I felt that the American system offered more opportunities. Despite my uncertainty, I remained committed to the system here.

The surgical hierarchical training program at the prestigious Brigham began with the selection of categorical residents. Following an internship and two years of postgraduate residency–the PG-2 and PG-3 years—as a junior resident, the vertical program transformed into a trapezoid for the fourth year, PG-4, and continued into the PG-5 year for Senior and Chief residents.

Several disciplines, including anesthesia, orthopedics, plastic surgery, and urology, require their residents to complete one or two years of exposure to general surgery; these residents are classified as provisional within the program. Once they fulfill these requirements, they can pursue their specialties. Dr. Moore offered me a position as a PG-2 provisional resident.

He suggested promoting an exceptional *provisional resident* to the chief residency level to complete their training at Brigham if a position became available. As a junior resident, I felt like a hopeful ballerina waiting in the wings, because sometimes, a more senior categorical resident would drop out of the training program due to illness, a change of heart, or the misfortune of being called to serve in the war. Dr. Moore was the sole decision-maker; therefore, he was the Chief of Chiefs. I would step out of the wings and fill that position to finalize my training. It was a dream only possible in the United States. Nevertheless, it was a dream I clung to.

Each year, we were asked to list the rotations for which we wished to be considered for the following year. The first time I was asked, following the British custom of "keep the best for last," I placed my heart's desire last—a mere sign of modesty. When I didn't get it, I asked, "Why?" The answer was, "You put it last. If you wanted it, you should put it first!" Another American lesson I learned was to adapt to American thought processes and psyche: ask for what you want.

To fulfill my aspiration of becoming a categorical resident and completing my training at the Brigham, I had to become uptight, super-competitive, turbo-compulsive, and hyper-efficient, molding myself into a forceful, aggressive resident. These personality traits felt unnatural, but I had to cultivate them to outperform my competitive categorical partners.

Residents are supervised by attending physicians who have completed five years of training and passed their surgical boards to become independent surgeons. Those interested in academia typically become assistant professors at medical schools. They are expected to conduct research, teach medical students, and perform surgeries. An attending physician appears on a patient's official medical record. He holds final medical and legal responsibility for a patient's care and billing, even though many of the minute-to-minute decisions are made by residents rotating through the service under the attending's supervision.

The duration of each service rotation depended on the training level. Interns typically stayed for one month, residents for two to three months, and chief residents for three to six months. Each rotation included a team of residents at various levels of learning. Everyone was expected to perform with increasing capability and responsibility, acquiring the skills and qualities necessary for promotion. Throughout my residency, all surgical personnel were male. However, this began to change during my second year when Dr. Moore recruited the first female surgical intern, Dr. Robin Goodfellow, who graduated from the Brigham program.

As a PG-2, I had to demonstrate a strong work ethic, great attention to detail, independent learning, efficiency, trustworthiness, and personability to advance—while steering clear of 'tripping over a blade of grass' that might derail my reputation and promotion.

Before residents sit for their written American College of Surgeons exam, they submit a list of all the operations they completed during their five years of training. As a PG-2, I was eager to operate each day. Common wisdom suggests that it takes 1,200 operations of as wide a variety as possible to gain adequate operative skills and surgical knowledge necessary to pass the written and oral exams. So, that's what I did: I claimed 1,200 cases to meet the requirement, despite having performed over 1,500 operations.

Transforming a naive medical student into a competent surgeon who can make rational judgments and perform successful operations requires a significant amount of time. This maturation process begins on the day a medical student starts dissecting a cadaver. Concurrently, the student learns about physiology—specifically, the molecular and cellular aspects of these organs and how they function. The subconscious psychological transformation, which involves distancing, detachment, and compartmentalization of feelings while working on another human being, becomes ingrained in their psyche. In my case, this distancing and detachment unintentionally carried over into my relationship with Victoria. Although I was aware of these defense mechanisms, I struggled to let them go once I returned home, experiencing varying degrees of success.

As a resident, assuming the surgeon's role involves a shift in responsibility, as the surgeon hands the scalpel to the resident for the skin incision. Each surgeon has a slightly different approach. The quality of teaching significantly impacts the transition of a surgical trainee into a surgeon in the operating room, along with the essential pre- and post-operative care and apprenticeship with senior colleagues, where teaching junior staff is a key aspect of education. While surgical techniques are learned through observation in the O.R., much of the etiquette, ethics, and information are shared during rounds and in discussions with a patient's family.

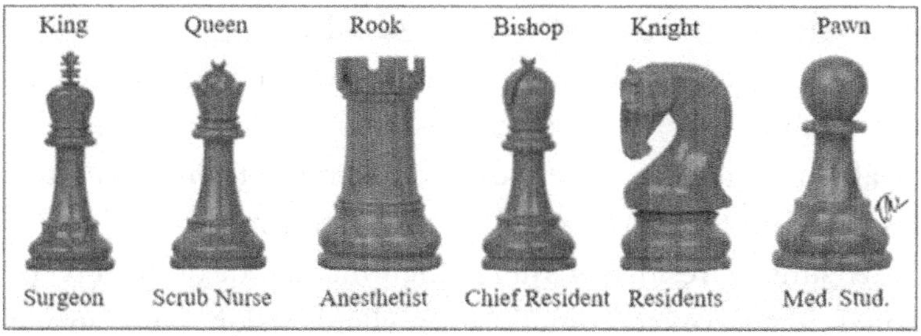

In the O.R., the patient remains the most central figure, even while anesthetized. Similar to chess, the surgeon is the King—an experienced surgical technician wielding the scalpel. He holds all the power, makes all the decisions, and everyone defers to him. The scrub nurse acts as the Queen, exercising authority over everyone except the King and the Rook. Next in the hierarchy of power is the Rook anesthesiologist, who maintains a close and vital collaborative relationship with the King. Anesthesiologists, referred to in England as anesthetists, possess the supreme skill and ability to keep patients alive. Yet, they do not receive appropriate recognition for their crucial work.

In the King's absence, whether he is delayed or called away from the O.R., authority passes to the chief resident, known as the Bishop, while the residents function as Knights. The medical students serve as Pawns, assisting the operative team as directed.

Surgical training begins with the intern or the PG-2 participating in part of the operation. From there, one progresses to a more advanced procedure, such as an appendectomy or an umbilical hernia repair, which involves entering the abdominal cavity and learning to suture fascia.

Once the craft of surgery is ingrained, trainees must practice establishing and refining the natural skill patterns that transform competence into mastery. During the procedures, residents become familiar with the various types and uses of instruments, needles, and suture materials.

Apprenticeship does not merely mean being allowed to watch and assist; it involves absorbing the essence of the invaluable hand-me-down pearls of operative technique, often discussed and demonstrated in the operating room.

A surgical resident requires high manual dexterity, exceptional hand-eye coordination, excellent vision, and strong visual-spatial awareness. Maintaining physical stamina is crucial to meet the demands of surgery. In addition to physical fitness, residents must enhance their emotional resilience, possess a calm temperament, cultivate the ability to work well under pressure, and develop the capacity to lead a multidisciplinary team. They should have keen diagnostic skills, the capability to solve problems and prioritize, practical decision making skills, and strong time and resource management to benefit patients, along with excellent communication skills to manage relationships with colleagues, patients, and their families. Recognizing and accepting that an effective anesthesiologist willing to contribute to your education and become a valued colleague is also beneficial. Another great asset is having an understanding and supportive spouse and family.

The Anesthetist

by Karin Cotterman

Doctor, the crow's feet by your eyes run deep, and I am grateful for that.
Doctor, I hope your baby slept through the night, that your lover didn't leave you yesterday, that it is not the anniversary of a parent's death.
Please hold tightly to all that you have learned.
Let the sight of stainless steel and fluorescent lights please you.
Hold to all the nights you stayed close to books and measurements and labs.
Recall your love for math, the feeling of falling in love with chemistry.
Don't think about the grocery list, or the pull of the tides off Ocean Beach.
Just measure and calculate, and measure again, and watch me breathe.
The ocean will be there. Your lover will make you dinner tonight; your baby is healthy and well rested.
Just put me under, enough not to feel and hear, and pull me up in my new body, pieced together with fat and sutures and threads that dissolve over time.
Let me open my eyes and see both questions and answers, both nightfall and dawn, the stars I always wish upon, the questions on my children's faces.
Bring me back for yet another moment at the too long red light, where I can run my left hand through a fistful of hair, tangles from the smallest knots tugging the roots, a strand caught between my fingers.

11

HIERARCHY, ROUNDS, & CONFESSIONS

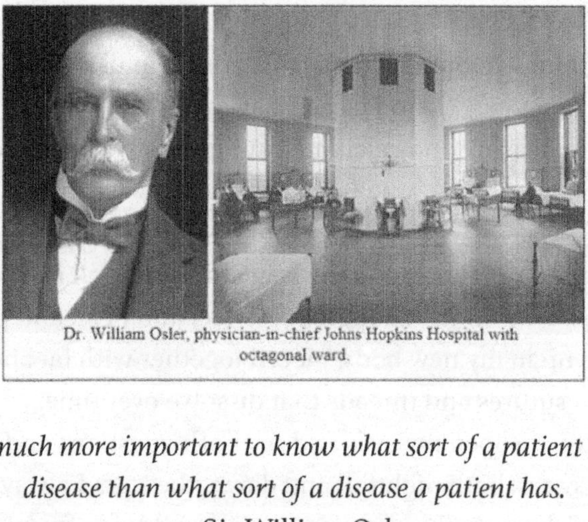

Dr. William Osler, physician-in-chief Johns Hopkins Hospital with octagonal ward.

It is much more important to know what sort of a patient has a disease than what sort of a disease a patient has.
—Sir William Osler

Many credit the genesis of the term "rounds," used when a doctor or team visits patients in hospital wards, to Sir William Osler. At the original Johns Hopkins Hospital, there was an octagonal ward, and in 1889, when Dr. Osler and his team of physicians toured patients' bedsides, they referred to this practice as "rounds." The term stuck. Dr. Osler believed that the patient was the source of medical knowledge. He and Dr. William S. Halsted, the surgeon-in-chief, are credited with establishing the first formal residency program.

Following their lead, the training for principal medical and surgical specialties elsewhere became formalized and institutionalized by the early 20th century. By mid-century, residency had become a standard part of in-hospital medical education, and resident doctors lived at the hospitals where they underwent training, hence the term "residency."

In surgery, *daily* rounds are usually held around 6 a.m. before operations begin. The most senior resident leads the team, which may include medical students and other healthcare professionals, such as nurses. The team examines each patient to ensure continuous improvement and reviews their status, progress, and care plan. Attention includes evaluating the four P's: pain, placement, the condition of the intravenous catheter, potty, and patient positioning to prevent decubitus ulcers or bedsores. The primary focus is to provide immediate care for the patient's surgical condition, with the ultimate goal of outlining the steps toward discharge. Sharing observations and asking questions during rounds promotes a valuable exchange of information that impacts treatment and care planning.

At the Brigham and, in general, at many teaching hospitals, more *comprehensive rounds* occur after the day's surgeries. Led by the attending surgeon, all patients are visited, starting with ICU patients, post-operative patients, and those scheduled for operation the next day. We formed a large group that followed the attending, who used rounds to teach medical students, interns, residents, and the staff involved in the patient's care, fostering cohesion among team members. Rounds are the cornerstone of medical on-the-job training and education—teaching one another is critical. The absence of formal daily rounds on the orthopedic service had left me adrift.

Grand rounds were scheduled for Saturday mornings at 9 a.m., with the entire medical faculty and staff in attendance. Dr. Moore typically presided, or another senior surgeon would step in during his absence. The front row of the auditorium was filled with a group of wise, gray-haired attending surgeons of professorial status, dressed in tweed jackets with leather elbow patches and gray flannel trousers. The resident staff—those eager to go home for their weekend off and those just starting their shift—were seated behind them in the tiers of seats that sloped gently toward the back, where most medical students and a few Research Fellows gathered. Almost every seat was occupied.

Sitting at a table in front of the auditorium, Dr. Moore stated from time to time, "These educational rounds are the major, joint hospital teaching staff meetings. Attendance is mandatory for each member of all services except for orthopedics, whether engaged in research or patient care." Looking around to check whether a particular resident or service was in attendance, he continued, "We will discuss all the complications and deaths to learn from the mistakes and successes of the week. They achieve their greatest usefulness when there is free discussion by *many* people and the entire staff is in attendance."

Initially, grand rounds functioned as a medical forum where patients with unusual symptoms or illnesses were presented in person to fellow physicians to educate them about diagnoses and treatments—similar to my experience when Dr. Goode took me to Queen Square, Institute of Neurology, London, during my time as a medical student. Over time, this spectacle format evolved into the Morbidity and Mortality—famous M&M conferences. Subsequently, at 10 a.m., a distinguished speaker of national or international renown delivered a lecture on a topic of novel interest in surgery. An intellectual discussion followed, the results of which were met with politeness.

During M&M, my fellow residents and I sat in apprehension as the chief resident presented a complication experienced by one of our patients, detailing the patient's diagnosis, the operation, the subsequent complication, and its management. More experienced chief residents developed techniques to present the complication engagingly, often deflecting blame to anesthesia or steering the discussion toward an intriguing aspect of the case unrelated to the complication. A cardinal rule was never to blame the attending surgeon, even if the fault lay with them. Lastly, they muddied the discussion by suggesting techniques that could have prevented the complication. Like the Pied Piper, they guided the audience to follow a different thread of conversation that sidestepped both the complication itself and accountability.

Once everything that needed to be said had been articulated, a few anxious moments followed. At the same time, we awaited Dr. Moore's deliberation on the error classification and, by implication, who had made a mistake. Like Moses descending from Mount Sinai, judgment loomed. In tense anticipatory silence, the audience awaited the inevitable moment of censure, akin to an accused standing in the dock, awaiting the jury's pronouncement of their verdict. Dr. Moore's pronouncement would bring some degree of discomfort, if not unintentional humiliation and embarrassment. Before the guillotine fell, he was sure to face a group of students and repeat what I had heard many times: "You want a surgical team including the anesthesiologist that squarely faces each mishap, straight up, and names it, and takes steps to prevent it from happening again!" Some students would nod, acknowledging the message. He would then announce one of four general errors:

Error in Technique: The wrong procedure is performed, or an error occurs during the procedure that is not identified and addressed. Although the goal of the discussion is for the younger generation of surgeons, anesthesiologists, and medical students to learn from mistakes and avoid repeating them in the future, the resident to whom the error was attributed would sink into their seat, feeling worthless and wondering about their future in the surgical program. The attending surgeon responsible for the mistake sat in uncomfortable silence, watching his resident being sacrificed. I always thought that such a surgeon lacked integrity—no courage. I decided that **when I became an attending, if the error were mine, I would stand up and admit my mistake instead of letting my resident take the blame.**

Other errors included:

Error in Diagnosis: The wrong diagnosis is made, and consequently, the inappropriate treatment is provided.

Error in Management: When a patient's care is mismanaged.

Error in Judgment: There is a misjudgment of a clinical or operative situation.

Patient's Disease: When no culpability is found, yet the patient still dies, what we euphemistically refer to as a "Harvard Death."

Studies show that the litigation rate is significantly lower when surgeons inform families of mistakes, rather than hiding them and allowing the errors to be discovered later. Yet, I have repeatedly been surprised by seasoned and otherwise responsible surgeons who refuse to tell families about their intraoperative mistakes, only to face serious legal consequences afterward. I consider this a violation of trust and ethics. The only surgeon who never makes a mistake does not operate!

Some Surgical Faculty—1972

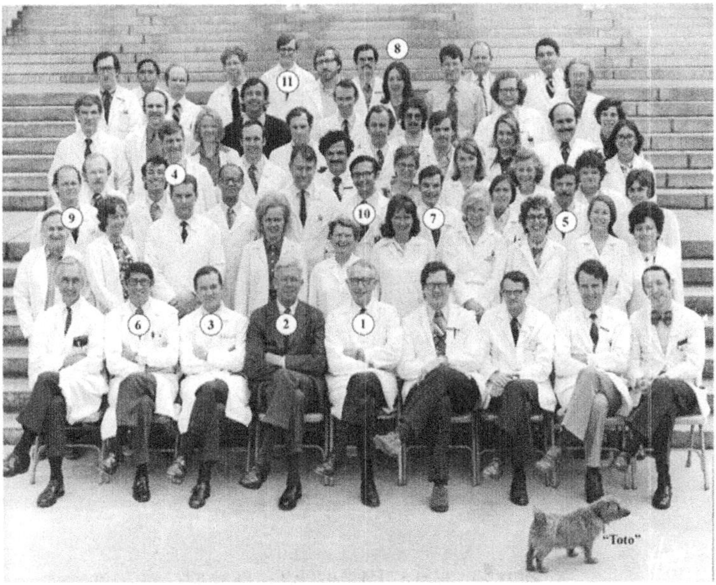

1. Dr. Francis D. Moore. 2. Dr. John Brooks. 3. Dr. "Jack" Collins. To the right of the number: 4. Dr. Lynn Peterson. 5. Dr. Richard Burleson. 6. Dr. Lawrence- 'Larry' Cohn. 7. Dr. Lawrence- 'Larry' Henry. 8. Gail—One of Dr. Moore's secretaries. 9. Dr. Murray Brennan. 10. Dr. Michael Meguid. 11. Dr. Robert Osteen

12

FIG LEAF SERVICE

Seek consultation even if it is not sure to help.
Never be a lone wolf.
—Francis D. Moore

I gradually adjusted to the new system of managing rather than caring for patients, which facilitated my transition, mainly because patients didn't seem to object. My fellow residents on the Fig Leaf service were Mort Kahan, my PG-2 partner, and Dr. Hillel Laks, the PG-3 resident. I had hoped that my chief resident on the Private Service, Dr. Lynn Peterson, would be a more ethical, humane, and patient-centric intellectual—instead, a PG-5 resident filled in for Dr. Lynn Peterson during his one-week vacation.

A majestic walrus mustache dominated most of his face, accentuated by a receding hairline. He barely made eye contact or shook hands when greeting Mort and me. Wasn't the Mustache a tiny bit curious about his junior? He spewed staccato sentences like an uncontrolled tardive dyskinetic tic. The only topic he discussed in his American Italian accent was last night's ball game, whether the American or National League. He voiced his opinion about the umpire making a wrong call, a player making an incorrect move, and on and on. Mort didn't care for baseball, and I didn't yet understand the game. The Mustache talked about the ball game when we entered a patient's room and while we stood at the patient's bedside. He completely disregarded the patient who lay there expecting some medical news.

I was flabbergasted that he continued the monologue over the patient's prone body. The rant didn't end even as we nodded in an attempt to cut off the discussion and redirect his focus to the surgical business at hand. One male patient became visibly irritated, sat up, and interrupted the ongoing chatter, asking, "Hey, Doc, does this have something to do with me or my operation?"

The Mustache stopped mid-sentence and looked at the patient as if to say, "Hey man, you're interrupting my Monday morning quarterbacking." Pausing, he collected his thoughts before addressing the patient, and we were back in the medical world for a brief moment.

When it was one of my patients, I'd immediately start presenting their progress. The Mustache stood across the patient's bed with a look of surprise as if to say, "You cut me off."

He asked the patient how he was doing, and then, as soon as we left his room, he resumed his obsessive monologue about last night's ball game. His insensitivity to the patient's awareness was unbelievable! This incredibly unprofessional behavior peaked when, on several occasions, he walked into a pre-operative fasting patient's room holding a steaming cup of coffee.

I had transitioned from a position where I had been reduced to a scut boy to a role where patients rarely needed operations because it was August. The private surgeons were vacationing at the Cape. All I seemed to do was more scut work with a couple of bedridden, long-term patients suffering from chronic bowel conditions. In England, the nurses appeared to excel at this custodial care. Here, I was a surgical resident starved of the chance to operate, and all I wanted to do—and dreamed about doing—was to cut, cut, cut.

Mrs. O'Connor was what American residents referred to as a high-maintenance patient. She was constantly buzzing the nurses and having us paged to see her. She and her husband had just returned from Ireland. This 54-year-old Bostonian claimed she was served eggs Benedict with less-than-fresh "hollandaise sauce that infected my gut," repeatedly complaining, "That's why I have the runs."

"That must be uncomfortable, Mrs. O'Connor, but you know your attending physician has treated you for many years for your long-standing Crohn's disease. Now, we are working to manage your flare-up."

"It was the Spanish waiter who served me the hollandaise sauce. Imagine a Spanish waiter in Ireland. When is my doctor coming back?" The reassurance and attention she required were both endless and exhausting. I understood why my fellow residents were prescribed medications to treat anxiety.

Mrs. Dombrowski, in the next bed, suffered from chronic constipation and constantly asked for laxatives. "That doctor, you know, the one who was just here. I can't remember his name, but it was something like Ex-Lax."

"Oh, you mean Dr. Laks."

She blushed. "Yes, that's him. He said he'd write me for a laxative, but so far, the nurses haven't given me anything, and I feel, you know, really bunged up."

"Well, no doubt they'll bring you something soon."

Finally, the new PG-5 chief resident, Lynn Peterson, arrived. As we had hoped, he was more cerebral, patient-oriented, and focused on surgical diseases and his residents. He was charming, well-read in various fields of surgery, and eager to teach as we conducted rounds.

I had expected many patients on the Private Service, so I'd be operating up a storm. My contrary experience reinforced the feeling that I wasn't doing or learning enough about surgery. My unhappiness intensified once more, verging on depression.

With only a few patients, we finished our rounds one day in the midafternoon when my pager squawked, "Call the operator."

"You have an outside call."

"Hello?"

"Dr. Meguid," came the voice over a crackly international line. "This is Charlie Clark, the new professor of surgery at University College Hospital." He asked me in his Scottish accent if I would return to London. I need a junior registrar. Are you interested?"

Taken aback by the invitation and enticed by the illusion of long waiting lists of patients in the National Health Service needing surgery, along with my aspiration of operating every single day, I responded impulsively, "Yes, I think so."

"Send me your curriculum vitae and drop me a line confirming." The line went dead. Returning to London seemed to offer me more general surgical options than continuing to be unhappy in Boston.

I ran home. Breathless, I told Victoria, "We're returning to London. Charlie Clark offered me a job at University College Hospital." She looked startled. Once I calmed down, I expressed my discontent and profound unhappiness with the position in Boston, my lack of sufficient cases to operate on, and my sense that I wasn't thriving in this environment. "I just don't feel I fit in here. I'd do better in London, where I'm wanted."

Her reply stunned me into disbelief.

I just started my residency, and I like it here. I have everything I need, so I'm not going back!

I felt trapped.

I fell in love with a strikingly beautiful woman, my Victoria, during her first year of medical school while I was a second-year student. We spent nearly every moment together during the intense four years of medical school, living a life filled with deep love and passion. However, the stressful periods of being apart for two years, as we each completed our internships in separate hospitals, strained our emotional and relational needs. This separation awakened and intensified my childhood fear of insecurity and abandonment, which is rooted in irrational emotional recall.

In her absence, when we were back in London, I eased my anxiety and loneliness with the comfort of another, leading to a brief romantic liaison. Although Victoria didn't know about my infidelity, I was aware of it, and it troubled me. I had wronged her. After graduating, we spent ten days making rounds, saying goodbye to family, and enjoying some sightseeing together. Free from stress, I rekindled my deep love for Victoria. I believed that leaving London for Boston and putting my emotional turmoil behind me would lead to a rebirth of our marriage. After all, wasn't America the land of second chances?

The stressful orthopedic rotation that deprived me of surgery reignited the emotional insecurity I had experienced in London. The woman I married, the woman I chose to stay with, now obstructed my path to becoming the surgeon I aspired to be. I also suspected she feared becoming the caregiver for her mother back on the Isle of Wight; as Shirley aged, her manic depression worsened, and she was living alone. Her brother lived in England—the land of social services—and contributed to her care. Victoria repeated, "I'm not going back!"

My unhappiness at the time prevented me from realizing

that Victoria was also pursuing her path. Without surgery to make me feel useful, the old demons of feeling unwanted, unworthy, and unloved resurfaced. That festering abscess of childhood healed when my self-esteem was strong—when I felt needed, deserving, and loved. But when Victoria, whom I cherished, rejected me, it removed the scab from the healing wound, and I drifted into despair. I would have to stay.

As August approached, tanned and relaxed, the attendings began returning to Boston. New patient referrals had accumulated during their absence, and hospitalized patients required surgery. The patients' chorus of "Where is my doctor?" grew progressively louder and must have reached the waters off Cape Cod. The Private Service became increasingly busy.

I admitted Mr. Gomez, a twenty-one-year-old Panamanian pilot for Pan Am—once an American global airline that has since ceased operations. Mr. Gomez's popularity at the company stemmed from his ability to pilot his propeller-driven Constellation aircraft over long distances for extended periods without needing a bathroom break. After taking off from San Francisco, he would land in Boston almost seven hours later without leaving his seat.

Instead of a blessing, it turned out to be a chronic surgical problem. When I reviewed his history, I discovered that he had experienced constipation since childhood. He mentioned he was the seventh son of poor farmers.

A doctor passing through town told my mother that it could be megacolon and prescribed cascara syrup, which he said would help because it was a laxative for constipation.

"And did it work?"

"Sort of, but it was expensive. I found dilating my rectum regularly using a candle I took from the altar of our village church worked even better." Looking around, he lowered his voice and added, "It was cheaper, of course."

"Really? So, the candle was more effective than a laxative?"

He nodded.

Mr. Gomez was a tall man by any standard, as he lay in bed, ready for me to examine him. He was slender and had well-developed upper body strength. His abdominal wall was so thin that I could see and palpate a swelling resembling the large colon filled with stool—a sausage that started in the right lower quadrant, swept up toward his liver, curved around the umbilicus to his left side, and then down to his lower left quadrant where the prominence faded. The mass felt like clay under compression and retained the imprint of my fingers—the famously termed "university tumors." These tumors were only feces. In addition to feeling doughy, I observed several waves of peristalsis rippling toward the rectum, accompanied by bowel sounds. With his consent, I performed a rectal examination. It was challenging to insert my well-lubricated and gloved index finger. I understood why he'd found the use of an ecclesiastical candle helpful. Since it came from the altar, perhaps it also possessed saintly curative properties for him.

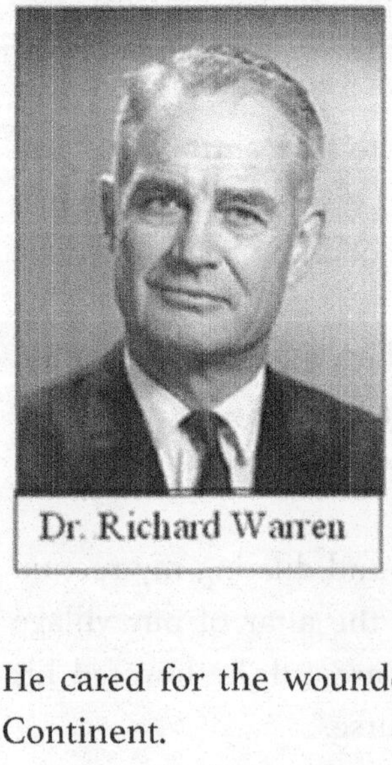

Dr. Richard Warren

Dr. Richard Warren, a tall, lean, middle-aged New Englander with thinning gray hair and a Boston accent, had obtained a series of abdominal X-rays for Mr. Gomez. As a Harvard professor, he specialized in gastroenterology and vascular surgery. Like many of his peers, he joined the Fifth General Hospital, known as the "Harvard Medical Unit," and rose to the rank of Lieutenant Colonel at the outbreak of World War II. He cared for the wounded, first in England and then on the Continent.

After lunch, Dr. Peterson, Mort, a few medical students, and

I went with Dr. Warren to view the films. Even without contrast, the films showed a dilated, distended large bowel, similar to my findings, along with a few loops of small bowel above it that were filled with air and feces.

Dr. Warren said, "Well, boys, this is an interesting case of Hirschsprung's condition. For those who don't know, Dr. Hirschsprung was a Danish surgeon who first described 'megacolon' in 1885. Still, it wasn't until 1901 that it was recognized that the real problem wasn't the impressively dilated large bowel, the megacolon, but the lack of nerve ganglia in the muscle walls of the rectum below the dilation." Dr. Warren hesitated and looked around the dim X-ray viewing room, then refocused on his motley audience of male residents and medical students. "The constipation is caused by missing nerve cells in the walls of the end of the colon—the rectal muscles just above the anus." He continued to explain that the genetic lack of ganglia leads to the nerves' inability to relax the rectum, preventing the patient from defecating. The absence of these nerve ganglia causes a spastic rectum. Consequently, stool collects above it, dilating the colon and causing the megacolon.

"Now, isn't that interesting?" he said with an air of amazement and authority. He was the editor of a prestigious surgical journal, The Archives of Surgery, which had recently published a paper on this very topic.

As he continued his teaching, I nervously checked my pager to ensure it was working and that I wasn't missing a call to examine an expected special patient I was to prepare for surgery the following morning.

Dr. Warren continued, "When the colon gets so dilated," and he made his point by separating his hands, "it gets ulcerated, infected, and painful. As a result, they used to cut out that piece of large bowel." He hesitated, allowing us to imagine the operation. Dr. Warren came to the punch line, "Some surgeons weren't up to speed with surgical pathology and were obsessed by their absolute power and their conviction that the problem was the megacolon. This was unfortunate. The poor patient would always have his normal dilated mega-colon cut out. The surgeon was satisfied each time that he was doing the right thing for the patient." Dr. Warren paused for the message to sink in.

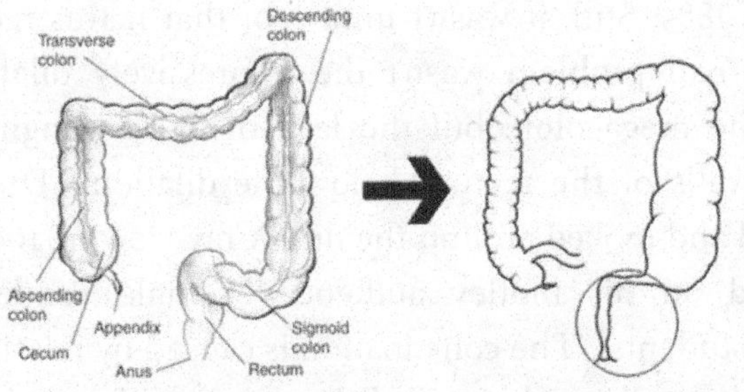

Left: normal large bowel with labeled segments. Right: Circled diseased segments of rectum and colon with no nerve area causing spasm resulting in dilated large bowel above it. The circled areas are resected.

"A saying comes to mind: Most doctors are prisoners of their education and shackled by their profession." We have to guard against our scientific misinformation and prejudices."

We began to understand that the real problem was not the colon but the obstruction in the rectum below it.

"If the surgeon had asked the patient what their problem was, if they saw that they suffered from rectal spasm, if they knew that the patient dilated their rectum, if they had attempted to perform a rectal exam, and if they'd kept up to date with the surgical literature about this disease, then perhaps they would have recognized that the problem was their inadequate knowledge and their incorrect conviction, and not the mega-colon."

I could anticipate his conclusion: "The patient's input would have raised doubts about the origin of the illness—the site of the pathology—and thus the type of operation to perform." When would patients become their advocates? This reinforced my early training in London, which emphasized the importance of taking a comprehensive history from the patient rather than relying solely on X-rays.

The field of surgery has often been dominated by misguided yet self-assured, well-intentioned, domineering, bullying, intimidating, and sometimes pompous men. They frequently muscled their way into leadership roles, held zealous opinions about which operations should be performed, and wielded immense influence over generations of fellow surgeons. They conducted surgeries with a firm, self-righteous conviction that they knew what was best, insisting they were acting in the patient's best interest. Their Achilles' heel was a lack of self-doubt—a quality every surgeon should possess. Unfortunately, they were often mistaken, as indicated by evolving scientific findings. As Dr. Warren spoke, I became convinced that basic or applied surgical research is an essential component of surgical training—necessary because research instills the vital element of doubt in surgeons. Every surgeon should question their actions and ask, "Did I do the right thing for this patient? After all, I'm not God." As William Osler said, "One special advantage of the skeptical attitude of mind is that a man is never vexed to find that, after all, he has been in the wrong."

Dr. Peterson asked Dr. Warren, "What do you plan to do?"

"We'll fix him in stages," he replied. "First, we'll do a rectal biopsy to confirm the histological diagnosis that he lacks nerve ganglia in the muscle walls of the rectum." He hesitated to make us understand that we couldn't perform an appropriate operation without an accurate diagnosis. "Once we have that," he continued, "then during the next operation, he'll need a colostomy, pretty low, I'd imagine, to get him cleaned out of all the accumulated stool. Then, when I'm satisfied his colon is clear of feces and I've endoscoped him, we'll excise the rectum and perhaps the lower part of the colon. After mobilizing the remaining colon, we'll pull it down and anastomose it to the anal cuff. Lastly, we'll close the colostomy."

My pager squawked. Through the static, I heard that a new admission was in the ward, ready to be clerked and examined. I hurried off to examine her.

13

A HOLE IN MY CHEST

Even the knowledge of my fallibility cannot keep me from making mistakes.
Only when I fail do I get up again.
—Vincent Van Gogh

During early morning rounds, the buzz was that a very important woman was coming to Boston. It was all hush-hush. Not even Mort Kahan knew the social details. It was whispered that she, "you know, that woman . . . that special patient" has a suspected diagnosis of breast cancer. When she was assigned to a private room, the system would inform the professor, a man I respected and admired. That evening, he asked me whether I was on call that night. Satisfied that I was, he told me with a gleam of delight in his eye that her surgeon in Chicago had referred this patient after consulting him.

I felt a slight pang of envy; it must be an excellent compliment to have a fellow surgeon think so highly of you that he would refer a patient. I was too naïve to understand the various reasons why a patient was passed on to a surgical colleague—

sometimes, the original surgeon didn't want to operate for undisclosed reasons. Dr. Moore's philosophy was to seek a consultation, even if not to assist, so that one was never a lone wolf dealing with a complex disease or patient. At other times, a consultation clarified the type or magnitude of an operation in the surgeon's mind, but a larger one wasn't necessarily better.

Far from being a secret, all the nurses at the nursing station were tittering with rumors and brimming with excitement, speculating about various names of famous fashion superstars and celebrated women featured in numerous fashion magazines. I concluded that she must be a model or a fashion editor—a celebrity up close!

When I entered the VIP's room to examine and prepare her for a breast procedure the next day, I was engulfed in Chanel No. 5. She sat in bed wearing an elegant mink bedjacket over a frilly nightgown. At the same time, her hospital gown still lay neatly folded at her feet. Despite her regal grace, she looked apprehensive and held her husband's hand.

"Who are you?"

"I'm Dr. Meguid, the resident who will care for you and prepare you for your operation tomorrow."

"Do I detect a British accent?"

"Yes. I went to medical school in London. And you must be Mrs."

"Mrs. Leonora Philbey," replied her gray-suited husband, who let go of her hand but remained standing closely by her bed, clasping his fedora.

As I began to take a history from Mrs. Philbey, she requested that I address her as Leonora. Still uncomfortable with the American practice of using first names, I continued to refer to my patients by their titles throughout my career. Using their given names felt like an excessive degree of familiarity for a professional surgeon-patient relationship. Additionally, I appreciated that her husband remained in the room. The discussion between the patient and me was equally important for a partner to hear. However, I remained mindful of asking specific questions that the patient might prefer to answer without her husband present.

Mrs. Philbey was in her late forties. Rather than having her children, she successfully raised three of Mr. Philbey's. Her slender, well-proportioned body attested to her past as a runway model.

Given her mink bed jacket and subtle yet shimmering makeup, I did not doubt that she always appeared sophisticated, wore the latest fashions, and exuded chic elegance. Stylishness served as her signature. I learned that she organized fashion shoots, met with couture designers, oversaw the weekly layout of the magazine, and routinely traveled to Gucci, Chanel, Dior, and other fashion houses across Europe. As the fashion editor of a weekend magazine for a major national daily newspaper, her career and lifestyle choices could be impacted by her medical journey.

Mr. Philbey's job as a stockbroker in Chicago rarely allowed him to travel with her on these trips, but I was sure she had a network of associates and possibly even a model who accompanied her. With Mr. Philbey's children grown they were now empty nesters, it was evident that the world of style and fashion consumed her entirely, just as stocks and bonds did for him. When time permits, they unwind for long weekends in their simple Frank Lloyd Wright home, where they appreciate the beauty of each season in the vast woodlands surrounding them.

When I took her history, I learned that she had never been pregnant or breastfed, and that her periods had become irregular. As she was an adopted child, she did not know her mother or any medical history about her "lost family," except that they had immigrated from northern Europe, possibly Sweden or England.

Two weeks earlier, she noticed a lump in her left breast

while showering. A mammogram confirmed a small 2 cm mass in the lower quadrant of her left breast, which triggered a referral to Peter Bent Brigham Hospital. During my examination, I gently palpated the mass, which was discrete and surrounded by relatively little fatty tissue. Her breasts were relatively small but not disproportionate to her slender physique, consistent with the typical model's build. I did not feel any lymph nodes in her armpit or above the clavicle. The rest of her physical examination was unremarkable.

With my notes in hand, I sat next to her and said, "Mrs. Philbey, did the professor mention to you or explain what he was planning to do?"

"Mr. Philbey and I haven't met him yet. Shouldn't we call his office and let him know we are here?"

"No doubt the admissions office and the nursing station have already informed him. He's probably doing his rounds and is on his way."

"I really must meet him before the operation tomorrow. The nurses mentioned I was first on his operative list."

The professor, dressed in his starched white coat, walked in as if on cue. Medical students and the head nurse trailed . Radiating the aura and dignity of an eminent surgeon, he greeted the Philbeys with a most congenial smile.

His appearance dramatically changed the mood in the room. The Philbeys, showing great deference, greeted him with a solemn air of gratitude for accepting Leonora as his patient. In the ensuing intellectual and social banter among the three, the professor admired Mrs. Philbey's status as an editor, noting, "My wife reads your magazine each weekend." Mrs. Philbey blushed. Shifting the subject as he approached her hospital bed, the tall professor looked down into Mrs. Philbey's face and asked, "How are you feeling?"

"I'm feeling quite nervous. Can you assure me that it's not

cancer?" she asked, her voice trembling with fear and uncertainty.

"That's what your doctor told me on the phone when he was referring you to me. But when you're asleep, we will biopsy areas of concern. This allows us to examine it microscopically." The surgeon's choice of words and approach to the situation were carefully considered to provide reassurance while conveying the seriousness of the problem. He continued, "Frequently, it's benign, you know, not cancerous." Observing his approach, I learned to handle such delicate medical issues with empathy and clarity.

"That would be good news. I have this intuition that it will not be a tumor. There is an important meeting coming up in Italy that I cannot afford to miss." Her hopeful tone and determined expression were palpable in the room.

The professor looked at her. Were they both on the same page? I got the impression that there were two parallel conversations: one attempting to gently ease the patient into accepting reality—that it was cancerous and all its sequelae—while the other continued to dwell in her world of fashion, fantasy, and magical thinking.

"Yes, as I said, the pathologist freezes and examines it under the microscope. Now, if it's cancer," he took a deep breath; there was a momentary calm in the room as we all held ours, "well then, we'll take care of it. You'll be asleep for the biopsy and any other procedures we need to perform until we finish. That way, you won't require a second operation. Once you're awake, you'll be moved back to this room."

"If it's cancer," she hesitated, "what will you do?" He patted her shoulder gently and said, "Don't worry. I'll take good care of you. We want to ensure it's all gone so it won't bother you again." His words brought a wave of relief over her, and she managed to offer a small, grateful smile.

At this stage, I expected the professor to clear the room,

asking the head nurse and me to stay so he could examine her breasts in relative privacy, enabling him to gather the necessary clinical information vital for forming a pre-operative impression that might influence the type of operation he would perform.

But he didn't.

The gathering remained in the room.

Turning to me, the professor asked, "Is everything otherwise in order?"

"Yes, sir, except I haven't been able to locate her mammograms." He turned to the patient. "Did you bring these with you?"

"No. Was I meant to?"

"We'll find it. Failing this, I have the report. Our pathologist will decide whether it's nothing to worry about or something we'll take care of." I admired how the professor deftly answered her questions about cancer and what he'd do to help her. By gently patting her shoulder to bolster her confidence while saying, "I'll take good care of you," he projected the image of a technically proficient surgeon, embodying the essence of an esteemed gentleman.

At the same time, I heard what the professor had told his patient. If it were cancer, he'd take care of it. What I understood was clearly recognized by most surgeons trained in America: a time-honored Halsted mastectomy. Yet, did the patient know what we meant in an era before the internet?

Worse, the professor had assumed a paternalistic role, believing he knew with absolute certainty what was best for the patient without sharing his thought process with her. He also neglected to discuss other options she might have had, such as McWhirter's lumpectomy with radiation therapy, given her small breasts.

Turning to me, he said, "Don't forget to match her for three units of blood." I understood that he had decided to proceed with the standard Halstead radical mastectomy, a procedure traditionally performed in America at the time.

As surgeons, we often speak to our patients almost in the code of surgical jargon to reassure and comfort them. However, I have frequently wondered with a sense of unease and concern whether what the doctor says matches what the patient understands and imagines. Inherent in the ambiguous phrase "take care of you" is "I'm the surgeon, the authority, and you are my patient. You must trust that I'll do what is best for you."

Mr. Philbey anxiously asked the professor, "Will she be all right?" His affirmative answer was encouragingly vague and unqualified. The nurse helped the patient change into her hospital gown as Mr. Philbey and I entered the corridor.

The operative consent form I completed that evening stated, "Left breast biopsy and radical mastectomy." Mrs. Philbey read the consent and signed it.

"Do you have any further issues you wish us to address?"

"No," she smiled. "Will you be at my operation?"

"I'm sorry, I've been assigned to help another surgeon, but when I'm finished, I might pop in to see how you're doing."

"Oh. That's good."

Like lower limb amputations on the orthopedic service, I found any disfiguring operation on the human body emotionally unsettling, even though I understood intellectually that we had to perform these procedures.

As a medical student, I spent a vacation with Victoria at her home on the Isle of Wight, lying on a blanket in her sunny garden, reading Larrey's 1815 Memoirs of Military Surgery. Dominique-Jean Larrey was the chief surgeon of the French army and a favorite of Napoleon. Larrey wrote about his surgical experiences during Napoleon's major military campaigns. He described the most common surgical injuries that soldiers sustained, numerous amputations he performed on limbs to save their lives, the use of warm coal-tar pitch to control bleeding, and, curiously, the guillotine amputations of a woman's breast injured as an innocent civilian.

Despite Larrey's descriptions, or perhaps because of them, I sensed that such operations—including procedures like Halsted's radical mastectomy—wouldn't be agreeable to perform. I never assisted with or was exposed to a radical mastectomy during my training in London, choosing to avoid this very operation described in 1894 by William Halsted, which had become surgical dogma in the treatment of breast cancer in America. The surgeon made large incisions, removed the breast along with the subcutaneous tissue of the skin flaps, excised the underlying pectoralis major and minor muscles, and removed the entire axillary lymphatic tissue up to the axillary vein. The resulting defect was closed when the flaps were brought together to cover the rib cage. Occasionally, this left a gap that required closure with skin grafts. The extent of the resection during the operation often led to complications, including paresthesia, numbness in the inner arm, and lymphedema, or swelling of the arm.

Thousands of these operations have been performed since Halsted described the procedure, which he named a radical mastectomy in 1898, while he was chief of surgery at Johns Hopkins. It became the standard of care for treating breast cancer until the 1970s, when our understanding of tumor biology changed, and we began to learn that there might be other options.

In 1966, I read the Scottish physician Robert McWhirter's paper in the British Medical Journal, which my mentor, Professor Pilcher, had given to me while I was an acting intern at University College London, where I was a medical student before he retired. I was impressed that the removal of the tumor alone, followed by radiation therapy, as McWhirter advocated, had similar survival rates and fewer complications than Halsted's radical mastectomy. In a randomized study comparing the two procedures, the survival rate at ten years was 52% for both operations. Although not entirely accepted in America when I was training, McWhirter's procedure appealed to me more. Given Mrs. Philbey's petite body type and profession, perhaps more thought should have been given to her options. Even though the professor may not have handled such a case, it was well within his technical abilities, though not within his comfort zone.

Although I never wanted to be involved in a Halsted-type operation as a trainee, I learned how to perform them while assisting on several cases because this was the accepted standard of care.

The next morning, after the 6 a.m. rounds, the team split into two groups. The chief, Mort, and several medical students assisted the professor with Mrs. Philbey's operation. I joined Dr. Warren in another operating room, where, with his help, I performed an extensive rectal biopsy on Mr. Gomez's rectum and drained a perirectal abscess. Operating in the general surgical domain, rather than the orthopedic field, was exhilarating. I loved it. Thoughts of quitting vanished like smoke.

Our operation was much shorter, so we finished while the procedure on Mrs. Philbey was still ongoing. Curious about the progress, I entered the operating room. They had completed the mastectomy, dressed the chest wound, and were wrapping six-inch elastic ace bandage dressings around the chest and upper torso of a semi-sitting, anesthetized Mrs. Philbey.

During evening rounds, the professor and his entourage crowded around Mrs. Philbey's bed. She sat up, looking slightly paler in her hospital gown, relieved that the operation was over.

Mr. Philbey stood by her side. He had previously shared the news with his wife that the professor had done a mastectomy due to cancer, to which she had wept softly.

"You did well," the professor said. "Everything went smoothly."

"Did I need a lot of blood?" she sniffed.

"There was no need for that."

"When will I know about the lymph glands?"

"The final pathology report should be ready in a few days."

Tugging at her ace wrap, she said, "These are quite tight."

"That has to stay on for at least three days." Looking up at me and the ward nurse, he emphasized, "I'll change the ace dressings myself, so leave it on."

We moved on to the next patient.

Three days later, the professor and the nurses unwound the ace dressings from around Mrs. Philbey's chest. Once the dressings were off, we saw that the professor had made a neat chest incision extending from the top of the left axilla or armpit toward the edge of the midline, exposing the breastbone of the chest wall. Through this, he had removed the breast, encompassing the skin cut off the biopsy site, plus the axillary nodes and both chest muscles in a single en bloc mass to prevent the spread of cancer. Given her slight build and paucity of subcutaneous fat, the chest wall skin flaps were thin, explaining why he had wrapped her chest with light-pressure ace wraps to ensure the flaps stuck to the underlying chest wall. No skin grafts were needed.

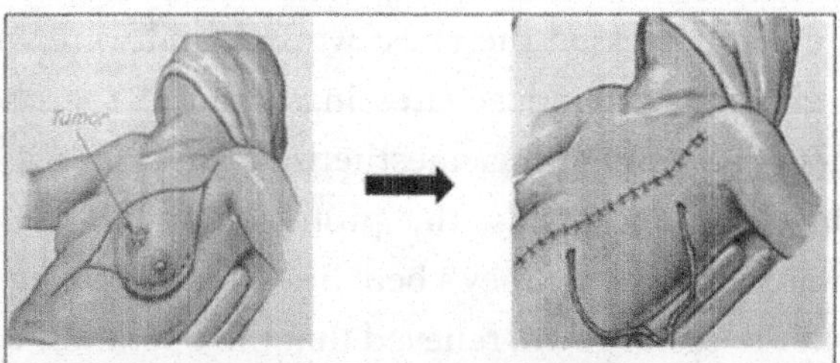

Picture of patient with breast tumor and following Halsted radical mastectomy.

Stepping back while the nurses redressed the wound with a fresh, lighter dressing, the professor nodded, pleased with the result. By any standards, he had conducted a careful procedure, and it was technically a perfect wound. However, throughout the dressing removal, Mrs. Philbey had averted her eyes. While her hospital gown was changed, the professor and I stepped out of the room to provide her with a modicum of privacy and to speak with her husband. "It looks good. I'm pleased that none of the twenty-two lymph nodes were involved."

"You're saying the cancer has been taken care of?" said Mr. Philbey. "Is that right?"

The professor nodded. "She will still need some radiation therapy to her chest wall, the mastectomy scar, and the two surgical Hemovac drain sites," he said. "That can be done in a facility near your home."

"For how long?"

"Typically, five days a week, for about six weeks."

Mr. Philbey beamed, shook the professor's hand, and entered his wife's room.

I departed.

As I was on call that night, the rest of the team left, leaving me with a long list of tasks to check and complete for our service patients. Mr. Gomez was doing well, and I continued my evening rounds, assessing the other patients in the service and coordinating discharges.

Suddenly, my pager squawked. I was being paged to Mrs. Philbey's bedside. When I stepped into her room, she was alone, wailing loudly. Curious as to what her wound looked like; she had taken the dressing down.

"Look what he's done!" she almost screamed as tears rolled down her face. "I'm no longer a woman. He mutilated me. Look, I'm lopsided! How could he have done this to me? How will Mr. Philbey love me? How can I continue my job? What will people say about me?"

She covered herself, her whole body convulsing as she wept. I pulled up a chair and took her hand, fearful she would touch and contaminate the wound, yet partly to comfort her, knowing I really couldn't. She made no effort to withdraw her hand. Instead of calming her, she sank into a torrent of self-loathing. Words spurted out incoherently, ". . . incomplete woman . . . less attractive . . . work and social communication." She wouldn't stop. When I tried to explain that the operation was necessary to ensure her longevity, the rage, fear, and expressions of anxiety started anew, mixed with waterfalls of tears and writhing in her bed. The noise drew a nurse into the room, who attempted to calm her down.

I picked up the phone beside her bed and had the operator page the on-call psychiatry resident, Dr. Chris Gates. He arrived promptly when Mrs. Philbey had exhausted herself into a catatonic state. I realized I didn't possess the skills to address my patient's psychological reaction to her radical mastectomy, but Dr. Gates was highly qualified to manage the situation.

This event made me realize that this type of operation may not be optimal for all patients. In Mrs. Philbey's case, we had not considered or asked what her expectations were regarding the operation or, given her profession, how she envisioned her physique would change. We didn't reflect on how this operation would impact her life. Her figure was the bedrock of her womanhood, and at that moment, she was at the pinnacle of her career. We may have cured her of cancer, but we crushed her spirit, the essence of her being, maybe even her soul, leading to profound depression, grief over the loss of her breast, and possibly even her job.

In this patient, perhaps a McWhirter's procedure—removing the tumor without excising the breast—followed by radiation therapy, would have been more appropriate. Could we have considered the possibility of immediate reconstruction with the help of the plastic and reconstructive surgeons, given that her body was her currency? I wondered whether we had treated the patient or merely the disease.

I found the surgeon's statement, "Don't worry. I'll take good care of you," unacceptable. The patient had the right to know what was to be done and the alternatives. It was too paternalistic a statement, like telling a little girl, "Daddy knows best." From this experience, I learned to discuss the operative procedure more fully with the patient in the presence of a family member, covering the pros and cons of each procedure and listening to the patient's input.

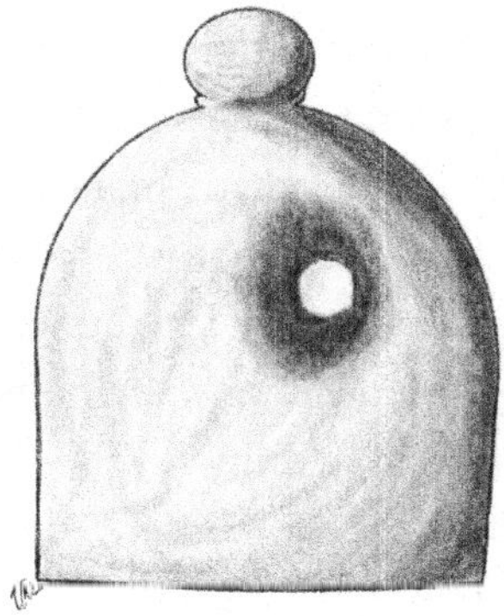

Months later, I received a package mailed in Chicago. On opening it, I saw a three-inch terracotta figurine showing an undistinguished head, shoulder, and the upper half of a torso. Through its left side, a pencil poked a hole through the torso. I was shocked. In an accompanying handwritten note, Mrs. Philbey wrote:

> Dear Dr. Meguid,
> I'm so very sorry not to have had a chance to say goodbye and thank you before I left the PBBH. But I do want you to know how much I appreciated all you did for me during my stay in hospital (I wish I could say you cured me!) I'm now receiving radiation therapy. You were more than kind—
> Sincerely, Leonora

In the future, I would explore with my patients the significance of their breasts, what they meant to them, and how they contributed to their psyche as women. While I understood the biology of the disease, it was important to me to understand their expectations regarding how the operation would affect their figures. Listening to what they had to say would occasionally change my approach, keeping their survival in mind. Sometimes, I would need to re-explain why I considered what I intended necessary for their health care. These conversations would empower the patients, allow them to feel involved in what I and my surgical team had planned, and prevent them from being surprised by the outcome—perhaps decreasing the incidence of malpractice lawsuits.

Victoria began receiving an advanced copy of a weekend fashion magazine mailed from Chicago to our home each Tuesday. We believed it reflected Mrs. Philbey's ongoing productivity. Despite the fatigue we experienced on the nights we finally returned home after being on call for 36 hours, we thumbed through it, drawn by the interesting articles we wanted to read. However, we couldn't do so because the magazine competed with our sleep needs.

A couple of months later, Mrs. Philbey wrote again, inviting us to lunch. They were visiting her sister in Connecticut, and she wanted to "pay her respects." I replied that we didn't have a car, but that Victoria and I would be delighted to meet her and Mr. Philbey.

A brief, unexpected snowstorm blanketed the northeast over the recent free weekend as temperatures dropped. On Sunday morning, the Philbeys picked us up in their Lincoln and drove us for a couple of hours to a charming, rustic restaurant, The Mill, by a stream somewhere in Connecticut. A cheerful Mr. Philbey stated, "Isn't the weekend fashion magazine a work of art? Mrs. Philbey is doing a terrific job, don't you think?" We simultaneously agreed with his comment and apologized for not having time to write a thank-you note. She smiled and waved her hand dismissively.

The conversation remained within the limits of socially acceptable politeness. There was no mention of her cancer, her hospital ordeal, or her visible disappointment with the outcome.

The truth in this case was that, considering her career, a lumpectomy with radiation or a McWhirter operation would have been a better fit for this patient than the radical Halsted procedure. What was done devastated her life, and she ultimately needed radiation anyway.

As only an affluent, perceptive, and empathetic fashion editor could, Mrs. Philbey wore flattering outfits that concealed her injured body. Yet she had changed. Gone was the air of confidence she had projected upon her hospital admission. She seemed more subdued. It slipped out that she was no longer the fashion editor of the weekend magazine but now worked at the editorial desk for the newspaper. Mr. Philbey gently guided his wife's conversation in other directions.

During lunch, I shared how the setting, sitting by a window of a mill next to a brook, reminded me of George Eliot's "The Mill on the Floss." I continued by saying that George Eliot was a pen name for Mary Ann Evans.

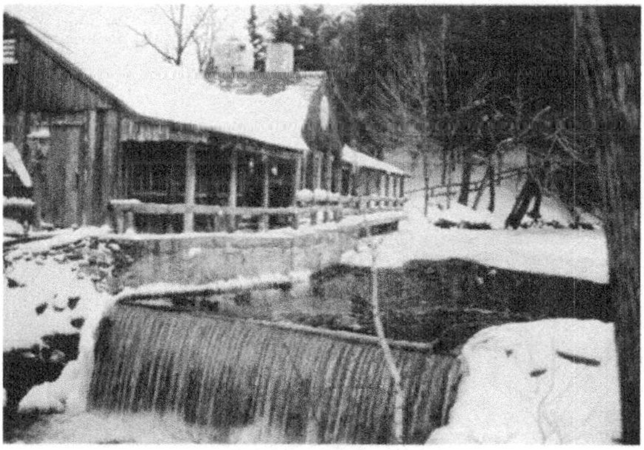

I suddenly realized I was walking into a sensitive minefield and wished I could stop the rest from coming out of my mouth. "She was a British novelist in the early 1840s who wisely adopted a man's name in a male-dominated society, as female authors were not accepted." The parallel didn't escape Mrs. Philbey. Looking at me intensely, she nodded. It was the nod of a sadder, yet wiser, woman.

Ten years later, she likely would have had a female surgeon who understood her career and lifestyle. That female surgeon might have also performed an alternative procedure that wouldn't have drained her spirit.

14

HUNGRY, BOLD, & UNLEASHED

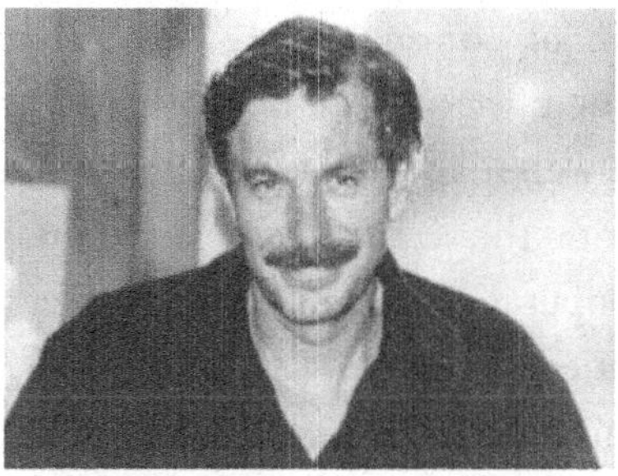

My dear friend, Dr Richard 'Burley' Burleson

A good chief has always been a good assistant.
—Charles F. M. Saint

In 1946, Congress passed the Hill-Burton Free or Reduced-Cost Care Act. This legislation provided hospitals and other healthcare facilities with grants and loans for construction and modernization. In return, they agreed to offer free medical services to all indigent individuals residing in the facility's area, including patients without medical insurance or resources, for necessary healthcare. The Brigham, like Mass General during my time as a student there, along with many other major district hospitals, had a "Ward Service," a large room designated for patients in this category.

Burley, the mature, energetic, and caring chief resident, known for his reputation as an experienced surgeon with strong technical skills—many of which were acquired in Vietnam—was responsible for the patients admitted to the Ward Service. Dr. Hillel Laks, a third-year resident, along with two second-year residents, Mort and I, assisted him. A dedicated cigarette smoker, a habit Burley developed while working in a Mobile Army Surgical Hospital Unit in Vietnam, he was also a passionate teacher with a positive, can-do attitude. He inspired us with his no-nonsense, resolute, and cheerful leadership style.

Unlike the unclear leadership of the resident Ortho Service, this team's chain of command was very clear. To my great delight, I'd be operating on the beloved abdomen once more. As residents, we were expected to see new patients referred to the clinic or from the E.R., diagnose them, prioritize their issues, and then operate on them. Perioperative care was part of our responsibilities. I learned early on that caring for the patient from beginning to end—the perioperative period—was as important, if not more so, than the technical procedure itself.

I suddenly experienced the joy of being independently responsible for patients again. Mort Kahan recognized that I was a provisional resident and thus didn't pose a threat. When we met, he asked me, "How old are you? Did you and Dr. Moore make a special deal? How much are they paying you?" I was flabbergasted. I found these very personal questions to be ones that would never be asked directly in any other culture I had lived or worked in. I perceived them not as inquiries intended to evaluate me as a colleague, but as a challenge from a competitor for one of the PG-4 slots in the training program, which had been contracted and changed from vertical to trapezoidal shape. Essentially, he had thrown down the gauntlet. To complete the five-year program, I would have to outperform him and become one of the provisional residents selected based on performance.

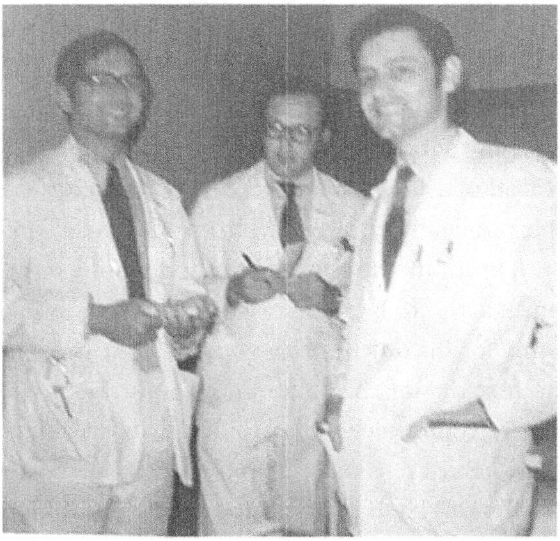

Drs Michael Meguid, Mort Kahan and Hillel Laks

Our chief's exuberant reputation preceded our meeting. Legend had it that one night in the E.R., the nurses were setting up for the pelvic exam for a wife who had contracted the clap from her husband. Burley was to do a surgical evaluation of her lower abdominal pain. The drunk Irish husband, swaying unsteadily on his feet in the corridor, threatened Burley. "If you so much as lay a finger on my wife's pussy I'll punch you in the face," he belligerently slurred.

Burley was a Texan who proudly wore cowboy boots into which he tucked a pearl-handled pistol "given to me by my daddy." He pulled out his pistol and threatened to shoot the drunk laborer, yelling, "Get this white trash out of my E.R."

The man fled.

We knew where we stood with Burley. No nonsense.

He assisted us as we operated on and cared for these needy patients. When confronted with surgical issues outside his expertise, he had the benefit of seeking opinions from or consulting with faculty members regarding complex cases. He could draw on any professor's wisdom and experience to enhance his surgical skills and occasionally ask for their assistance in improving his operative proficiency.

I learned the subtle politics of consultation through observation. Instead of asking for an opinion, which places the questioner under obligation, I learned from him to seek a senior's suggestion. This didn't carry the obligation to follow the recommendation exactly. If I chose my own course of action, the responsibility for the outcome lay with me.

On the first day of the rotation, a senior faculty member, Professor Carl Walter, needed a resident to assist him with an unusual case. Burley asked me if I wanted to scrub in. Of course, I said yes! "Then hurry to the O.R., he's waiting." After quickly changing into my greens, I entered his operating room.

"Hi, I'm Michael Meguid. May I assist you, sir?"

He nodded.

On the operating table lay 84-year-old Louise Bottomley, who was already under anesthesia. I gently placed my hands on her left breast and felt a small tumor. Given the age of the patient, Dr. Walter chose a simple mastectomy—merely the removal of the mass—instead of a radical Halsted operation. He recognized that dying from a heart attack was more likely than surviving the complications and lengthy recovery associated with a radical mastectomy. I agreed with his decision: the patient's overall physiological condition and existing comorbidities, such as heart disease, hypertension, and diabetes, had to be considered in the evaluation. Furthermore, Dr. Moore always said, "The surgeon, like the ship's captain or an aircraft's pilot, is responsible for everything that happens. His word is the only one that can't be contradicted or contravened."

Dr. Walter had a gentle demeanor, reminiscent of a lovable grandfather. In age and physique, he reminded me of Mr. Rodney Maingot, the most distinguished abdominal surgeon in London with whom I had previously operated. I was so awestruck by working with one of Brigham's surgical giants that I neglected to ask about the patient's history or the reasons for the operation. Eager to participate, I was shamelessly excited, and he was an experienced surgeon who moved quickly, his steady hand gliding between tissues like a maestro intensely focused on his violin while performing a concerto.

Once we were both gowned and gloved, I stood on the patient's left, ready to assist Dr. Walter, who stood on the right. He lifted the left breast and drew a circle around the base with the purple medical skin marker. To my surprise, he addressed the scrub nurse and said, "Give him the scalpel."

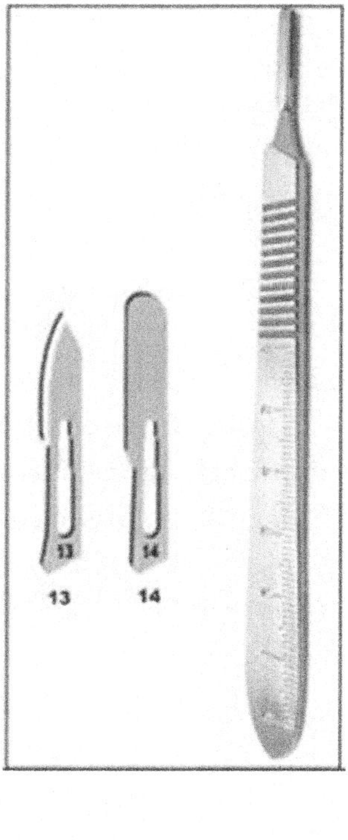

She passed me the sharp, pointed knife with the #13 skin cutting blade. I scored the purple line of the surgical marker, cutting through the skin into the underlying subcutaneous fatty tissue. Dr. Walter controlled the small bleeders. We continued to work with minimal talk, which I liked because I could concentrate on the task and see the motions he intended me to do next without distraction from extraneous chatter or noise. I liked that Dr. Walter clamped off the sucker when we weren't using it to silence the continual hissing and sucking noise. As the Egyptian proverb says, "The fruit of silence is tranquility." To this, I'd add greater serenity.

In surgery, the general term 'cutting' is a misnomer. Aside from cutting the skin, surgery separates tissue planes within the body. In the case of the breast, after I had cut through the skin and subcutaneous fat, I entered a tissue plane that separated the small fat globules of the subcutaneous tissue, which looked a pale yellow, from the larger, more yellow-looking fat globules that encased the breast. I placed a lap pad over the breast, gripping it and pulling it downward as I started at the top of the incision. Dr. Walter applied countertraction with two-prong, sharp-tipped skin hooks beneath the skin flaps, exposing the tissue plane. Peeling the fruit reminded me of the pithy layer around an orange or a tangerine.

Using a #14 scalpel blade, whose tip is rounded for dissecting between tissues, I beveled my blade and swept the knife's tip from left to right and back again within this space, separating the subcutaneous tissue from the breast. Dr. Walters electrocoagulated the bleeding vessels crossing the plane that nourishes the skin. Continuing, I moved deeper around the breast until I reached the underlying fascia of the chest wall muscle.

"Give him a fresh #13 blade," he murmured to the scrub nurse. This command was the only interruption of our focused silence. She passed me the knife.

Having dissected in the fascial plane from the top of the wound, around the sides of the breast toward the bottom of the wound, I now dissected the breast off the chest wall fascia, leaving the pectoralis muscles and axillary lymph nodes in situ. At the same time, Dr. Walters clamped the large bleeders. I placed the breast with its embedded, firm cancer and the moist, bloody lap pad into a dish held out by the scrub nurse. We briefly made eye contact—her hazel eyes gazing at me between her hat and mask—and her eyes aroused me. What sensual pleasure—the moment she became more than a shadow that stood next to me. There is something sensuous, almost erotic, about the scrub nurse and me in the surgical moment as we move silently alongside the operation, like three lovers dancing a tango—aware that one hesitation or misstep can create a dangerous dynamic tension. No wonder the scrub nurse has often been referred to as a surgeon's second wife.

Dr. Walters instructed her to provide me with a straight needle threaded with cotton to close the wound after I placed a single Hemovac drain beneath the flaps to drain any blood or fluids that might accumulate or seep into the tissue space I created.

I started to close in the middle of the wound by approximating the flaps, as I was taught in London, and kept bisecting the two flaps to get a neat horizontal wound. Dr. Walter nodded his approval as he cut the knots above each stitch and then steri-stripped the wound edges together. The resulting incision satisfied me because it looked quite neat in an elderly chest, which would heal nicely into a slender scar without distorting her figure from a radical mastectomy. We completed the task in thirty minutes.

"Nicely done," was all he said.

While we were operating, Dr. Moore slipped into the O.R. like a shadow and stood watching for a moment without saying a word. He and Dr. Walter were old friends. Was he there to talk to him?

However, I knew Dr. Moore was watching me as I continued working. Dr. Walter looked up and said, "Dr. Meguid, here, is a born surgeon." Just as suddenly as he appeared, Dr. Moore vanished. It was the first time I had seen him since he interviewed me three years ago. I thought he was trying to remember our interview and who I was, especially since I suspected I might have received a poor evaluation from my previous rotation.

Dr. Walter dressed the wound and noted the date on it. Together, we removed the sterile sheets that had covered Louise Bottomley.

"I'll dictate the op-note," he said.

I thanked him.

As I left the O.R., I ran into a fellow resident. When he asked me about my day, I told him what I'd done and with whom.

"Do you know who he is?"

"A clinical professor, right?"

"He's a surgical pioneer, an entrepreneur, and a business tycoon."

"You mean not really a surgeon's surgeon?"

"No. He's a surgeon, but one who looks over the horizon, if you know what I mean. He developed and established Brigham's blood bank in 1937 and introduced vinyl bags to replace the fragile IV glass bottles that often break."

"Wow. I admire such innovative men."

"Not only that, but he also helped develop an early artificial kidney for dialysis and set up a manufacturing plant with a friend," and lowering his voice, added, "It's said that he's into developing monitors, you know, like the ones we're beginning to use in the ICU. I imagine he is a multimillionaire."

I was honored to have worked with him. Unfortunately, I never saw Dr. Walter again, which is a pity because I would have liked to discuss his many innovative accomplishments with him.

15

THE SKILL NOT TO KILL

But I will restore you to health and heal your wounds, declared the Lord.
—Jeremiah 30:17

During my residency, I didn't receive formal instructions on the techniques for opening or closing wounds. However, based on the complication rates, I believe these procedures deserve specific and intentional emphasis in training. I learned these skills by assisting and observing experienced surgeons during operations. Observing means noting what to do and, equally important, what not to do.

To access the abdomen through the skin, an incision must be made. The consequences of cutting into the abdominal wall vary depending on the incision's location. These effects are not related to the intra-abdominal disease but to where the incision is made and how well it is closed. Although there are no specific statistics on injuries associated with accessing the abdomen, data from the American College of Surgeons indicates that, due to inadequate closure, approximately 15% of patients develop an incisional hernia, and this percentage rises to 60% during the first to third years following surgery.

The musculature of the anterior abdominal wall is fascinating. In the front midline, two longitudinal muscles called the rectus abdominis connect the ribs and the pubic bone. These two muscles bulge when contracting, producing the "six-pack." The nerves supplying the rectus muscles enter from the sides. Consequently, any incision that cuts through these muscles denervates and weakens them. The sides of the abdominal wall consist of three major overlapping anterolateral muscles, whose nerves originate from the sides and enter from underneath.

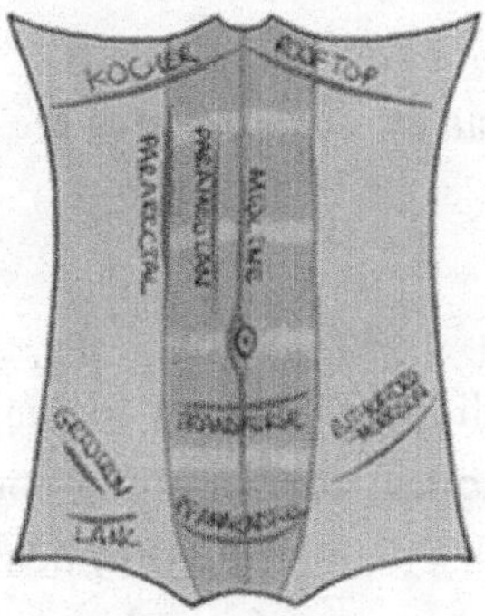

Common Abdominal Incisions

On the ward service, Burley and I used several different incisions. The most common was a midline incision that cut through the fascia between the two rectus muscles to access the general intra-abdominal contents. We used a subcostal (Kocher) incision if we performed a cholecystectomy, which involved cutting the right rectus muscle and the lateral abdominal muscles.

We would have used a rooftop or Chevron incision if we had operated on a pancreatic issue. This would involve cutting through both rectus muscles. I disliked performing a longitudinal pararectal or paramedian incision because it would sever the nerve to the muscle fibers beyond the incision, weakening the front abdominal wall and causing a high rate of hernias.

When Burley and I performed an appendectomy, we made a McBurney or gridiron incision in the abdominal wall, which allows access to the three oblique muscles that intersect at right angles. We then spread the muscles along their fibers to prevent cutting the muscles and their nerves.

If a patient has a history of surgeries that resulted in multiple abdominal scars, the combination of these previous incisions significantly weakens the abdominal wall and the patient's core posture, especially when the tough fascial covering encasing the abdominal muscles is inadequately or improperly sutured together.

Many issues surround the details of successful wound closure, and inattentiveness to them can lead to disastrous results. There are unspoken cardinal rules. Start by closing the peritoneum. Next, close the fascia of the muscle that provides wound strength. It's a fallacy to believe that muscle itself has strength. A common mistake is placing stitches through the muscle, which cuts off its blood supply and eventually leads to muscle necrosis, weakening the overall closure. I used a continuous proline suture, a non-absorbable, sterile synthetic fiber. The ratio of suture to wound length should be about 4:1 to ensure the wound isn't closed too tightly. A closure that is too tight can lead to wound breakdown, known as dehiscence. In one or two percent of cases where a midline laparotomy wound begins to fail, the small bowel may protrude through a defect or weakness in the abdominal wall.

Rarely does an abdominal wound begin to deteriorate in the immediate postoperative hours. This catastrophe of a burst abdomen or an abdominal wound dehiscence due to a poor closure results in the guts spilling out of the abdomen and onto the bed and is a severe postoperative complication that is often fatal.

Men dehisce their abdominal wounds three times more often than women; the cause remains speculative. Wound dehiscence is a major complication and is associated with a 20% death rate. Because the incidence is relatively low, despite the devastating outcomes for the patient, awareness of the early signs of impending wound dehiscence is not consistently recognized.

Burley and I had performed surgery on Abraham Otis for an infected pancreatic cyst. When we examined his wound on the third post-operative day, a peculiar pinkish, foul-smelling, serosanguinous discharge stained his dressing, and a droplet oozed out from between the edges of his wound. The wound appeared red, inflamed, and tender to the touch.

No alarm bells rang as they should have. The discharge was the pathognomonic telltale sign of the impending wound bursting open. Instead, I cultured the fluid after not observing any signs of wound separation and continued with the same antibiotic. On the sixth post-laparotomy day, Mr. Otis mentioned that he had felt a pop some time ago in his wound. We removed his dressing and witnessed, as if in slow motion, a loop of small bowel worm its way out of the end of the inflamed wound.

We quickly covered the protruding loop with moist sterile pads. I held these in place to prevent additional loops from forcefully meandering their way out. Other team members increased the IV fluids, administered a dose of different antibiotics, and inserted a nasogastric tube to decompress his stomach and intestines, all while informing Mr. Otis that he had a serious complication that we needed to address. Meanwhile, Burley notified the O.R. desk about our in-house emergency, which required immediate reoperation. It was the surgical equivalent of "mayday, mayday" or a flashing SOS. We were facing a type of surgical emergency that had priority for the first available O.R. room because the condition could be fatal.

The patient was quickly moved out of the room, the scheduled case was postponed, and we wheeled our patient in his bed even while the floors were being mopped. A new O.R.

nursing team prepared their instruments, and an anesthesiologist was on standby.

A member of the anesthetic team skillfully and swiftly inserted an IV catheter into a neck vein, providing direct access to the central venous circulation and the heart. They then expertly anesthetized Mr. Otis while he lay in his hospital bed. Relaxed by the drugs and anesthesia, Mr. Otis was transferred onto the operating table by several attendants using his bedsheet. After his hospital bed was removed, the anesthesiologist administered an additional relaxant, causing his abdominal muscles to relax and reducing pressure on the bowel. The nurses cleaned the wound with warm saline while Burley and I scrubbed, gowned, and gloved efficiently.

According to the culture report, the wound was infected with a mix of bacteria. The anesthetist administered a more specific antibiotic while assisting the circulating nurse in covering Mr. Otis with sterile hospital drapes. As we gathered around our patient, Mr. Otis's protruding bowel was cleaned further.

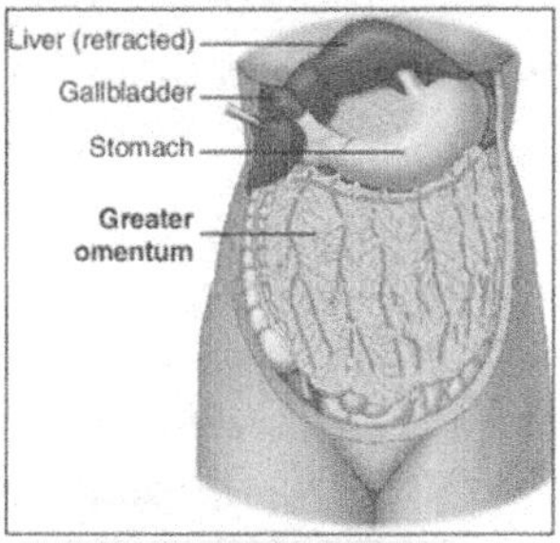

Abdominal Content

Burley instructed me to remove the old suture. I gently separated the inflamed, angry-looking edges of the wound with my index finger. The wound fell apart like overcooked ham detaching from a bone. I recognized the suture, cut it in several places, and carefully removed the bits and pieces as we opened the wound.

The old sutures had been placed too tightly, strangling the blood supply to the wound edges and tearing through the tissue. This technique error, combined with the infection, ultimately led to the wound's failure to heal and subsequent breakdown or dehiscence. We checked for any source of infection or abscess within the abdomen, and then we covered the small bowel with the greater omentum, a large fold of tissue that protects the small bowel like a pinafore.

Later, I would say aloud: "Approximarè, non strangularè." It sounded good, but God knows what languages I had mixed up to convey my message. Nevertheless, a generation of residents heard it over the 35 years I assisted them in closing belly wounds.

After approximating the muscles, we thoroughly irrigated the wound with warm saline. We brought the remaining wound edges together by placing heavy sutures through the upper layers of the abdominal wall a few inches apart, lightly binding the wound. Each stitch is first passed through a piece of red rubber catheter to serve as a bolster before the suture is tied.

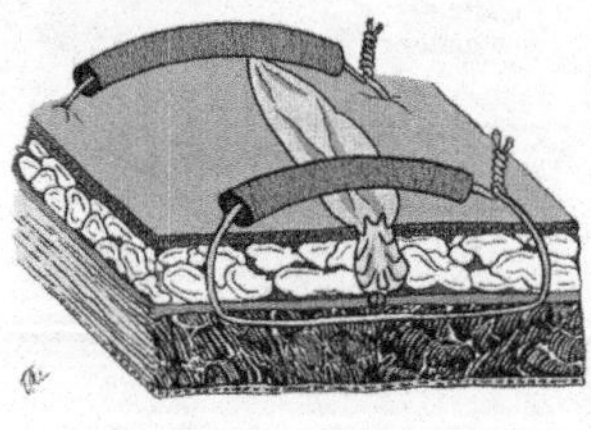

The bolster prevents the suture from cutting through the skin when the wound swells, as anticipated, after the operation. These stay sutures are left in place for ten to fourteen days until the abdominal incision heals. After that, it is safe to remove them without risking the wound falling apart.

Finally, we placed moist gauze pads between the exposed skin and the wound. These must be changed with each nursing shift. As the moist gauze dries and is removed, it pulls away tissue debris, effectively cleaning the wound.

The wound will heal by secondary intention, meaning it closes from its depths upward to the skin through the process of granulation. An invaluable lesson I learned was to always invest the appropriate time in closing a wound, paying attention to the abovementioned points. Closing an incision correctly became my obsession. I reasoned that the skin incision and the invoice were the only things the patient saw.

Another complication of poorly closed wounds is the development of an incisional hernia. Over time, the skin stretches and becomes very thin, forming a hernial sac filled with bowel loops. The sac can then open, creating a ring that may strangulate the bowel, leading to peritonitis. If not operated on promptly, bowel strangulation accompanied by peritonitis can result in a patient's death.

As always, in the case of Mr. Otis's surgery, the danger of repairing a large hernia lies in closing the defect too tightly. As surgeon Matt Oliver stated, "If it looks all right, it's too tight." The patient would experience difficulty breathing, much like women in the French courts during the 1500s and 1600s, who often fainted when wearing tightly fitted corsets to flatten the stomach and emphasize their narrow waists.

16

ACKERMAN'S ABDOMEN

Nothing is impossible to him who will try.
—Alexander the Great

Not only was Burley 'Ein Mensch,' but I also met two surgeons on the Ward Service who were of the same ilk, deserving of my love and respect. Both eventually became mentors. Dr. Joseph Murray and his talented fellow, Dr. Mutaz Habal, were members of the Plastic and Reconstructive team, with whom Burley consulted about our patient, John Ackerman.

Mr. Ackerman was a patient with a significant abdominal wall defect caused by an incisional hernia, which primarily involved weakened skin and subcutaneous tissue that compromised his abdominal wall. Unfortunately, this issue was quite common in surgery. I didn't realize at the time that, throughout my many years of practice, I would frequently encounter failed surgical incisions. It became essential for me to thoroughly understand the causes of this issue, how to prevent it, and how to address it in severe cases, through the reconstruction of the abdominal wall. As I gained experience, I nearly always performed the closure myself, contrary to the practice of allowing the most junior member of the team to handle that task.

John Akerman's giant ventral hernia, or hernia sac, contained not only most of his small bowel but also part of the stomach. Because he had only minimally healthy fascia and viable muscles to close the enormous hernia, we would need to mobilize lateral muscle flaps along with the skin on the right and left sides of the abdomen. Once these were pulled together to close the defect partially, a piece of mesh would be placed over the remaining gap to seal the hole in his abdominal wall. We would use the excess skin from the hernial sac to cover the mesh.

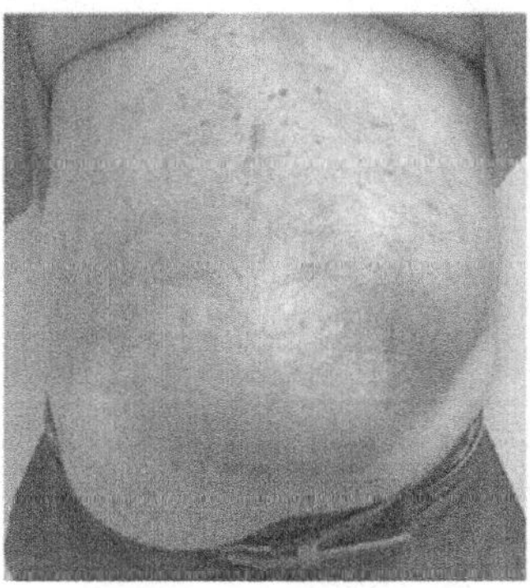

Abdominal Incisional Hernia

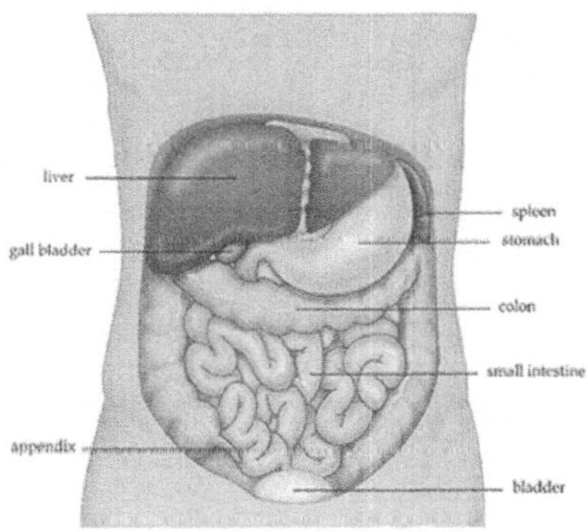

Schema of Abdominal Organs

Was there another approach to this problem that we could use?

There were two surgical dilemmas: the first was what material to use for closing the defect. In 1970, the availability and the size of the mesh were limited. The second issue was how tightly we would have to close the wound so his guts were returned to their normal domain without compromising his ability to breathe or the blood flow from the legs and guts back to the heart.

Burley, Dr. Murray, Dr. Habal, and I stood around John Ackerman's bed, his belly exposed, discussing various possibilities and devising a surgical plan.

They listened as I presented the patient's history of numerous surgeries and my physical findings regarding the abdominal wall. Their eyes focused so intently on me that I became self-conscious as I spoke. Was it my English accent? Dr. Murray was soft-spoken and exuded humility and kindness. He asked the patient, "Do you mind if I examine you?" John Ackerman nodded before Dr. Murray placed his hands on the abdomen to assess the hernia's size and the strength of the surrounding muscles. Dr. Habal also examined the patient. In his gentle voice, Dr. Murray then spoke to us. He discussed the various options for constructing a new abdominal wall, as well as the pros and cons of each. "In essence, the bowel has to be returned to its abdominal domain. Coverage has to be optimally fashioned from the surrounding abdominal wall tissues."

Before we dispersed, Dr. Habal and I briefly exchanged words in Arabic, which helped establish our national identities. He came from the American University in Beirut, Lebanon, where few individuals of Arab heritage worked and contributed to America's growth and wealth. Burley, along with Dr. Hillel Laks, chose to have Drs. Murray and Habal assist with John Ackerman's challenging ventral hernia. I wish I had the chance to work with them on this case, not only because I heard from Burley that both were skilled surgeons, but also because, throughout my years of active surgical practice, incisional hernia repairs ranked alongside appendectomies in both the challenges they posed and the joy I derived from fixing them. Little did I know at the time of the consultation that I would be working with Drs. Murray and Habal and would publish a couple of medical scientific papers with them in the coming months.

My indefatigable chief, who keenly ensured that his juniors

participated in as many varied operations as possible, often assigned us to assist other attendings and services that needed an extra pair of hands when the Ward Service was slow. He arranged for an attending to help me in performing surgery on a patient with an indirect inguinal hernia, followed by my assisting the gynecological attendings, either Dr. Goldstein or Dr. Taymour, with hysterectomies.

As was the practice then, my indirect inguinal hernia patient was admitted the night before so I could take a history, examine him, and make sure he was ready for the next day's operation. On evening work rounds, Mort asked me if I had obtained a barium enema before operating on my patient's hernia.

"Do a barium enema for a hernia repair? What for?"

"A recent article in the New England Medical Journal reported a higher frequency of rectal cancers in patients with hernias. Rectal cancer obstructs stooling, so for the patient to evacuate, he has to strain a lot, more than usual, causing an inguinal hernia. They'll frown on you for doing an incomplete pre-operative hernia work-up," he said, shaking his head.

"Don't be ridiculous. Most rectal cancers are found within a finger's length during a rectal exam. If there is blood in the stool, I'll use a rigid sigmoidoscope to examine the rectum and distal sigmoid colon, where remaining rectal or colon cancers would be found. His rectal exam was normal and showed no trace of occult blood."

Mort looked at me, disappointed. Before he could comment, I added, "You know, by doing recitals on the patients we saw in GPs and clinics, the incidence of rectal cancer was almost wiped out. It's unusual to come across them now, thanks to . . ." Looking at Mort, I waggled my index finger around.

"But seriously, my patient has an indirect inguinal hernia. He was probably born with it, and it's become bothersome now. I see no indication of doing a barium enema." William Osler, the most outstanding clinical diagnostician, said, "One finger in the throat and one in the rectum make a good diagnostician." And Mort, my friend, if you fail to perform a rectal exam, which I know you'd never skip, then you and the patient will be fine. Now, as medical students and their mentors continue to fail to perform rectals as I've seen on the ortho service, well then, expect an epidemic of rectal cancer to rise.

Although I liked and respected Mort, his statement reinforced my understanding of the significant differences between British and American medical school training. In England, we relied on taking a patient's history and conducting a physical examination to obtain a working diagnosis, which we supported by performing selective tests. In the United States, there was a greater reliance on technological marvels, including automated blood work, X-rays, and, years later, computerized tomography (CT scans), as well as other innovations, such as MRIs and PET scans.

His statement also clarified two mysteries: the first was the orthopedic team's tendency to go to the X-ray Department to view films instead of initially visiting and systematically examining a patient. The second tendency was similar to not talking with and thoroughly examining the patient.

This happened while I was assisting Dr. Eddie Edwards with a procedure on a woman who had significant varicose veins in her left leg. Dr. Edwards was well known for his surgical expertise in the venous system rather than the arterial system. Varicose veins occur due to thrombosis or injury to the main central veins located deep in the leg. Walking helps the muscles pump venous blood back to the heart. When the central vein is damaged, blood disrupts the valves between the deep and superficial veins in the leg, causing it to flow upwards through the peripheral veins beneath the skin, which results in unsightly, tortuous varicose veins. The procedure with Dr. Edwards to correct varicose veins involved identifying these valves and tying them off to redirect blood up the central veins toward the heart.

During my pre-operative examination, I performed a Trendelenburg test. In this test, I elevated the leg above the patient's heart to drain the blood from the varicose veins and applied a tourniquet around the upper thigh to occlude blood flow in the superficial veins beneath the skin's surface. Finally, I lowered the leg so that the varicose veins became visible. This test assessed the competency of the valves between the deep and superficial veins.

Mrs. Innis had many incompetent valves, which I marked with a Sharpie so we could locate them during the operation, even after washing the leg with an antiseptic solution. I learned the Trendelenburg test as a medical student while working in the Surgical Unit at University College Hospital in London under the guidance of Mr. Hart. While operating on Mrs. Innis with Dr. Edwards, the essence of a grandfatherly gentleman, Dr. Moore, appeared like a ghost and strolled through our operating room. It always made me anxious, for Dr. Moore was the pinnacle of power at the Brigham and held the fate of my surgical future in his hands. Dr. Edwards looked up, and I heard him say, "Dr. Meguid did a very thorough examination and found many more incompetent valves than I did. With his help, we'll fix them." Dr. Moore nodded and then walked out of the room.

17

INCISION OF INDECISION

Remember, we all stumble, every one of us.
That's why it's a comfort to go hand in hand.
—Emily Kimbrough

The Ward Service under Burley's leadership transformed my outlook and life at the Brigham. Perhaps I could stay here after all. I was an independent-thinking surgeon, acquiring additional surgical skills. All I had learned in surgery from my various London surgical jobs came to the forefront. I was liberated from the endless scut work of orthopedics. Encountering new patients in the Ward Service allowed me to utilize my initiative in making a diagnosis, operating on them under Burley's guidance, and helping manage their pre-, during, and post-operative care. This was the reason I had come to the Brigham. With these surgical challenges came maturation. My spirits lifted; I was delighted to go to work. Thoughts of returning to London, once paramount, now receded. Did they disappear entirely? Not yet.

Working in the ward service was a time of significant personal growth. I could rely on my ability to assess a patient's condition through examination without adhering to the rigid formal presentations required in ortho. I could make a diagnosis based on the history and physical exam, complemented by new and evolving technological results.

My basic training in England emphasized the importance of showing bedside interest in the patient, reflecting the humanity of caring for the sick, as championed by Frances Peabody, Sir William Osler, Sir Robert Hutchison, Bernard Lown, a physician and researcher at Brigham, and even my chief, Francis D. Moore.

Nineteen-year-old Ed White was brought in by ambulance, unaccompanied by a family member or friend. I found him on a gurney, clutching his belly and writhing in pain, suggesting he had biliary or renal colic from a stone too large to pass, or possibly spasms from intestinal obstruction or strangulated loops of bowel in a hernia. However, the squirming pain flitted around his abdomen, which was rigid and not distended.

That didn't match known abdominal pain patterns associated with the disease. He didn't have a hernia or fever, nor did he vomit or have diarrhea; however, his pulse was racing and his blood pressure was elevated. The pain left him breathless, making it impossible to obtain a comprehensive history of his condition. His blood work results were relatively normal, but his restlessness prevented me from performing an ultrasound or X-rays of his abdomen. He consented to the insertion of an intravenous catheter but resisted the placement of a nasogastric tube. He had a Foley catheter draining normal urine, with no red blood cells present. When I performed a rectal exam, it was also normal. After consulting with Burley, who also examined him, we decided that the only remaining investigation to solve the mystery was an exploratory laparotomy, knowing that it's safer to look and see rather than wait and see.

Declaring an emergency and entering the first available operating room, we bumped a scheduled case, which was never appreciated. Once Mr. White was anesthetized, Burley and I reexamined the abdomen. We didn't find any intra-abdominal masses, hernias, or indications of gross disease. Essentially, it was a routine examination, which deepened our quandary.

"Should we still operate on him? And if so, what is our preoperative diagnosis?" I asked. Burley stared at me, his gaze conveying uncertainty. What was the correct answer?

Burley picked up the scalpel.

As a medical student, I learned that examining the abdomen was challenging when the patient was awake and in pain from what appeared to be an intra-abdominal catastrophe. Anesthetizing the patient to relax the abdominal muscles was an accepted method for re-examining the abdomen and conducting a thorough pelvic examination in women. An anesthetic was considered a diagnostic tool. If the abdomen was soft and no visible masses could be identified, the patient was awakened and admitted to the ward. Subsequently, their abdomen was examined serially again by the same surgeon. If the symptoms did not recur, the patient was discharged. In the years that followed, CAT scans and MRIs replaced or supplemented the physical exam.

When we encountered Mr. White, we could only rely on our physical exam and what is known as a KUB, surgical lingo for Kidney, Ureter, and Bladder. A KUB is essentially a plain X-ray of the abdomen used to evaluate abdominal pain, searching for radiographic evidence of the hallmarks of bowel obstruction, renal stones, and even biliary stones.

"He needed a lot of meds to put him down," the anesthesiologist said, making a cogent observation. Both of us heard him, but in our anxiety over not overlooking an acute surgical abdomen, the meaning of the anesthesiologist's crucial statement eluded us. A couple of years later, after the E.R. Holding Unit had been built, I would have admitted Mr. White to the Holding Unit. Within three days, we would have discovered that his writhing abdominal pain was due to cocaine withdrawal symptoms.

Burley made a mid-abdominal skin incision around the navel—the infamous incision of indecision, as we sarcastically called it in London, since we had no definitive pre-operative diagnosis. We entered the abdomen through this incision, cutting through the fibrous ligamentous tissue between the right and left rectus muscles. This midline incision does not damage the abdominal musculature on either side of the midline.

Burley and I explored the abdomen: the stomach, duodenum, twenty-two feet of bowel, appendix, and five feet of colon were normal. There were no internal hernias or volvuli. We found a normal gallbladder, kidneys, and ureters. We discovered a Meckel's diverticulum two feet from where the small bowel enters the colon; however, it was normal, and this outpouching is an incidental finding in approximately 2% of patients.

Suddenly, the significance of what our anesthesia colleague had mentioned dawned on us; we had just fallen into a trap. We had operated on a drug addict experiencing withdrawal symptoms that manifested as abdominal cramps. When we operated on Ed White, we didn't realize he was the vanguard of a tidal wave of patients that would lead to America's drug crisis.

Our operation didn't classify as a diagnostic error, since we didn't have one. More likely, it was an error in judgment—hence the incision of indecision. Aside from having egg on my face, what harm had we done to this young man by proceeding with the operation? We had probably induced an intra-abdominal adhesion or two. These are a common development after abdominal or pelvic surgeries, occurring in up to 93% of patients, due to the small bowel coming into contact with a foreign body, like gloves. Most cause no ill effect, but in some patients, they may result in small bowel obstruction years later.

I reported our diagnostic error at the weekly M&M conference, wishing to prevent others from falling into the same trap after making a fundamental mistake. After some initial hesitation, a senior attendee admitted to having made a similar mistake several years earlier. Gradually, others joined in with similar confessions.

Another attending stated, "If an inappropriate incision is made because a pathological condition is found in another part of the abdomen or the pelvis, the initial incision should be closed, and another more appropriate incision should be made directly over the disease." After this cathartic discussion, Dr. Moore concluded the dialogue by saying, "That's a satisfying communal confession one day short of Sunday."

There were lighter moments during the service as well. In an emergency operation in which I wasn't involved, a man was admitted through the O.R. with a foreign object in his rectum. The abdominal X-ray revealed it to be a bottle. Removing foreign objects from the rectum was startling due to my naivete, but I encountered the need for such procedures throughout my life. What was a novel operation during my residency became routine in my early career and eventually a bothersome procedure in later years.

In this case, the pre-operative diagnosis was "Beer bottle in rectum." After dilating the rectum to its maximum diameter—usually the size of five fingers or a fist—the bottle's base became visible, and the entire object was deftly extracted. Burley pronounced the operation a success and declared that the post-operative diagnosis was "Heinecant Craft Pilsner beer bottle in the rectum."

18

BURLEY, BILE, & THE BUG

If there is a Creator, he must have an inordinate fondness for beetles.
—Charles Darwin

One mid-afternoon, I darted to the E.R. like a bee to a flower to see Joe Mackey, an obese 64-year-old man experiencing nausea, vomiting, and upper abdominal pain. My spirits rose; I was back in familiar territory. I took a focused surgical history and examined his abdomen as best I could while he lay on the gurney in pain. My diagnosis was acute cholecystitis with the potential for ascending cholangitis —the gallbladder infection causing waves of bacteria to spread up the biliary system to the liver and engulfing his body with sepsis. His high temperature rendered him almost delirious. An ultrasound of the gallbladder showed one large stone blocking the cystic duct. The findings confirmed my clinical diagnosis.

I admitted him to our ward service and inserted a nasogastric tube into his stomach, which was standard care at the time. I continued to hydrate him aggressively with intravenous fluids and provided antibiotics to fight the sepsis, along with a small dose of Demerol to ease his pain. Morphine, one of my favorite drugs for pain control, was contraindicated because it caused the gallbladder to contract, which would worsen the patient's distress. Despite the antibiotics and my aggressive hydration, he maintained a fever of 103°F and remained in great discomfort.

Burley was in the O.R. assisting another resident with an operation. I sneaked in and gently interrupted him to present the patient. He agreed that, based on my findings, Joe Mackey would require an emergency cholecystectomy (gallbladder removal) that night, once the last ward service case was finished in the O.R.

While the anesthesiologist assessed Mr. Mackey, Burley led the team, which included a few medical students, during our evening work rounds. We checked on all our patients, and fifteen minutes after our rounds concluded at 8 p.m., Joe Mackey was moved to an operating room.

"Since I admitted Mr. Mackey, I want to operate on him. While in London, I assisted in this operation a dozen times. It's now time I did one."

"Are you on call tonight?" Burley asked.

"No. But he's my patient, so I'd like to do the operation, and Mort doesn't object." I didn't mention that this operation also had very personal and sentimental value.

He hesitated for a minute before agreeing. "You know it's already 8 p.m. You'll go home late, and you're on call tomorrow."

"That's OK. I want to operate," I repeated.

The gallbladder is a bag-like structure located beneath the liver. Bile flows through the common bile ducts from the liver to the gallbladder, where it is stored until it is released during eating, particularly after fatty meals. Eating causes the gall-bladder to contract, squeezing the bile down the cystic duct, which joins the common duct on its way to the duodenum. Its purpose is to emulsify dietary fat, much like soap washes fat off one's hands. When a patient consumes a consistently high-fat diet, excessive bile is produced, leading to the formation of bile or cholesterol stones and sludge in the gallbladder, similar to pulp settling at the bottom of a bottle of orange juice. The contracting gallbladder then ejects these stones. When a stone is too large to pass down the cystic duct, it blocks it, causing the remaining bile to become infected, which can lead to general sepsis in the patient.

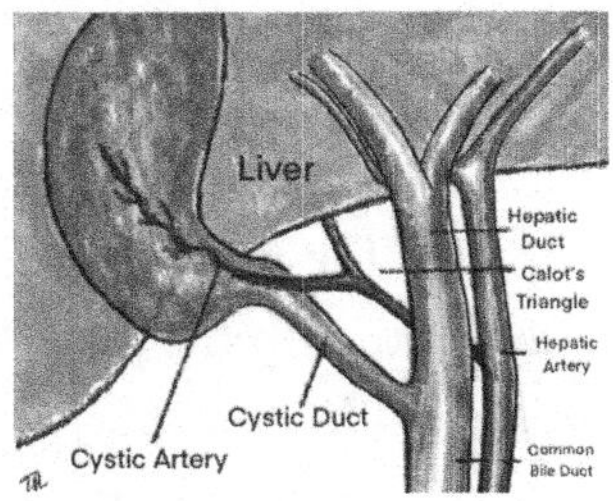

The anatomy in this area is quite tricky. To avoid injuring the vital structures during acute inflammation, patients were previously sent home for six weeks while the inflammation subsided. However, in most cases, the patients never returned because they were operated on right away elsewhere. And rightly so. After all, one wouldn't send a patient with appendicitis home to wait for the inflammation to subside. Consequently, the trend shifted to operating on the "hot" gallbladder.

The cystic artery lies within the hepatocystic triangle of Calot, an anatomical space defined by the cystic duct and an artery at the triangle's base. The common hepatic duct, closely bound to the hepatic artery, forms the left side, while the undersurface of the liver defines the right side. Calot's triangle is an important landmark for locating and tying off the cystic artery during a cholecystectomy. When this area is encased in bleeding and raw inflammation due to a severe infection, dissecting out the cystic duct and its artery becomes challenging. The surgeon needs to identify the cystic duct, which joins the common bile duct and cystic artery, without confusing it with the right hepatic artery, which supplies blood to the right half of the liver. Once these structures are identified, they should be independently tied off and cut. Failure to accurately identify these structures amidst inflammation has led to countless injuries to the vital common bile duct, which is an unforgivable surgical error. Such an injury results in life-altering complications for the patient and brings sorrow, shame, and possibly even the derailment of a surgeon's career. A lawsuit is sure to follow.

The most notorious injury occurred in 1953 when Sir Anthony Eden, then Prime Minister of Britain, had his common bile duct transected—divided in half—during a cholecystectomy. Although this was surgically corrected, Sir Anthony suffered from recurrent pain. He was prescribed Demerol for pain relief, barbiturates to manage the anxiety associated with his pain, and amphetamines to keep him alert. This combination may have influenced his political judgment in planning the Suez War, which involved England, France, Israel, and Egypt in 1956. The war prompted my decision to leave Egypt, pursue my medical education in London, and ultimately undergo my surgical training in Boston.

Once Mr. Mackey was anesthetized, Burley and I prepared him for the operation. I made a subcostal incision, starting at the midline below the lower part of the sternum and extending it outward, parallel to the lower edge of the ribs past the 9th rib, which serves as the topographical landmark for the gallbladder, to provide easy access to that organ.

For a brief moment, I had a flashback of Victoria as a first-year medical student, lying on my dorm bed, partly clothed, letting me draw the various organs on her skin. I clearly remember the position, including the gallbladder under her right breast at the tip of the ninth costal cartilage. We were intoxicated by love, enchanted by each other's prospects, and heading towards marriage. It was a wonderful way to become familiar with the topographic signs of organs. I love Victoria, but surgery was and remains my mistress.

Deepening the incision, I entered the abdomen. The dome

of the gallbladder appeared from under the edge of the liver; it was black and smelly. Burley held the big liver retractor while, with his gloved hand, he tried to prevent the writhing, small bowel from creeping into the wound. This provided a clearer view of the liver and the green-black, necrotic gallbladder embedded in its underside. Regrettably, we didn't have a medical student to hold another retractor to prevent the small bowel from constantly creeping around Burley's retractor like a series of octopus tentacles into the space where I was working.

I asked the anesthesiologist to raise the head of the table so the liver would fall further into my view, and I requested a green surgical towel from the scrub nurse, which I placed above the dome of the liver. This helped to position the liver and gallbladder within the operative field, allowing me to see the anatomy more clearly. Burley expressed his surprise at the two maneuvers, noting that they improved the visualization of the gallbladder. He retracted the liver upward so I could work on its underside to dissect the dome of the gallbladder free. I continued dissecting from the top downward toward the midline, following the duct and its accompanying artery, navigating through a significant amount of thick, gelatinous of inflammation—the consistency of marshmallow—that surrounded the area where the two key structures, the common bile duct and the major hepatic artery, were located.

Burley was doing an excellent job as an assistant, helping me as much as possible since this was a three-person task. Suddenly, I encountered a potentially dangerous issue. Typically, the gallbladder's artery branches off the hepatic artery to become the cystic artery by passing above the common bile duct. However, I couldn't locate the cystic artery in Joe Mackey's inflammatory mass. A mild panic gripped me—it had to be there. Yet, without seeing it, I couldn't tie it off. Was I operating beyond my capabilities in this very treacherous anatomical area, where renowned surgeons had ruined their careers by blindly tying off the wrong structure? My blood sugar was low, and I needed a better view of this critical area. If I asked Burley to take over the operation, I would lose face or damage my self-worth.

The cystic artery had to be there! Hadn't I seen it in Fred, my cadaver, and in the countless cholecystectomies I had assisted on? I believed it must be present. I just had to keep dissecting with great care until I found it. No, I wouldn't let Burley take over. As these emotions swirled in my mind, Burley mentioned he needed a break.

Backing away from the operative field, he stood in the doorway, lit a cigarette, inhaled deeply, and blew smoke into the corridor. "You know, I could smoke while operating. Any ash falling into the wound is sterile!" The thought horrified me. He was right. The ash is sterile, but he must be joking.

The exposure of our anatomy, which we had so diligently worked to establish, had collapsed: the liver fell onto itself, hiding the partially dissected gallbladder, and the small bowel rushed into the operative field like a tsunami, obscuring my view. I stepped back and rested for a moment. The circulating nurse slid a straw under my mask, and I took a long drink of cold orange juice. Ah! Glucose! I felt fortified. Burley re-gowned and re-gloved. The break provided me a moment to gather my emotions. Despite the challenges, I was determined to push on.

We reestablished our optimal operative view of the anatomy. I dissected through the inflammatory mass that obscured the critical structures using a cotton peanut attached to the tip of a dissecting clamp and bluntly separated the tissues. Despite feeling tired, I noticed that the cystic artery passed below the common bile duct; it only passed under this duct 25% of the time. I tied it off and finally removed the gallbladder, which had a single large stone wedged into the cystic duct. The liver bed oozed a mixture of bile, lymph, and blood.

We removed the towel, the anesthesiologist straightened out the O.R. table, and in accordance with the standard practice of the day, we laid a drain under the liver by the raw gallbladder bed to exit at the patient's right flank as an exit track for the oozing blood.

Burley excused himself once more, removed his gown and gloves, stood in the doorway of the operating room, and smoked again. He then re-scrubbed, re-gowned, and re-gloved. His actions, though unconventional, demonstrated the mentorship he provided.

Based on the discovery of a single large stone, there was no indication for performing an intra-operative cholangiogram, where contrast material is injected directly into the common bile duct in search of small, missed stones that could block the bile duct and exacerbate the sepsis.

By now, it was almost 10:30 p.m.

"Why don't you go home, and I'll close up," Burley volunteered.

"If you don't mind, I'd like to help close the wound since this is my patient. Then I can walk home a happy man."

Burley looked up from the open wound, staring across his mask at me. "Walk? Now? At night? Where do you live?"

"Near Coolidge Corner."

"That's dangerous. Why don't you drive?"

"We've only been in Boston for eight weeks. I don't have the money to buy a car."

"Wow. It's dangerous," he repeated. "Go tomorrow to the chief and ask him for a loan so you can buy a car."

"To Dr. Moore?"

"Yeah. Tell him you don't have a car and that I think it's too dangerous for you to walk home so late at night in the dark. People have been mugged and stabbed around here."

"Seriously? I'd be too embarrassed to ask him."

"You tell him I suggested it."

As I walked home, I remained vigilant. Victoria was asleep, and as I lay down beside her, I realized that the operation had been a success—a testament to our hard work and dedication!

I was hesitant to ask Dr. Moore for a loan, especially since I hadn't formally met him. I felt quite uncomfortable. A couple of days later, I walked into his office suite.

Timidly and a bit embarrassed, I greeted him and asked my question about a loan while standing and facing him as he sat behind his desk. It was obvious that I was interrupting his work. As he looked up, he asked, "What type of car?"

"A Volkswagen."

"How much does it cost?

"Two thousand dollars."

"Let me see what I can do."

With a "thank you, sir," I left. It was an odd feeling. Our meeting was transactional—nothing personal. I had no clue how I stood with my Chief of Chiefs. I would soon find out because Labor Day weekend was approaching.

The next day, I was called to his office. Gail greeted me with a broad smile and handed me an envelope. In the privacy of the basement stairwell, I discovered that Dr. Moore had written me a personal check for the full amount, which I repaid a year later. After depositing it at The First National Bank of Boston, located across from the hospital, I withdrew the same sum in twenty $100 bills.

Carrying cash, I walked along Huntington Avenue toward Route 9 to the VW dealership in my white hospital uniform during the next day's lunch break from Brigham. A brand-new, metallic, pale blue car from the 1970s stood gleaming in the late afternoon sun. The salesman greeted me warmly and invited me into his office. I handed him the cash.

"We can't take money. Don't you have a credit card?"

"No." I was baffled. Why wouldn't they take the money like they did in England and Egypt? As for a credit card, we hadn't been in Boston long enough and weren't sure how to obtain one.

"We'll need a cashier's check, then."

"What's that?

"We don't take cash. Go back to the bank and ask for a banker's check."

I was getting frustrated with this salesman. Didn't he want to sell me a car? Every time I visited the dealership, I had to walk quite a distance in the summer sun, and I was on duty every other night and weekend. I was chronically tired and on the brink of exhaustion. Who did this jerk think I was?

Monday, September 7, was Labor Day weekend, and I was determined to get the car. We were planning to attend Dr. Moore's clambake in Marion. Additionally, Victoria and I had the day off, and the thought of our freedom made us both euphoric. We'd been in Boston, or more precisely, confined to the hospital, for almost ten weeks. Without transportation after work hours, we were limited to our apartment. We hadn't seen any of America yet.

Victoria had managed to buy some food items locally, and our neighbor occasionally took her grocery shopping, but we were growing restless. The summer was slipping away. All we seemed to do was work 110 hours a week, leaving us consis tently sleep-deprived, irritable, and hardly in the mood for lovemaking. We desperately needed a break. We needed to socialize and better balance work with our personal relationships.

I returned to the bank, deposited the cash again, and paid $25 for a cashier's check. I learned that, unlike a regular check, the bank guaranteed payment. Armed with this document, I walked back to the dealer, sweating in the heat. The moment of elation came as I drove my new VW off the dealer's lot to 45 Marion Street in Brookline—a triumph of my determination.

19

DEAR MOTHER

Mother, have I told you
That you are the first woman
I ever fell in love with, that is what
I've always wanted in life is to hear
You say you love me, too?
—Kevin Powell

Boston, Thursday, Sept 3, 1970, 4:30 am

Hello Mother:

I returned from the hospital around 10:30 p.m. on my night off and found your lengthy letter, which took only three days to arrive. I can't comprehend your many newsy items from Egypt or England. Given my intense life here, the list of things you want me to do in Egypt is staggering—much beyond my ability. Living and studying here is all-consuming, making your Egypt seem far behind me. Some of your tasks are understandable for me, given your on-again, off-again life in Cairo, but many are non-sequiturs that I don't grasp and are best discussed when we meet in the future.

Residency is more intense and demanding than training in London. I'm barely able to keep my head above water. It is exhausting and stressful, and I work about 110 hours a week. When I come home, I am sleep-deprived, fatigued, and often unable to connect with Victoria emotionally. Surgery is a solitary way of life.

Victoria took the enclosed picture this morning, as my getting up early to write to you also disturbed her. The weather here is unusually hot. We have a built-in air conditioning unit, but we are more accustomed to sleeping with a partially open window, as we do in England. We think this photo is amusing. My day starts at 6 a.m. I'm busy all day, operating and caring for patients. I get to go home every other day. Last night, I assisted in an emergency until ten and then returned home. Nurses have less authority in the United States than they do in England. Residents have to handle more routine tasks—scut work. My meals are very irregular. However, by 11 at night, when the cafeteria closes to the public, we can eat as many leftovers as we want for free. There is little time to socialize. I miss the positive feedback from the faculty, which makes me feel like I'm not doing a good enough job despite the long hours. This sometimes makes the residency feel like a depressing task. I love operating on and helping patients, which makes the struggle worthwhile.

Victoria is completing her pediatrics residency at the Children's Hospital. We see each other occasionally. We have fewer vacation days than in the U.K. It's unrealistic for you to come for Christmas since we are both on call. Come over for the New Year when we are off.

We got a lovely, shiny, metallic blue VW car that you'll love. We go food shopping after work since the stores stay open late. Monday is Labor Day (like the First of May in England). Finally, we are both off duty. It's a time when Victoria and I can reclaim our humanity and each other. Let me know your travel plans so we can meet up.
Oma writes frequently. She's so sweet and loving. No letters from my sister Gulnar—not on birthdays or even Christ-

mas. In that sense, our relationship has remained unchanged over the years. So that I'm not always disappointed, I've considered her dead. Sounds frightening or bizarre, but in reality, one thinks so very fondly of the dead. Isn't it so?

We hope to see you in Boston over the new year, when we won't be on duty, or later in the year in London. Victoria says, "Hi."

Must go. Lots of love.
Your son.

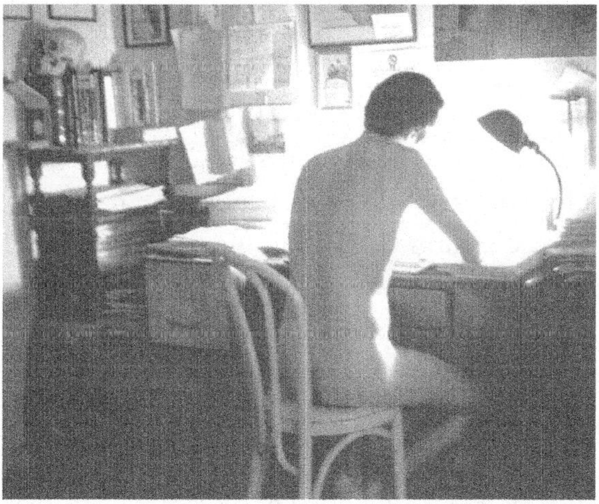

20

SURGICAL BOUNTY HUNTER

It's OK to move . . . surgery is a mobile sport.
—Bruce Schirmer

At the 11 p.m. free meal in the cafeteria, I sat and ate with the medical interns to seek unofficial referrals for surgery. On one occasion, an intern in the medical service informed me that one of his patients had pus coming out from around an intravenous catheter.

"Really? He'll soon become septic. Perhaps even develop septic endocarditis or osteomyelitis and die," I said, to scare him into letting me see the patient.

"You think so?"

"For sure, unless it's attended to right away. This is a crucial catheter because the patient receives chemotherapeutic drugs, followed by some saline."

He stared at his plates of food, seemingly weighing how much he could eat before his patient died. He ate with great haste. "Can it wait until tomorrow morning? My patient is asleep, and it's nearly midnight."

"I hope he'll survive until then," I said.

"Ok. We'll go and see him now."

We tiptoed through the dim medical ward to the patient's bed.

"Larry, hey Larry. Wake up. I brought a surgeon to see your painful arm."

Larry opened his eyes as we turned on the light above him. I examined the catheter, which had been inserted into the ulnar vein on the left flexor aspect of his forearm. This was an uncommon site for a standard hydration catheter, indicating that its use was necessary. After washing my hands and donning a face mask and sterile gloves, I noticed a two-inch segment of the vein above the catheter insertion site filled with pus, causing tenderness and inflammatory redness. Pressing on the vein made the pus, resembling Crème Anglaise, ooze out around the catheter. The intern watched.

"The catheter has to be removed, and the infected segment of the ulnar vein cut out because it is seeding bacteria into the rest of your patient's body," I murmured as a nurse closed a curtain around us.

The intern blushed, understanding the seriousness of having pus and bacteria seed the venous system—poison going straight to the heart.

After explaining everything to the patient and obtaining his consent, I called Burley at home and scheduled an emergency in the O.R. It was 2 a.m., and I informed him of the situation. "I think you can manage this on your own, or would you want me to come in and help you?"

"I'll call you when I've finished."

"Let's include him on our rounds in the morning," he added.

"O.K., boss."

In the O.R., under light anesthesia, the anesthesiologist inserted a new sterile catheter into the patient's right forearm after I removed the infected catheter. The anesthesiologist used this new catheter for sedation medication and strong antibiotic coverage. Eventually, the nurses on the ward would utilize the new catheter in the opposite arm for the patient's chemotherapy.

At the time, no one knew the outcome of inserting a new catheter into an infected patient. Would the infection from the old, infected catheter seed the new one? We assumed it would, but what was the necessary interval before that happened?

I made a mental note to experiment and determine the delay time for the body to clear the bugs and when it would be safe to insert a new catheter without risking infection. In rats, it takes 12 hours before it is safe to insert a new catheter, but for this patient, we didn't know this because he was on a chemotherapy protocol.

I incised the skin over the vein, removed the catheter and the infected venous segment that had developed into a pus bag, and sent a sample to the bacteriological lab. I stripped the ulnar vein up the arm and down toward the hand, well beyond the injection site, until blood flowed freely from both freshly cut ends of the vein, which I then tied off. I thoroughly irrigated the wound and injected 3cc of a broad-spectrum antibiotic into the open wound, uncertain if this procedure had any true benefit. Still, I had observed this in England when one of my registrars had removed a perforated appendix. I lightly approximated the skin edges of the wound after inserting a wick to facilitate drainage of exudate. The scrub nurse wrapped the arm, and we woke the patient. It was past 4 a.m., but my adrenaline had kept me awake. Fatigue set in after dictating the operation note.

This infection was likely caused by the intern not washing his hands before inserting the catheter, an avoidable mistake in 1971. The infection could have had serious consequences for this immunocompromised patient. Nearly two centuries earlier, in the mid-1800s, puerperal fever was common in hospitals after childbirth and often fatal, with mortality rates ranging from 10% to 35%. Ignaz Semmelweis, a Hungarian gynecologist, discovered that the incidence of puerperal fever could be significantly reduced through handwashing and disinfectant use when examining pregnant women about to go into labor. He advocated for this simple antiseptic procedure by having fellow doctors wash their hands, and they were surprised to find that this easy act greatly decreased women's mortality following delivery.

I view the lack of hand washing as an inexcusable offense. Residents and professors should not transmit germs among patients and throughout the hospital. It's not unreasonable for a patient to ask their physician to wash their hands before touching them. I insisted that my team members follow my example by washing their hands before and after interacting with each patient.

The ledger left in the X-ray department served as another potential source of surgical cases. After my 11 p.m. meal and rounds, I would visit the X-ray department and flip through the ledger pages. I was searching for patients who had undergone radiological investigations for gallbladder disease, gastric ulcers, or colon issues such as polyps or cancer, and who had been seen in the clinic or ER without an attending or private doctor. As a result, they wouldn't learn about their results until they returned to the surgical clinic.

I will arrange their admission to the Ward Service. Along with Burley, I performed more cholecystectomies than any other operation while on his service. Burley also loved operating on colonic cases and welcomed my "fishing."

When the radiologists realized that a surgical resident had been visiting their log notes, it raised the issue of patient confidentiality; the logbooks were consequently locked up at the end of the day.

Burley offered our assistance to the gynecological attending on hysterectomies. The gynecologist appeared relatively young, which led me to wonder about his level of experience. He hesitated frequently during the operation, as if he weren't entirely comfortable with pelvic anatomy. This made me feel quite uneasy. Each time the young gynecologist worked in the pelvis, I experienced distressing moments when he blindly clamped a "blood vessel" in its dark, narrow depths, which the O.R. lights didn't adequately illuminate. Had he clamped off the ureter?

I remembered a solemn sermon given by the seasoned Professor Larson during preparation for the Primary Surgical Fellowship in London just a few months ago. He warned us about "tiger country," an area of anatomically crowded complexity. He stopped to face the class to emphasize the danger. "The ureters course downward from the kidney on the psoas muscle to cross over the iliac artery as it enters the pelvis into tiger country. Then, the ureter crosses further down into the deep pelvis. Then it goes underneath the uterine artery, a branch of the iliac, as it passes a mere 1.5 to 2 cm lateral to the cervix before it hooks up to enter the bladder from its undersurface."

Pausing to listen to the auditorium hush as the students sat in suspense with pens in hand, he continued, "The name tiger country is well deserved because when operating in this tight space, the ureter is often accidentally cut, tied off, or injured while blindly clamping tubular structures such as the ureter or fallopian tubes. And boys, I know you wouldn't do that."

There followed a unanimous cheer from the thirty would be surgeons!

At 11 p.m., the residents and interns from various services flocked to the cafeteria for the day's leftovers, reminiscent of animals in Africa heading to the watering hole. The first to arrive piled as many dishes as he believed his stomach could hold onto his tray. Latecomers faced fewer choices. It was common to trade one food item for another. We all sat at the tables and ate, initially indulging ourselves after a day of fasting. Conversation began as we became satiated. After our fill, I recounted the excitement of the beer bottle escapade. The story elicited general laughter.

"That's nothing," yelled another resident down the long table. "We had a patient with a vibrator stuck up his rectum. When we told him that we'd try to remove it, he objected, saying, 'I just want you to change the batteries!'" We laughed at the apparent absurdity.

The surgical residents watched the clock, as most of us still had to do night rounds with the 11 p.m. nurses coming on for the night shift before we could lay our weary bodies on mattresses and get some sleep. Did I say my prayers? You bet. I'd say, "God, please let me sleep uninterrupted for six hours."

This prayer didn't depend solely on the Almighty; it relied on how well I organized the service and supported the night nurses in caring for my patients. For an intern or resident, the nurses could truly make your nightlife miserable. They deserved the utmost respect. Our positive working relationship, based on mutual trust, reduced their need to call me.

GENERAL HOSPITAL, USA

by American Lore

CHIEF OF STAFF

Leaps tall building with a single bound
Is more powerful than a Jumbo Jet
Is faster than a speeding bullet
Gives policy to God

ATTENDING STAFF/PHYSICIAN
Leaps short buildings with a single bound
Is more powerful than a DC3
Is just as fast as a speeding bullet
Walks on water if the sea is calm
Talks with God

RESIDENT
Leaps short buildings with a running board and good winds
Is almost as powerful as a DC3
Is faster than a speeding B-B bullet
Walks on water in a swimming pool
Talks to God if special request is granted

INTERN
Clears a small hut
Loses the race with the 1903 Wright Flyer
Can fire a speeding bullet
Swims well
Is occasionally addressed by God

MEDICAL STUDENT
Runs into small buildings
Recognizes a glider 2 out of 3 times
Frequently wets himself with a water pistol
Dog paddles in a kiddie pool
Mumbles, mostly to imaginary puppies

NURSE
Lifts buildings to walk under them
Kicks Jumbo Jets off the runway
Catches speeding bullets in her teeth
Freezes water with a single glance
SHE IS GOD!

21

THE NIGHT BEFORE

The best bridge between despair and hope is a good night's sleep.
—Anonymous

After a long day, I wearily climbed the stairs to my on-call room and flopped into bed in my O.R. scrubs. I don't even recall falling asleep.

At 2 a.m., I whizzed by the ICU, checked on my two post-op patients, and addressed the nurses' concerns. Then, I climbed the stairs to enjoy three more hours of uninterrupted sleep before returning to the ICU to extubate my patients. It was the Friday of a holiday weekend, so we didn't have any operative cases lined up, nor M&M or Grand Rounds scheduled for Saturday morning. The team would gather for rounds at 7 a.m.

I had just fallen asleep when the phone rang. It was a nurse from the cardiac ward informing me that she had removed Mrs. MacArthur's intravenous catheter because it wasn't working, and I needed to come and reinsert a new one. I pulled myself out of my bunk bed and went down to Mrs. MacArthur. The nurse stood beside her bed, waiting.

"Please get me a #18 small Butterfly catheter, a tourniquet, and tape."

Off she went. Mrs. MacArthur looked up from her bed. "I'm so sorry to disturb you," I said. "You need your IV. It looks like you have great veins. This won't take long." Looking sleepy, she nodded.

I washed my hands, and the nurse reappeared. In my hazy state of sleepiness, I didn't particularly notice her. She brought all the items I needed and laid them on the patient's bed beside me. Within minutes, the patient had a new IV catheter, securely taped in place, and her hydration fluid flowed through it. "That was slick," Mrs. MacArthur murmured, having perked up during the procedure. I acknowledged her compliment and wished her a good night. I wrote a dated and timed note in her chart, documenting the insertion.

Twenty minutes later, I climbed the stairs to my room and fell asleep again. Victoria always admired how quickly I would drift off and wake up.

The floor nurse called me an hour later. "What?"

"Again?"

"Really?"

"Have what I need ready," I said irritably and swung out of bed. Why were catheters falling out of patients? This was unheard of. They were disturbing my well-established sleep routine.

I was fortunate. Mr. Enid remained vigilant throughout my search for a suitable vein and didn't flinch when I managed to insert a new catheter, which I secured well with tape. Throughout the process, the petite nurse shadowed me and stood beside me as I recorded the event in the patient's chart. After closing it, I looked up at her and said goodnight.

By now, it was just past 3 a.m. As if on a train's schedule, I visited my ICU patients, checked previously ordered blood work, briefly exchanged reassuring words with their nurse, and went to bed. I was prone once more and closed my eyes, setting my internal clock for at least a bit more sleep.

Incredibly, the cardiac ward nurse woke me again. Another catheter needed replacing. "I have all the things you need by the patient's bed," she said. After inserting a new catheter into my third patient, I looked at her with wide eyes. "What are you doing, pulling out my IV catheters?"

Bashfully glancing at me, she said, "I lower the IV bottle. If blood doesn't flow back from the vein into the catheter, I remove it."

"What? You have no idea about catheter hemodynamics. Never touch the catheters unless the fluid is infiltrating. Is that clear? You're incompetent, and I'm reporting you to your super in the morning." I turned on my heels and rushed to bed, trying to salvage a bit more of my night's scant sleep.

At 6 a.m., I checked on the ICU patients. They were stable, and I extubated them. I was eager to begin Saturday's 7:00 a.m. work rounds, ready to pass the duty baton and the care of my eighteen cardiac patients to my partner and start my weekend.

Weary and irritable, I yearned to get out of this place—to escape, to connect with my inner self, to decompress from the ongoing stress, to enjoy the pleasure and leisure of my wife, the summer sun, and the sounds of nature in the surrounding New England environment. On my way down The Pike, the nurse supervisor intercepted me. "Do you really want to lodge a formal report?"

"Yes. She endangered patient care."

"She is a new graduate. She confessed in tears that she thought you were cute and wants to date you."

"Really?"

"So, do you still want to report her? She's young. Perhaps you'll forgive her."

I nodded. "OK. I'll give her another chance. Let her know

I'm happily married, and I greatly value my sleep over sex to perform my best for my patients."

I didn't even remember what she looked like. She was young and infatuated with me, but I saw her as a nurse, not as a woman. The credo states that Residents can be replaced, but nurses can't.

22

CRANE'S BEACH

LABOR DAY WEEKEND 1970

Of the delights of this world, man cares most for sexual intercourse, yet he has left it out of his heaven.

—Mark Twain

I arrived home earlier than expected, feeling much less grumpy. Labor Day weekend was sunny and beautiful, with temperatures ranging from the mid-70s to the 80s. Victoria and I drove north along Route 1 to Ipswich and Crane Beach, looking forward to the promise of soft, golden sand. It felt wonderful.

Route 1 took us through the suburbs north of Boston. In Saugus, we passed the iconic Hilltop Steak House, the hilarious plastic colossal cactus, and the larger-than-life cow—quintessential Americana. We were well on our way. Woodlands lay to our west, and Route 1 was busy with families driving north to see the early changing foliage.

With each mile from Boston, I felt increasingly more alive and human, bolstered by the warmth of the sun on our skin. I reconnected with my feelings, looking forward to a swim in the cold Atlantic and lying next to Victoria on the beach, just as we had on our Antigua honeymoon a little over two years ago.

Ipswich, founded in 1634, is one of the oldest English settlements along the Massachusetts coast. Its primary trade was cod until about 1970. As the fishing industry declined, the town transformed into a bedroom community for Boston's growing population and emerging industries.

Veering off Route 1 and taking the exit to Ipswich, we drove along the charming Main Street, where buildings displayed their age with plaques stating the year the houses were built. In the bright midday sun, a faint path between two buildings, shaded by the boughs of birch trees, hinted at the direction of the beach.

The few hundred feet of paving soon turned into a rutted clay trail. I maneuvered my new car over tree roots and through soft, sandy potholes. The VW swayed from side to side as I drove in first and second gear, carefully guiding the car toward what I hoped would be an open beach. The path progressively narrowed as shrubbery, wild seagrass, and trees encroached. It shrank to the width of one car—a tight passage I still hoped would lead to the beach.

To my amazement, in the rearview mirror, some distance behind us, I noticed a police car following us. It was much wider than our VW, crawling along the track. There were no flashing lights or sirens; its mere presence scraped against the banks of sand and seagrass on either side.

I stopped.

It stopped.

I waited.

Nothing happened.

I could see through the mirror two very young policemen sitting in the front seat, staring in my direction and talking to each other. After a while, I got out of the car, barely able to stand on a ridge of uneven earth wedged between my VW and the tall tufts of grass. I must have looked quite a sight, for they continued to stare at me with even more intensity as I leaned against the car in my gray wool suit, which I had put on that morning without thinking in my haste to get on the road.

Nothing happened. They just sat there staring at me. I approached them, maneuvering along the uneven trail in my black Oxford shoes. I expected them to inform me that this trail didn't lead to the beach or that I was trespassing on private property.

When I reached their car, I leaned on the warm hood, continuing to inch toward the driver's window, where I peeked through the glass. It lowered. The officers stayed seated.

"Good morning, Officer. I'm Dr. Meguid. Can I help you?"

They seemed surprised by my friendly approach.

"Is that your car?"

"Yes."

"Do you have a driver's license?"

I presented my British and international licenses. They examined them curiously, passing them back and forth without saying much.

Pointing to the VW, one officer said, "How long have you had it?"

"I bought it last week, brand new, from the dealership on Route 9 in Boston."

"From a dealership? Really?"

"Yes. Why?"

"Where is the Motor Vehicle Inspection Sticker?"

"What do you mean by 'inspection sticker'?"

He pointed to the one in his cruiser's window.

"What is it for?"

"It's a required annual emission and safety inspection sticker for a vehicle needed to drive in Massachusetts."

"Where do I get one?"

"The dealer should have given it to you."

I shook my head, irritated that the dealer hadn't done his job.

"How long have you been in this country?"

"About two months. I'm a surgical resident at the Brigham in Boston." The mood and their tension lightened considerably.

You really must get one. Go back to the dealer and ask him to give you one. I'll give you four days to get it.

"OK. Thank you for bringing this to my attention."

He smiled. "If you're ever stopped again, Doc, stay seated in your car with your hands visible on the steering wheel."

"All right."

"Have fun at the beach." I nodded, glad for the confirmation that we were on the right track. They carefully began to edge backward. We moved forward, and a few yards farther along, the trees retreated, the grass gave way to turf, and I parked the VW.

We were the only ones on this fabulous, wide beach; in Europe, it would have been crowded on a holiday weekend. A cool breeze occasionally gusted, carrying stinging sand. Victoria spread a large red towel. I took off my shoes, socks, and suit, and under the cover of the towel, awkwardly shimmied into my swimsuit. She was already in her bikini. This was the first time we had exposed our bodies to the sun and elements since our honeymoon in Antigua. Now, breathing in the sea air felt like freedom, a release from responsibilities and the grinding schedule of hospital life.

"Can you put sunscreen on my back?" Victoria asked as she lay face down on the towel. Remembering how painfully red her sunburn had been after dozing on Antigua's beach, I undid her bikini top's strap as I lathered her skin carefully. I could not focus fully on my task, for it had been days interrupted by residency fatigue since we had touched each other with tenderness. I couldn't recall what her skin tasted like. What it smelled like. Her murmurs of enjoyment encouraged me to lather her from the shoulder blades to her loins. Stroking her felt exquisite. "Do you want me to put some on your tummy? I think you need it?" In reality, it was I who wanted to caress her belly, to feel what I desired as I grew hard gently.

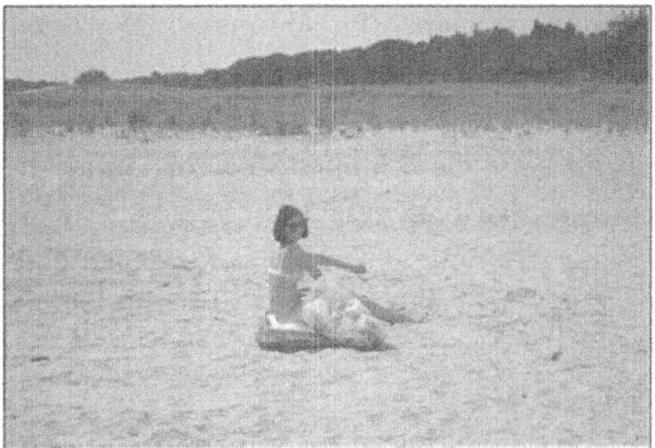

Crane's Beach- 1970

"No, I'll do that and my arms. But put some on the back of my legs." My hands drifted to her thighs, my fingers pushing under her pants to momentarily feel her soft bottom and to try and advance my eager fingers to her pubic hair and labia.

"Hey! What are you doing?'

"Sorry. Just being thorough. I confess I want you . . . it's been so long."

"We're in public. Just finish my legs."

"Spread your legs a bit more so I can put lotion on your inner thighs to protect that soft skin I love to stroke."

"No. Please stop it. People can see."

"What people? We're alone. I've always had this fantasy of making love to you on a beach. Why stop it?"

"Stop that."

"I want you. I need you. I want to touch every part of your

body. You know that's the sexiest part of you? Just touching that area stirs my parched, desolate soul. Is that what people will see? And I'm so hard for you, my dearest wife."

"I think you've already had too much sun!"

"No. I've not had enough of you. And now I can't lie next to you on my back. It's obvious to all. And it's throbbing for you." She leaned over and looked.

"Not here, sweetheart," she whispered. "Don't you think I want you just as much?"

"Then show it . . ."

She placed her wide-brimmed straw hat on her head. Her words were like salve to my soul; I craved more than just words. "Come sit on me. Come and ride me so we can end in each other's arms. No one will see us. And if they do, they'll be jealous."

"No. Not here."

"Then, let's go home."

"No. We just arrived."

"I'm told the Americans do it in their car. Let's try it."

She smiled, adjusted her bra strap, and sat up. "Look," she pointed to the crashing waves. Off in the distance, we saw an overweight policeman in a dark blue polyester shirt and pants, equipped with all his accouterments and a gun dangling from his belt, walking along the water's edge, patrolling in the midday heat. What a distraction. What a spoiler.

"He must be boiling in this heat." A cop, watching or guarding against what? Victoria and I in the gully? This is a recreational beach. We'd never seen a fully dressed cop on a beach in England.

After a while, we ate our sandwiches and cooled ourselves with a drink, satisfying my body but not my passion. The sun released my pent-up feelings of desire. I lay back and fantasized about what we could do until the passion faded like air escaping from a balloon. I took her hand, and we briefly dozed off.

"I dreamed of us, and when I awoke, I wrote a poem inspired by your closeness."

"Really?" She sat up. "Read it to me, for I love hearing your voice." Then she lay back down and closed her eyes.

"It's called '*When You Awake.*'"

"Sounds interesting," she murmured.

I recited.

"When you awake,
Know I have watched
Over you
And seen you like
A breathing child
Move your eyes
As you dream—dream of me,
And move your lips,
Seeking mine.

Know I have watched over you
And longed for your every feature.
Your beautiful face
And lusted for your body,
Beholding it in the glow of
The sun and the waves on
Crane's Beach, where
I want to make love to you.

We will be free
To delight in each other's company,
And do what our minds
Tell us and our bodies yearn for it.
And you will have your way with me

As I with you, again and again
In the essence of pure passion,
In tolerance, respect, and spirituality.
And . . .
You'll be mine forever,
to hug and to hold."

Then I adlibbed, "And fuck the residency!"

She opened her eyes. "Did you really say that? Did you?" She smiled, looking at me with curiosity.

"No. But it's a good idea. I loved the freedom—you and me—where we could 'fuck up a storm,' as D. H. Lawrence once said."

She smiled and drew my head down to kiss me . . . on my lips . . . so tenderly, so fervently.

23

MEASURING THE PULSE

Your wounded inner child has valid reasons for the pain they feel,
But your wounded inner child also doesn't deserve control over your decisions and narrative as an adult.
—Billy Chapata

The next day, we headed to Cape Cod for the departmental clambake at Dr. Moore's cottage in Marion. Victoria was dressed and ready. I changed my clothes repeatedly, switching from jeans and a sheer see through shirt to shorts with a casual shirt and street shoes since I had no sandals. No, I told myself, dress more formally! A shirt without a tie, my gray suit, socks, and shoes for the formal meeting with Dr. Moore would be appropriate. I'd look ridiculous on the beach. It didn't help that Victoria approved every outfit. In the end, I don't remember what I wore, but time forced me to decide apprehensively, and we left, following the printed instructions to Marion.

Traffic was heavy, making me irritable because we would be later than we wanted to be. According to British etiquette, one arrives a little later than the time specified on the invitation. It is polite to allow the host a few more minutes to put the finishing touches on the party—perhaps even to finish dressing. Americans are prompt and on time, a habit I began to appreciate and tried to adopt.

The weather was perfect for a sunny day social gathering on the beach. On the menu was a seafood picnic—a New England tradition adopted by early settlers who learned it from Native Americans on the Atlantic coast. This would be a new culinary experience for us. Local clams, lobsters, chicken, sausages, potatoes, and sweet corn were baked in a pit in the sand over heated stones and under a bed of seaweed—food fit for a king. It was promised to be appetizing, scrumptious, mouth-watering, and enjoyable.

I respected and venerated the man to whom I owed so much for finding a place for Victoria and me in America, and I looked forward to reintroducing my wife. At last, I would meet and greet him in person instead of just nodding to a shadow that repeatedly appeared and disappeared in the O.R. The car loan business had been purely transactional. I was eager to socialize with fellow residents I would train and work with.

Dr. Moore would be surrounded by the categorical residents he had committed to train fully from intern to junior, senior, and chief resident for five years. As a provisional resident, I envied that they would be branded 'Trained by FDM' at the prestigious Brigham. These young men rarely tripped over a blade of grass, and when they did, they were forgiven. I imagined that this brand of approval opened many doors to success, glory, power, and fortune. I wanted to be one of those residents, one of his boys with his stamp of approval.

On the other hand, I viewed myself as being on probation—a junior assistant surgical resident on trial for 24 months to prove I could overcome obstacles, fit in, and gain acceptance. These were long odds: 730 days in which to avoid mistakes, unintentional blunders, or damaging my record.

As I drove toward the Cape, I considered the pros and cons of taking the British Primary Fellowship exam versus arriving in Boston on time, an issue I felt had set me back. I didn't have a choice. To have a backup plan, I needed to complete the Primary. Was I fully committing to a residency in the American surgical field? I was, but if things didn't work out, the Primary still provided England as an option.

"You're very quiet," said Victoria.

"I'm deep in thought. How are you getting on in your residency?"

"Well. Why do you ask?"

"Just wondering . . . "

My unwavering clinical skills and my successes in operating or managing surgical patients may have outweighed the mistakes I made. They fostered my growth. Was all of this merely a mental construct because we only heard from management when errors occurred, but seldom received praise for our successes?

We arrived late, as expected. No one was there to greet us as we entered his open front door. We walked through the empty house, following the sounds of voices to the beach. Most of the residents were playing an informal game of football. A few wives were sunbathing on beach blankets and quilts. We didn't recognize anyone. Neither Mort Kahan nor Howard Snyder was there with whom I'd be working. Dr. Moore was out on his sailboat. We returned to the house, changed into our swimwear, and went back to the beach, where we awkwardly mingled with the others. Beer was the beverage of choice, and I didn't drink.

"Where are the chief residents?" I asked someone on the beach. "They and the attendings are taking care of their services so that we can visit with Dr. Moore," came the answer. This gathering was for the new interns and the new residents. Despite the circumstances, we decided to make the most of the freedom the day offered. We took deep breaths of cool, moist, salty sea air and felt the warm sand beneath our toes.

Dr. Moore greeted me cheerfully and warmly, clearly delighted that we were finally in Boston. He looked so different from what I remembered. Relaxed and sun-kissed, he wore shorts, a sailor's shirt, and old loafers. There was a sense of curiosity in his banter as he chatted with Victoria and me about our trip across the Atlantic on the QE 2. Had we been seasick? Had we rested? Were we ready to join the Brigham family?

We shook hands enthusiastically. I thanked him warmly for assisting Victoria in finding a pediatric residency, funding our car, and joining such an exclusive group of residents.

Pleased, he offered to take me out on his sailboat. With Dr. Moore at the helm and me in the bow, there was enough distance to prevent a lecture, a discussion, or a casual chat as a light breeze billowed the sails and the boat sliced through silver seas. We relished the surrounding elements. He'd glance at me much like he had when, ghostlike, he entered the O.R. Had Drs. Walters and Edwards' praise made him comfortable enough with my surgical knowledge and operative skills to move past my review of the orthopedic service, or was our past disconnection in Cambridge, England, in 1968 still on his mind and troubling him?

For a brief moment, I found myself responding in fear to the evocative ghost of my father, the man who had demanded more of me than I could deliver when I was a young boy. But Dr. Moore wasn't my father, and although he had taken on some fatherly qualities in my mind, I refused to allow Dr. Moore to assume that role in my life. Daddy, you are dead, and I'm well ahead of your expectations, career-wise. So, let me find my way.

Finally, Dr. Moore said, "Do you sail?"

"No. I like flying a glider and soaring. Victoria is a sailor. She was raised on the Isle of Wight, but I never considered it."

"Come and take the helm here and head toward the prominence across the bay." I nervously complied, grateful for his brief moment of trust in me.

I wasn't a sailboat lover, so I held firmly onto the helm, feeling the vibrations of the sea as we skimmed across the bay. Prone to seasickness, I almost didn't continue dating Victoria because, on free weekends, we'd leave our medical studies in London and train down to her home on the Isle of Wight to see Shirley, her widowed mother, who was an incredible cook and a social butterfly attracting young people who loved to eat and sail.

Having been raised by the sea, Victoria was a Class A helmsman, and we young people would sail in the Solent almost every free weekend. Everyone contributed drinks or food, while I generously offered my vomit to the English Channel.

If God had wanted us to sail the seas, some say he'd have made us fish. Instead, I emanated genetically from the dinosaurs that evolved into birds as I progressed to becoming a glider pilot. To soar above the land and sea, above authorities and experts, to feel the buffeting of the wind, the rush of air in my hair, the sun on my face, and to get sucked into a vortex of rising air to fly with the birds was akin to reaching heaven. But I didn't tell Dr. Moore about my biases.

When we docked, the clam bake was ready. Victoria and I balanced a delicious variety of seafood and corn on the cob on wobbly paper plates and sat with the others on the sand. Corn was new to us and eating it off the butter-covered cob was sublime.

I heard my name called to come to Dr. Moore's office. I chose a hard chair with a straight back opposite my Chief of Chiefs. He had showered and changed into more formal clothes, which changed his behavior and the atmosphere in the room. Now, it was business, and I was unprepared for the sudden shift in mood, which felt more like an interrogation.

"Tell me, what services have you done so far? What new papers have you written? What are your surgical goals in life? Any specific ideas about research?"

I trotted off the rotations and mentioned that I liked the Ward Service best, where I was the essence of a clinical surgeon. "Bones and I aren't compatible, but I learned a lot and mastered the art of amputation." He tilted his head as if he thought I would add more. "I like abdominal surgery best, although I'm fascinated by the evolving surgical management of breast disease and gaining some experience in pediatric surgery before going into your lab to study the metabolic effects of operative injury and trauma."

His question about published papers told me he valued inquisitiveness and intellect, so that I would pursue this activity more aggressively.

In my role as editor of Potential — Journal of the Physiology Society, University of London, I wrote an editorial entitled, 'Application of pure science to clinical medicine,' and a paper entitled 'Megaloblastic anemia associated with the oral contraceptive pill,' which was accepted by the Postgrad Medical Journal. I'm awaiting the galley proof. Its basic message is that the first generation of the oral contraceptive pill led to high levels of estrogen and progesterone binding to folic acid in the gut. Suppose a woman becomes pregnant after several years on the pill. In that case, she might become folic acid deficient, which may relate to brain abnormalities and neural tube damage in the fetus. I couldn't figure out what he was thinking as he bent over the notebook into which he was writing.

I emphasized my belief and supported his views that a surgeon should conduct approved clinical studies on patients to enhance our knowledge and apply or modify therapy for subsequent patients. I want to continue writing papers to contribute to the body of surgical knowledge. When we have this interview next year, I intend to share more published papers with you.

"I look forward to working with you on the metabolism of traumatized patients."

"Do you have any projects in mind?" he asked.

"I think two potential research areas are important in advancing our understanding of metabolism."

Looking at me inquisitively, he asked, "And these are?"

"Studying fat tissue or fat cells is quite important when it comes to the energetics of injury and trauma."

"For that, you'll have to go to a lab in Sweden," he said definitively. From this, I sensed he didn't believe it was possible in his lab, but he didn't rule it out. Later, I considered that he might be interested in supporting me to gain experience in a Swedish lab and bring my expertise to his lab. He may have thought that, but he certainly didn't make any commitment to me, an unknown entity.

"And?" he questioned after a pause.

"I've always been intrigued by how the fetus can lay down muscle tissue at such an incredible rate to support growth. What are the secrets?"

"Probably the hormone milieu. Don't you think?" Adding, "that's a complex situation beyond my lab's immediate interest."

A silence ensued as he kept writing his notes. His capacity to shift from personal warmth to apparent aloofness or detachment made me uneasy.

"Do you and Victoria want to immigrate to the United States?"

The question was unexpected. "Frankly, I don't know the options and opportunities ahead of me and my wife. But I strongly feel that a good research scientist must also be a solid clinician to fully comprehend the clinical problems fueling research."

He continued taking notes. I expected him to say I'd messed up ortho. Maybe I didn't. Nor did he commit to completing my five years of clinical training, which I would have appreciated hearing. Instead, he mentioned that residents should aim to publish two papers each year as part of their surgical maturation process. These shouldn't be case reports, which are frowned upon as trivial endeavors not considered serious research.

He stood up. The interview was over, and the next candidate was brought in. I didn't find it to be a warm or friendly exchange, which left me with that familiar, uneasy feeling from my father's days that I hadn't performed well enough. I despised the anxiety it stirred within me—no words of praise. I may have mentioned it before, but I repeat it to emphasize that a list of one hundred words of encouragement was created to uplift junior residents and research fellows.

I would post these encouraging words in a future office and apply them both clinically and in my research endeavors. A genuine word of praise would be both welcomed and a significant moral boost.

After interviewing the residents, he invited us to gather around the piano. He played beautifully, his fingers dancing over the keys with ease. In a rich baritone voice, he led the gathering in song, most of which I didn't know. I tried to mouth the words and hum along.

Shortly thereafter, I told Victoria it was getting late, and we should take our leave. The traffic to Boston was unbearable, stalling and crawling, made worse by the unpleasant taste left in my mouth from the uncertain interview. I was also irritated to be invited to a party and then cross-examined. I drove in brooding silence, contemplating the discussion I had experienced. Two papers and passing a highly competitive exam in anatomy, physiology, and pathology—wasn't that worth a word of praise? But I was determined that next time, I would have more substantial papers and reports of my clinical performances for my Chief of Chiefs.

"What did he say to you?" Victoria wanted to know as we drove north.

Not much. I hoped to hear that he didn't say what bothered me.

"Such as what?'

"Well, something to buck me up would have been nice. I get the feeling that may never come."

"Are you expecting too much from the man?"

Victoria had a point.

24

SOCIAL LIFE

Emotions are not just the fuel that powers the psychological mechanism of a reasoning creature,
They are highly complex and messy parts of this creature's reasoning itself.
—Martha Nussbaum

Social life? We had none in the conventional sense. Victoria and I still had no friends. We both had acquaintances—fellow residents we worked closely with—whom we liked and wanted to get to know better. We invited half a dozen colleagues and their spouses over for a typical English Sunday morning get-together featuring snacks and drinks, similar to what we'd often done in London. We placed the invitations in their mail slots at the hospital.

On Saturday, Victoria was busy preparing typical English sandwiches: cucumber on well-buttered whole wheat bread with the edges cut off, salmon sandwiches on white bread, and others with Marmite. I bought a bottle of gin, several mixers, and a single malt whiskey. The choice of alcohol was limited since I was unfamiliar with the different types. The store manager flattered me by asking to see my driver's license to ensure I was old enough to purchase such libations. We also bought a bag of ice and some Budweiser.

Sunday came.

Our table was covered with plates of sandwiches, cutlery, and napkins.

We wondered who would arrive first as we waited.

Minutes passed, and we could hear Victoria's carriage clock ticking in the morning's hush. Perhaps they were delayed.

We continued to wait, but no one turned up.

At noon, the church bells rang in Brookline as usual, and the sun slowly swung around to the front of the house, shining directly into our living room. As we waited with no one arriving, I felt increasingly foolish. Weren't we told that Americans were friendly? What was the problem?

By 2 p.m., we had packed away the glasses and napkins, started eating the finger sandwiches and pickles, and finished our meal with slices of jelly roll that Victoria had baked, topped off with whipped cream. To lighten the moment, we joked that they hadn't received the invitations, or worse, that Americans didn't use the Latin R.S.V.P.

No one had told us that drinking starts at 5 p.m. in America. It was embarrassing to go to work on Monday and look at the faces of those we had invited. Had they not received the invitation? I didn't ask.

Part of our acclimation process involved socializing, and our progress was slow. A few weeks later, I invited Lynn Peterson, my chief resident of the Private Service, and his wife to have tea on Sunday afternoon. They arrived punctually and were charming and polite. He, too, was puzzled by the lack of operative cases during August and the start of September. He reasoned that most attendings were on vacation at the height of summer. "We'll have plenty of cases after Labor Day."

Once we had a car, we spread our wings. Some evenings, we

went to Cambridge to visit Harvard College and the shops in Harvard Square. We bought a white kitchen table that I squeezed into the back of our VW to avoid a delivery fee, a concept unfamiliar to us.

On Longwood Avenue, there was a co-op; the head of the record section had an encyclopedic memory of various versions of the classics and limited knowledge of current pop songs. Consulting him was necessary before buying an LP of a piano concerto or another classic! He became my music sommelier, my Google before it existed. His recommendations were outstanding. I walked out with a classical music record that he suggested, and when I could do so without feeling guilty, I added Roberta Flack's latest LP to my purchases.

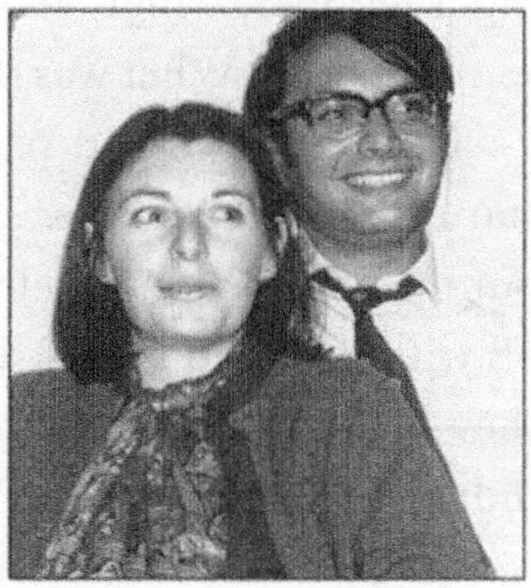

On the few evenings we were off and at home together, or on a Sunday afternoon, we'd lie in bed and get lost in the music while listening to "The Very Best of Roberta Flack's L.P.," starting with the melodious love song "Killing Me Softly with His Song," followed by "Feel Like Makin' Love," "The First Time Ever I Saw Your Face," and moving on to the mind-blowing songs "If Ever I See You Again" and the sad, melancholic melody of the story about Jesse. Lying in each other's arms, skin to skin, reinforced our role as the nucleus of a family, and until children joined us, we, like so many couples who ventured to America . . . were family.

The reviews and raves of "Upstairs, Downstairs" induced us to purchase a small 9-inch RCA black and white TV. Sunday nights were magical, transporting us back to England with the silver-haired British raconteur Alistair Cooke's suspenseful stories, followed by an episode of "Masterpiece Theater," which rounded off our blissful domestic weekends. Gradually, we became accustomed to dining with Walter Cronkite's version of the news.

We became friends with Elissa and Dan Aarons, who were fellow residents with Victoria at the Children's Hospital. They took us to a tailgating party before a football game. Unlike soccer, the teams seemed to have sub-teams on the field, each with a different role. While it was entertaining, I found the rules difficult to follow. In contrast, when the hospital gave us tickets to a Red Sox game at Fenway Park, I fell in love with baseball. What an artistic, athletic game.

Alongside our new friends, we explored the eateries of Boston's Italian quarter, discovering unique restaurants like Durgin-Park, where the steaks overflowed from our plates, and the upscale French cuisine at Maître Jacques, where our budgets determined which dishes we could choose from the tempting menu.

The period between Thanksgiving and Christmas was party time at most hospitals, courtesy of the nurses. They decorated the conference room and arranged lunches featuring Kentucky Fried Chicken, pizzas, and occasionally a fancy salad with marshmallows or Jello, pies, Dunkin Donuts, and numerous plates of cookies—each nurse contributing something, including sodas. Between operations, the nurses issued siren calls to ever-hungry interns and young residents in their quest to feed them and perhaps find a suitable husband. After all, the stomach lies contiguous to the heart, separated by the thin veil of the diaphragm. I avoided these eating events primarily due to the high caloric density, sugar, and salt, and because I was often lured to a pressing surgical clinic, an emergency, or an operation, which, in my book, took greater precedence. There were spicy rumors of a nurse and resident discovered in a linen cupboard and whispers of the discipline meted out to the resident.

Victoria's brother Tim and his wife visited us, and we loved having family around. They were easy-going and were delighted to spend a day at Crane's Beach enhancing their tan.

One of Victoria's attendings, John Lloyd-Still, an English physician, and his wife hosted an elegant soirée at their home before Christmas. This event complemented his role as an attending physician. We thoroughly enjoyed the delightful evening.

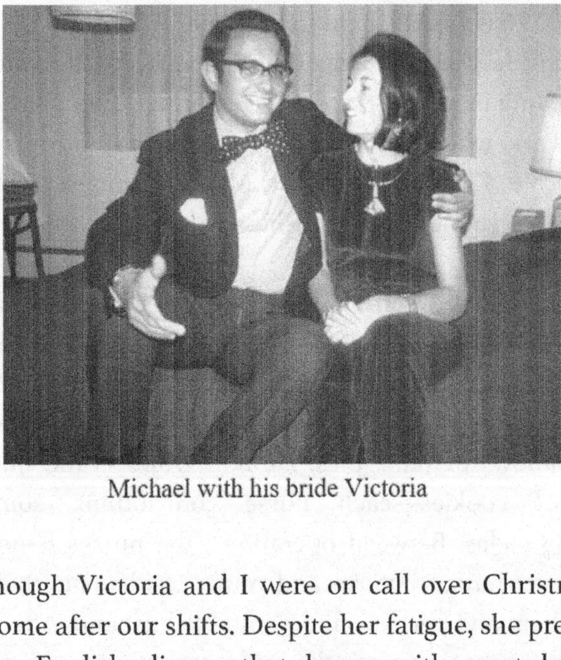

Michael with his bride Victoria

Although Victoria and I were on call over Christmas, we came home after our shifts. Despite her fatigue, she prepared a delicious English dinner that began with roast beef and concluded with generous servings of iconic Christmas pudding and custard. She was a fantastic cook. Neither of us was called in to work. We called our mothers in England to wish them a happy holiday.

Mother visited over the New Year. Our relationship had always been strained. I never got over her leaving me in

Germany when I was four years old, abandoning my sister Gulnar and me with her elderly parents. After my father suddenly died, ongoing tension developed, leading to numerous arguments about money between Mother and Gulnar—arguments that lasted for years. I tried to mediate, but Gulnar accused me of siding with Mother, while Mother felt equal distrust toward me, undermining any effort I made to arbitrate. A stalemate persisted throughout their lives and likely contributed to Mother's untimely death.

Still, a son's blood connection to his mother obligated me to entertain her to the best of my ability, despite her endless criticism of Victoria. Regardless of the frigid, biting winter cold and the daily snow showers, we walked the Freedom Trail, wandered around Faneuil Hall, and visited the Isabella Stewart Gardner Museum.

Mother mainly wanted to shop and seemed more interested in complaining about Gulnar, who lived in Hamburg. She repeatedly brought up the issue of her daughter taking money from their joint account. I listened once again to her version of their troubled relationship. My suggestions for resolving the issue were once more ignored. I recognized that this was a problem she lived with; she accepted it and had no desire to fix it. A classic folie à deux, because what would she talk about if the issue were resolved? Moreover, if she confronted or solved the problem to her satisfaction, she feared she would lose her daughter's friendship. While she didn't ask for money, she expected me to cover everything, including her clothing purchases, which strained our household budget.

Her four-day visit was manageable. After that, she flew off to visit a German childhood friend who had immigrated to Calgary, Canada, after WWII. Once Mother left, we breathed a huge sigh of relief and resumed our busy lives, feeling less relaxed than we had before her arrival.

When spring arrived and the weather turned milder, Victoria's brother, Tim, came to visit with his girlfriend. Hailing from the land of eternal rain and overcast skies, they were drawn to Crane's Beach. Being young, they kept themselves entertained while we worked. On our free weekends, we introduced them to the abundance of steak meals at Durgin Park and other charming Boston eateries.

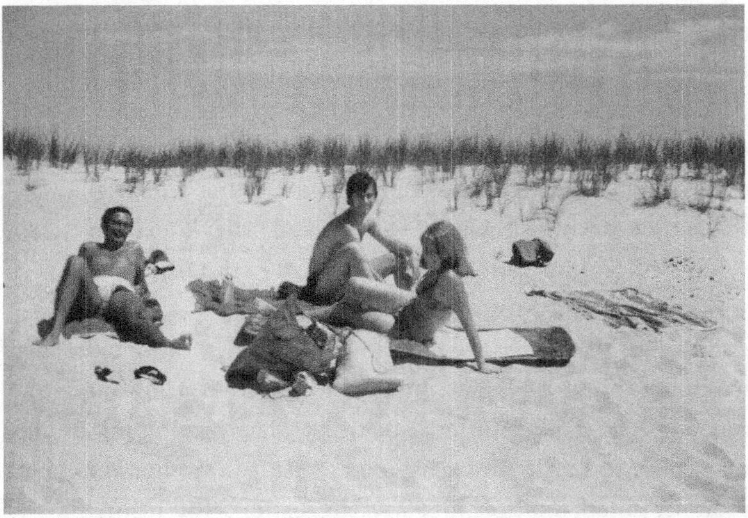

25

BEATING HEARTS

Criticism of pioneering is always the tool of men frustrated by their inability to create.
—Dwight E. Harken

Dr. Dwight Harken, a pioneer and visionary with an illustrious history, served as the chief of the Thoracic Service. During WWII, he extracted shrapnel and bullets from the bodies of 134 soldiers, saving their lives without a single fatality. Operating on a beating heart was considered impossible—this was a miracle. He also gained fame for developing a technique to correct mitral-valve stenosis using closed-heart surgery, as cardiopulmonary bypass had not yet been invented. Such challenges excited me because they evoked the spirit of my early childhood in Germany. When facing adversity, I had to summon determination and daring to succeed and overcome obstacles.

He resembled Theodore Roosevelt's Man in the Arena: "It is not the critic who points out how the strong man stumbles. The credit belongs to the man who is in the arena . . . because there is no effort without error and shortcoming . . . who knows

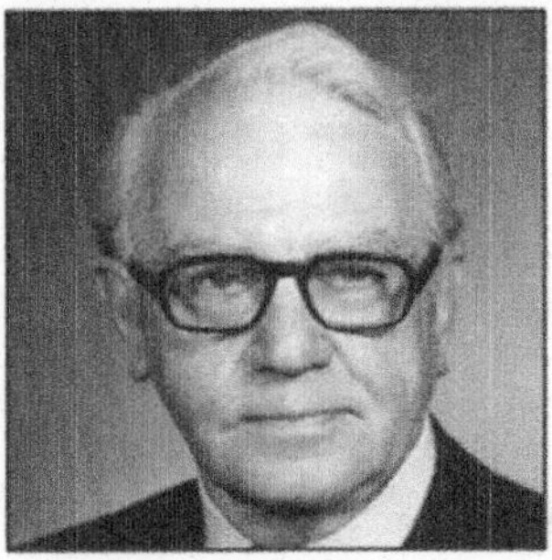

great enthusiasms . . . who at the best knows in the end the triumph of high achievement . . ."

I scrubbed for my first thoracic service operation at the Brigham with great wonder and curiosity. To my amazement, I was the only assistant standing on the patient's right opposite Dr. Harken at the operating table. Once the patient was anesthetized, the chest was washed with antiseptic solution and draped. Dr. Harken had the patient's torso elevated so that blood pooled in the lower half of the body. He gave me the knife, and I confidently made a two-inch horizontal incision above the sternum or breastbone. He inserted the sternal bone cutter and cut straight down the middle, opening the patient's chest like dividing a watermelon in half. I was ecstatic, seeing the rhythmic beating of the heart and the pulsating large vessels.

The sight took me back seven years to when I was a first year medical student in 1963. There, together with my five other colleagues whose last names began with the letter M, I dissected the chest of Fred, our formaldehyde-pickled cadaver, to expose the heart and great vessels. They looked dull and gray, without vitality. In contrast, this patient's vital signs were beating with life. Fred's organs served me well, for I knew the anatomy of this critical area.

In the third to fourth week of conception, the heart develops from a simple round tube of cells via the most elegant origami folding; the tube is shaped into four recognizable chambers.

In adults, the heart muscle is approximately the size of a clenched fist. This remarkable tissue contracts intrinsically. The primary energy source for cardiac muscle is fat, which is

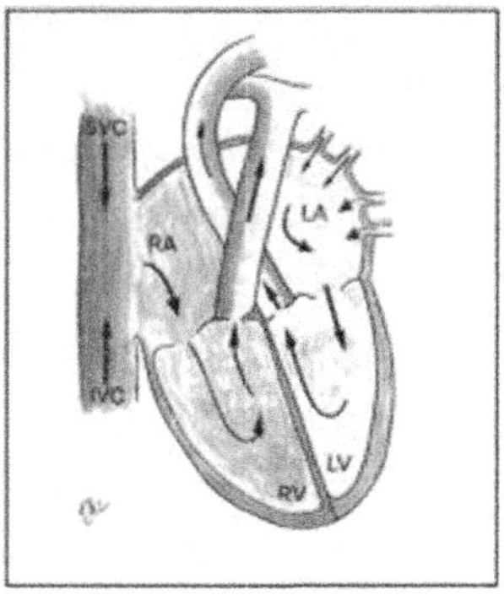

regulated by a special enzyme, Co-Q-10, designed specifically for the heart muscle. This allows the ventricles to contract around sixty times per minute, totaling about 2.5 billion heartbeats over an average lifespan of 66 years.

Receiving oxygen-poor blood from the body, the right chambers of the heart pump this blood through the lungs for oxygenation, and then, through the left chambers—the left atrium (LA) and left ventricle (LV)—it is sent to the brain and the rest of the body. This ensures that oxygen-rich blood flows in one direction through the one-way mitral valve into the aorta. The mitral valve between the LA and the LV is susceptible to debilitating diseases and damage as it ages.

After Dr. Harken opened the chest, he placed a purse-string suture around the beating left atrium above the mitral valve. He then created a small hole in the center of the purse-string suture while I used a suction device to capture the blood that escaped with each heartbeat. He began inserting his index finger to feel for the calcifications on the edges of the mitral valve.

"Ah," he said, his face lightening up. "Come on this side." I did and stood next to him while he kept the suture cinched to minimize blood loss.

Surprisingly, he said, "Insert your index finger and feel the calcifications along the valve's cusps. Also, seek the pinhole opening between the cusps, which are stenosed by calcium. Then crack the valve open and note the increase in the stroke volume as you push your fingertip through the valve into the left ventricle to open it wider."

"Really?"

"Yes, yes," he said eagerly. "But first, let the nurse fix your glove."

When I showed her my gloved right hand, she lifted the tip of my latex glove over my index finger, stretched it into the air, and snipped off about an inch, leaving my index fingertip bare. Astounded, I looked at him, thinking, "Are you sure I should put my ungloved finger into this patient's heart?"

"Ready?"

I inserted my bare finger through the purse string while Dr. Harken sucked the blood. As if I had an eye at the tip of my finger, I could see the ridges of calcification at the edge of the mitral valve cusp. As I pushed my finger through the two leaflets, I swear I heard the cracking open of the valve, as loud as splitting wood. Blood squirted with each contraction, becoming a steady flow. The anesthesiologist nodded as if to say, "Harken, you old magician, you've done it again." I felt great satisfaction as Dr. Harken's and the nurse's eyes smiled at me above their masks. I felt initiated into some venerable, time-honored fellowship.

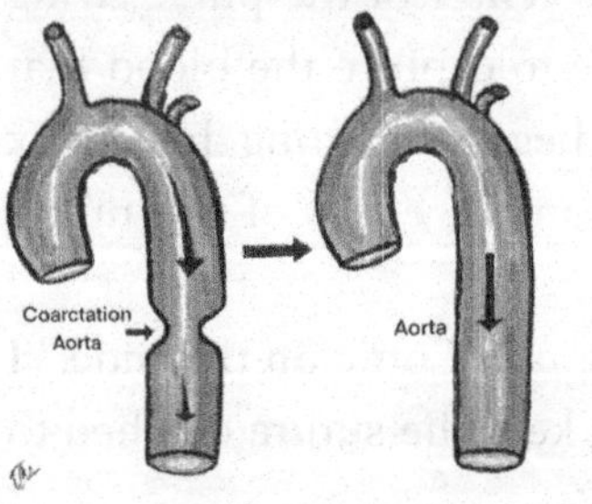

On another occasion, I was fortunate to assist him in performing surgery on Josiah Pollak, a 24-year-old Jehovah's Witness with mild coarctation of the aorta. This condition, which is characterized by a narrowing of the aorta, forces the heart to pump harder to move blood through the aorta to the body, leading to persistent high blood pressure for the patient.

After I'd taken his history and conducted a physical examination, I said, "This is quite a serious operation. We may lose a lot of blood, which may risk your health."

He looked at me, waiting to be asked the obvious question. "Can we transfuse you to save your life?"

"No," came the reply. "I have an advance decision document that the nurse placed in my chart. It clearly states no blood transfusions."

I noted this in the chart, feeling very uncomfortable because no one had ever refused blood. I understood his religious reasons and wanted to argue that Dr. Harken was going to operate on the main artery in his body and that we would likely lose a lot of blood, which could affect his life. But I didn't know how futile it would be. Instead, I cross-matched him for three units of blood just in case we needed it to save his life. Any death on the operating table was a tragedy and created a lot of paperwork for everyone, but this one was avoidable.

With the patient positioned on the table and the left chest prepped with an antiseptic solution and draped, Dr. Harken made a long posterolateral incision on his left chest wall. At the same time, as his assistant, I electro-coagulated the bleeders or clamped off larger torn arteries. Dr. Harken was a swift, assured surgeon. He entered the chest cavity through the fourth intercostal space, the muscular gap between the fourth and fifth rib. He placed a self-retaining contractor between these two ribs to keep the wound wide open. The left lung deflated, as the anesthesiologist only ventilated his right lung, and we saw the descending end of the aortic arch as it took blood to the rest of the body. He next mobilized or freed up the aorta, placing tapes around it so he could bring it fully into view. This was a new type of surgery to me, way over my head so that I couldn't help much. I felt like a medical student again, unable to follow his fast moves to assist him. His primary assistant was the scrub nurse. The short segment of the aorta with the coarctation or narrowing came into view. I was impressed by how quickly he clamped branches on either side of the narrowed aortic segment. With these in place, he cut out the narrowed portion of the aorta. We lost a fair amount of blood, as some blood leaked past the clamps.

Dr. Harken turned to the anesthesiologist and told him to transfuse the patient.

"Sir," I said. "He's a Jehovah's Witness who told me he would refuse blood. He has an advanced decision document." Dr. Harken looked at me briefly, as if to say, "What do you know? You've never been responsible for a patient's life." He then nodded to the anesthesiologist.

I felt torn between two perspectives: a religious one, which I respected, and a surgical one that I valued. Weighing the conflicting ethical issues, the decision to give blood from the surgical standpoint prevailed. After all, had I already ordered three units of blood?

Physicians strive to interpret the Hippocratic Oath, "First, do no harm," even though it does not appear in the oath verbatim. However, one could argue that such ideas are implied in the text. I encountered similar ethical conflicts during my surgical career, and despite respecting a patient's wishes, my higher calling was the surgical decision to save a life.

As these thoughts swirled and organized themselves, I lost focus on the master surgeon and his actions. When I refocused on the operation, he had sewn the two ends of the aorta together, re-establishing a complete aortic union.

I don't remember much about closing the wound, the incision, and restoring the anatomy of Josiah Pollak's body because I was preoccupied with how I would break the news about the transfusion to him. Maybe Dr. Harken would. To clear my conscience, I decided to confront the issue directly. Indeed, I would want to know the truth if I were the patient.

In the ICU the following day, after I had taken care of his daily fluid and medication needs and he was wide awake, I mentioned to him that we had faced a life-threatening moment during his operation that required us to give him some blood to prevent his death. I emphasized DYING. I took a step back and held my breath.

He turned to me, and I saw great concern in his eyes. He paused, looked around the ICU, and then looked at me expressionlessly. Then he uttered the two words that made me inhale again.

"Thank you."

Dr. Harkin, the seasoned surgeon, had made the right call.

26

THE HEART TEAM

Till the tired heart shall cease to palpitate.
—Henry Wadsworth Longfellow

The new chief, Dr. John "Jack" Collins, changed the name of the service from Thoracic to Cardio-Thoracic to emphasize the new skills he was bringing to Brigham. The national death rate from heart attacks was approaching 100 deaths per 100,000 people. Worse, those who survived became patients with unstable angina, managed with digoxin, an extract from the foxglove plant. The drug had a very narrow margin between efficacy and toxicity. Some patients could not be managed on digoxin due to intolerance; they became cardiac cripples and had to limit their everyday activities.

Dr. Collins's talent lay in performing surgery on patients with completely blocked or critically narrowed coronary arteries due to fatty deposits (plaques). He would skillfully bypass the blocked arteries by suturing a harvested artery in front of and behind the plaque to ensure blood flow beyond the obstruction and prevent further damage.

On my first day in the Cardiac service, our first patient was an unscheduled, critically ill ad-on who was brought to the O.R. directly from the cardiac catheterization laboratory, displacing the regularly scheduled initial patient. In the cardiac catheterization lab, an interventional radiologist inserts a catheter into the patient's right femoral or groin artery and threads it up the aorta into the openings of the cardiac muscle or coronary arteries, which supply the heart muscle with the oxygen and nutrients it needs to contract and beat. By injecting a contrast medium into the coronary artery while X-raying, he obtains a visual outline of the anatomy, the blockages, and the plaques within these vessels, indicating which need to be bypassed to improve blood flow to the heart muscle. Occasionally, this procedure endangers the patient, nearly causing a heart attack and necessitating a rush to the O.R. for an emergency bypass procedure.

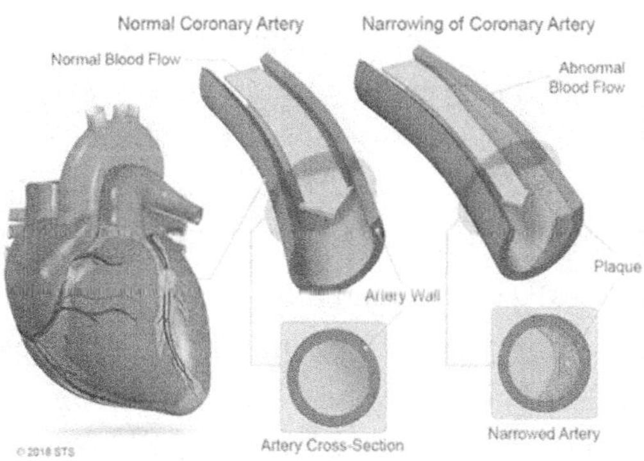

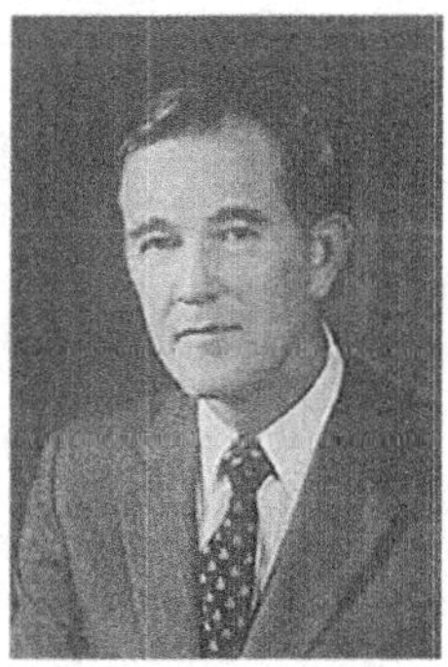
Dr. John Collins

The entire residency team rushed into the O.R. with Dr. VanDam, the Chief of Anesthesiology, his resident, Lorraine Comanor, and other cardiac team members. Along with a group of nurses, we transferred the patient from the gurney to the O.R. table.

My chief resident, Dr. Larry Smith, inserted an arterial catheter into the right radial artery so the anesthesiologist could continuously monitor oxygen levels during surgery and post-operatively in the ICU. A nurse inserted a Foley catheter into the bladder to measure the hourly urine flow, indicating whether the patient had sufficiently high blood pressure to ensure the kidneys were adequately perfused. Other nurses positioned pillows under potentially bony pressure points. I washed down the legs to harvest the superficial veins that would be used to bypass the numerous blockages in the heart.

The unique team of technicians operating the heart-lung pump-oxygenator quickly set up their machine, priming it with compatible blood and checking the valves to ensure that blood flowed through the machine in the correct direction. They calculated the amount of anticoagulant needed to prevent blood clotting while the patient was on the bypass machine. Once Dr. Collins arrived, the patient would be put to sleep, and the operation could begin. Until then, he received oxygen to breathe through a mask covering his face.

Suddenly, the patient emitted a mournful groan, a disturbingly loud sound that pierced through the low-level hubbub in the room. He stopped breathing. His drawn face turned blue-gray, and his EKG tracing showed a change in heart function, indicating ventricular tachycardia. He was immediately intubated and given oxygen directly into his lungs. At the same time, Larry Smith, the most senior member of the surgical team, shouted "cardiac arrest!" and began pumping the patient's chest. He alerted the charge nurse for cardiac meds, which he injected directly into the heart in an attempt to prevent the patient from dying.

Where was Dr. Collins? He'd been expected any minute but had not shown up. Since I had no specific duties in this new service, I left the O.R. in my blues and hurried to the Cardio-Thoracic Office. It was locked. I called the office and heard the phone ringing endlessly through the door. I had Dr. Collins repeatedly paged, "Code Blue. Stat O.R. one!" Like a shuttlecock, I dashed between the O.R. and his office, searching for him. I wrote a note with the same message and slipped it under his door. As I stood up, I encountered a man holding an office key.

"Dr. Collins, I presume?"

He gazed at me for a brief second.

"You're urgently wanted in Room One."

He spun on his heels and dashed off, with me following.

The patient didn't survive, despite Dr. Collins's presence. I felt a pang of sadness for the team and deep sorrow for the patient and his family. The case wasn't discussed at Saturday's Morbidity and Mortality conference, as it was considered a death resulting from the patient's disease.

Although my first encounter with Dr. Collins was a nonoperative event, I learned to admire him as his resident. He looked you in the eye, spoke softly, and listened intently. He was fit, with a ramrod-straight back, ears aligned directly above his shoulders, shoulders over his hips, and heels—posture acquired while serving on nuclear submarines. Well-dressed in an immaculately fitting suit and polished shoes, he embodied the Southern gentleman. When a situation in the O.R. turned critical, his military training took over; he remained calm and persevered. I admired his unwavering composure in emergencies and sought to emulate his behavior.

Larry Smith was an exceptional role model. He possessed a dynamic, individualistic personality and was willing to take calculated risks based on logic to improve patient care. He excelled under surgical pressure and cared for his patients both physically and intellectually. He was a dedicated athlete who ran five miles three times a week, barefoot through the streets of Boston.

"Seriously, barefoot? No running shoes?"

"Yeah. To toughen up my soles."

This idiosyncrasy aligned with his personality: lean and

tough. He told me it sharpened his focused mind. I was impressed by his no-nonsense "let's get things done now" attitude. He exuded confidence and laughed easily when the occasion warranted it, and I liked him from the start. He collaborated with his team and assisted with the scut work when he knew I had the evening off, allowing me to get home earlier. I tried to exceed expectations to make his job easier. Like Burley, calm and confident, he was a team leader par excellence. The affinity between Dr. Collins and Dr. Smith may have been that he, like Dr. Collins, was going into the Navy after completing his adult cardiothoracic training. He joined the crew of the aircraft carrier, USS John F. Kennedy, as one of their medics. The last I heard from him was that he ran around the perimeter of the carrier each dawn.

As the senior resident, Dr. Larry Henry was shorter than both Larry Smith and me. He was polite, introspective, and systematic in his problem-solving approach, but he was considered relatively rigid in his methods. When Larry Smith assisted Larry Henry during an operation on a Ward Service patient, a constant tug-of-war ensued between them over the height of the operating table, with Larry H. wanting it lowered and Larry S. preferring it raised. Initially, watching how it unfolded was amusing, but I soon realized that the issue was really about power. Since it was Larry H.'s case, he felt that he should decide on the table's height. However, Larry S. was the chief resident and senior to Larry H., so he believed he had authority over the table's height. I grew weary of this conflict and tried to avoid getting involved in such cases.

From time to time, we encountered patients in the service who required thoracic operations for lung cancer. Dr. Henry saw a patient in the clinic and approached me, "I've scheduled Mr. Adler for an 8 a.m. start tomorrow. Be there."

Later that day, after the O.R. schedule was printed, Larry Smith approached me. "I've rescheduled Mr. Adler's start time.

We will start at 7:30 a.m. I want to do the case, and you need to assist me. No need to tell Henry."

I fully understood what was happening. Larry Smith wasn't partial to Larry Henry. This was a personality issue, not a surgical one, and it shouldn't have influenced the situation. Or was it that Larry Henry hadn't consulted with his Chief Resident, Larry Smith? Was this a matter of politics or pettiness? I was in the O.R. before 7:30 a.m., feeling quite uncomfortable in the middle.

Personality disorders influence interpersonal relationships in medicine, much like they do in other fields. Surgeons sometimes act out, forgetting that they have matured and no longer play in the sandbox. The game's name is compromised before earning the label of a "disruptive personality." Such a characterization is difficult to shake. Regrettably, I have witnessed such behavior throughout my 35 years in surgical life, particularly when contending with the competitive egos of surgeons.

Despite this episode, I thrived in this service due to its positive leadership. There was a sense of security among the Brigham residents, a feeling of being safely situated in the midst of a meritocracy, privileged, elite, and part of an academic leadership league in the surgical world—the chosen few. Surviving residency was the name of the game, which I was gradually learning. I appreciated that feeling of belonging.

27

SEX & THE HEART

In love, it is no other than the frantic desire for that which flies from us.

—Michel de Montaigne

I informed Mr. Goldberg that I was a resident under Dr. Collins and that he would eventually meet several other residents, as we worked as a team. With Mr. Goldberg's permission, I took a history of his chief complaint. I examined him due to seven valuable points of consideration, a well-known adage that "Proper prior planning prevents piss poor performance." These seven "Ps" were important to remember in any surgical endeavor.

Mr. Goldberg, a 45-year-old jeweler from New Hampshire, smoked two packs of cigarettes a day and drank an occasional beer. He reported tightness in his chest and discomfort—cardiac angina—along with shortness of breath when climbing stairs or walking certain distances. He had been experiencing these symptoms for the past eight months, with two to three episodes each day, always relieved by sublingual nitroglycerin tablets. His medical history included hypertension, elevated cholesterol, and early-onset type 2 diabetes, with no history of heart attack. His medications included those for high blood pressure, high cholesterol, and diabetes management. His physical examination was unremarkable.

I reviewed his EKG, drew his admission blood, and had him sign a consent form for the operation. Afterward, I went to the X-ray department in the basement and examined all the X-ray films of the patient's heart and chest, going back as far as available, to evaluate the aggressiveness and progression of his disease.

During evening ward rounds, the team visited each patient. We started in the ICU and proceeded to see the post-operative patients and the pre-operative ones. Dr. Collins led the group, followed closely by Larry Smith and Larry Henry in quasi-rank order. Following were Dr. Collins's office nurse, his nurse practitioner, three members of the heart-lung machine team, a group of ward nurses, and finally, the medical students. At one point, I counted fourteen individuals crowding closely behind Dr. Collins and into a patient's room.

I pushed my way to the front of the crowd, straining to hear what Dr. Collins would ask Mr. Goldberg as we gathered around his bed. I stood next to Mr. Goldberg, across from Dr. Collins, who was on the patient's other side.

"This is Mr. Goldberg," I said, starting my presentation with a summary of his symptoms and what I had read were Dr. Collins's plans for tomorrow's operation. Dr. Collins listened to my presentation with patience and interest. He knew far more about Mr. Goldberg than I did, as I was not privy to all the referral materials or the details of the cardiac catheterization. I had not attended all the conferences where each patient was discussed in depth before surgery. Mr. Goldberg's coronary arteries had become clogged with fatty deposits. Dr. Collins understood where the critical disease was in Mr. Goldberg's coronary arteries and said to him,

"We plan to do two bypass grafts tomorrow morning."

"How long does the operation take?"

"About three to four hours," came the reply. "Do you have any further questions?"

Mr. Goldberg shook his head, and the team, like a writhing snake, filed out of his room.

The next day, after the morning ward rounds, we headed to the O.R. The room buzzed with activity, and the usual pre-operative teams were preparing everything to put the patient to sleep. Mr. Goldberg, already lying on the operating table, recognized my face in the crowd and greeted me.

Once the patient was anesthetized, the teams started working. I harvested the superficial leg veins, and Drs. Collins and Smith split open the chest and prepared the large vessels to connect to catheters for putting the patient on the heart-lung machine that replaced the heart function. The coronary artery bypasses were done on the still, non-beating heart. This meant that deoxygenated blood from the body and head was diverted to the heart-lung pump oxygenator, taking over the heart and lung functions. This machine was run by a team of skilled technicians working closely with the surgeon and anesthesiologists. The heart can be stilled for about 30 to 90 minutes.

Mr. Goldberg's heart was stilled by chemical injection to allow Drs. Collins and Smith to sew one end of the harvested vein before the blockage and the other end into the coronary artery, bridging or bypassing the blockage to increase blood flow to the heart. Once the harvested veins were sewn around the blockages, the patient's heart was electrically shocked using paddles to resume normal heart function. The patient was taken off the heart-lung machine when the heart was pumping effectively and functioning better.

This operation was executed in stillness and speed. Each team member understood their role in this complex procedure, which had the potential for tense moments if something went awry. With each step, our anxiety levels rose. Once these steps were completed, there was a collective sigh, and the tension in the room gave way to a quiet calm. To recover from the high stress I experienced during surgery, I retreated into a zone of inner calm, summarized by Herman Hesse as "A stillness and a sanctuary to which you can retreat at any time."

While Drs. Smith and Collins closed the chest, I tended to the leg wounds. Once my task was finished, I left the O.R. to address issues on the ward and prepare to present patients for the afternoon ward rounds.

When the first patient was moved into the Cardiac ICU, usually by 1 a.m., I was paged to meet them and take over their care. Working with the ICU nurses, we placed the patient on a respirator, and their cardiac status was continuously monitored by the arterial catheter, which reflected the patient's oxygen levels, and the Foley catheter, which indicated the adequacy of his blood volume. I wrote the post-op orders and ensured the patient received sufficient pain medication. Once the patient was fully awake and all vital signs were stable, the endotracheal tube was removed, and the patient was extubated.

I put on fresh O.R. greens and hurried back to the O.R., where Dr. Collins and the senior team prepared another patient for the day's second cardiac operation. Occasionally, during a cardiac emergency, a third or even fourth operation would be performed late into the night.

On one occasion, we operated late into the afternoon on a man described as "The King of the Gypsies." When the family visited the ICU after the operation, they noticed that the other two cardiac patients were on monitors.

"Why isn't the King on a monitor?"

"We only have two," came the reply. This was true.

On rounds that evening, we noticed that the King also had a cardiac monitor. It looked different from the other two. On the side of the monitor, in white paint over the beige enamel, were the initials CHMC. Without a monitor at the Brigham for their revered King, the family had crossed the road and taken a monitor from the Children's Hospital Medical Center. I hoped it would be returned when the King was discharged.

Evening rounds in the ICU began any time after 4 p.m. When I was the resident who had operated on that day's patients, I would stay overnight. While I was in the O.R., Dr. Henry admitted a few new patients, prepared them for the next day's schedule, and presented them during evening rounds. He would go home after writing me a detailed cut list.

As the only in-house resident for the heart service, I was responsible for patient issues. Despite my physical needs, including hunger and fatigue, I survived on adrenaline and continued to push forward. If I encountered a problem beyond my expertise or knowledge, I could reach out to my immediate senior, Dr. Larry Henry. However, I often called Dr. Larry Smith instead, as he encouraged it, and I felt that as Chief Resident, he was ultimately responsible for his residents. I may have done that twice in six weeks.

The hours after the rounds were filled with numerous chores. By 11 p.m., I needed to write prescriptions for the patients going home the next day and go down to the records room to dictate the discharge summaries. I ate as much as I could from the cafeteria, completed my night rounds, and tried to get some sleep.

By 5 a.m., I'd rise, and after a quick shower, head straight to the ICU to check all my patients' cardiac and breathing parameters. I'd detach each from their respirator, and if they were fully awake and could breathe on their own for ten minutes without it, I would suction the mucus out of their throats and, at the count of three while the patient exhaled, remove the endotracheal tube. Most patients smiled and were happy to breathe spontaneously and talk. Dr. Smith would be pleased if I effectively performed a task he'd need to do before the rest of the team and students arrived to start morning ward rounds at 6 a.m.

Mr. Goldberg's recovery was very satisfactory. On postoperative day four, the team led by Dr. Collins entered his private room. Knowing he would be discharged the following morning, I stood beside the chief to hear what he had to say. His words spurred me to action, which meant dictating a discharge summary and writing prescriptions.

We gathered around the bed. Dr. Collins asked Mr. Goldberg, "How do you feel?"

"I feel great. I've been walking up and down the corridors without any problems."

"The nurses tell me that your leg incisions are healing nicely, which is a good sign. Your heart is pumping well, and blood is getting down to your toes," explained Dr. Collins.

"You had a worse disease than we expected. We did six bypasses instead of the two we had planned."

"That explains why you took the veins from both legs," deduced Mr. Goldberg. Dr. Collins nodded. "Nevertheless, you've done very well, and I think you can go home tomorrow."

A broad smile crossed Mr. Goldberg's face. "That's good. That's good." Dr. Collins stretched out his hand and shook the hand of a smiling Mr. Goldberg. "I'll drop your doctor a note. Dr. Meguid will give you prescriptions, and the nurses will give you dressings to change for your various wounds." With that, Dr. Collins made a move to leave the room. As the Red Sea did for Moses, the crowd parted, and Dr. Collins headed for the door, with everyone closely following. I almost crossed into the corridor when Mr. Goldberg yelled, "Hey, doc. When can I have sex?"

Over my shoulder, I replied in a loud voice, "As soon as you get home."

Dr. Collins froze as the team crowded around him. He spun around, and the entourage parted. He took a few steps forward, his face purple and his eyes bulging. He prodded my chest through my white coat and said, "Don't you ever say that to my patients. He has six delicate anastomoses in his heart."

I was taken aback. As he stood facing me, I heard myself say, "Dr. Collins, every one of your patients asks me that question. From now on, I respectfully suggest you preemptively address the question with them."

I couldn't believe I had said that to the Chief. I fully expected to be fired. Sex could be the end of my career as a surgical resident at Harvard.

As a young man, I never imagined that elderly patients had sex, so my response was based on the understanding that after a major chest operation or any significant surgery, the accumulation of all the pains and aches experienced by a patient wouldn't be conducive to having sex right away. It was a safe bet that Mr. Goldberg's desire exceeded his ability to engage comfortably in a sexual act as soon as he got home.

As I grew older, I came to see the world differently and started to discuss the topic more frequently. Some patients were taken aback by my mentioning it, while others appreciated my brief comments and engaged in discussions about the issue with me.

We humans are driven by our libido. For some, it's making love; for others, it might be a passionate kiss, the embrace of companionship, the comfort of a pet, or even the touch of a hand. As Spencer Michael Free reminds us, "Tis the human touch in this world that counts, / the touch of your hand and mine, / which means far more to the fainting heart / than shelter and bread and wine . . ."

I appeared to have done reasonably well in the service since

I wasn't fired. I received a letter from the Chief of Chiefs stating that I could become a categorical resident. I loved the man! What exhilarating news! I was eager to continue the challenge and validate my positive feelings about eventually being branded "Trained by FDM."

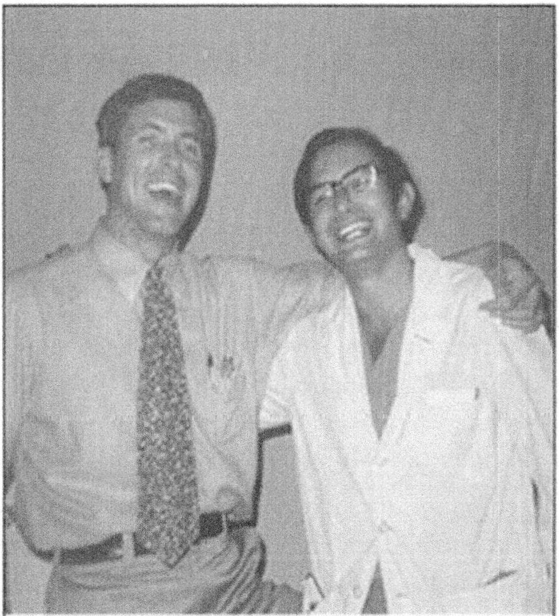

Dr. Larry Smith, Chief Resident & author

28

GOOD INTENTIONS OF TOMORROW

The road to hell is paved with good intentions.
—Bernard of Clairvaux

On my way to the O.R. that morning for the second coronary artery bypass operation, I was paged for an outside call. I briefly stopped, leaning against the wall of the busy Pike, and heard John Rackey's voice, the American friend I'd initially met in October 1963 when we started at University College Medical School in London. Some eight years later, he called me from Naples, Florida, where he was the junior partner in an OBGYN practice, having just completed his residency in Washington, D.C.

In 1963, we were part of a group of 12 foreign students, or as the British euphemistically identified us, "Oversea Students" (OS), in a class of about 100. Our acquaintance began on the third day of classes during a lively class husting related to my election, where a majority vote of the class members confirmed my chairmanship of the Physiology Society. A vocal minority of anti-foreign rebels, dissatisfied with the outcome, vigorously and noisily lobbied to overturn the vote. John, along with other

OS and open-minded colleagues, supported my candidacy, defeating the renegades. John and I became close friends.

Together, we completed the 2nd MB examination, a critical stage in our advancement toward becoming doctors. The exam evaluated our knowledge of anatomy, physiology, pharmacology, and pathology acquired over 18 months at University College. Passing the challenging examination ensured our progression across Gower Street to University College Hospital, ultimately allowing us to see patients and develop our clinical knowledge and skills. During the three years of clinical work, we occupied adjoining rooms in the Hospital Annex dorms on Gower Street, just a short distance from the hospital. We studied and dined together, shared our life stories, and reflected on his British love life. He had been a concert pianist in college, and we enjoyed evenings of classical music as a way to relax during the evenings and on weekends.

He met my girlfriend, Victoria Perfect, and attended our wedding reception at Apothecary Hall on Black Friars Lane in London, which is the headquarters of the Worshipful Society of Apothecaries. After graduating, we both secured residencies on this side of the pond. John's influence led to Victoria and me being in America.

"Can you talk?"

"Not really; I'm wanted in the O.R. for a cardiac case. Can I call you later?"

There was a slight hesitation in his voice. Not knowing if he had heard me over the noisy background traffic, I shouted, "John, are you there?" and repeated my initial response.

"Perhaps," came the hesitant and ominous reply. Then there was a buzz.

"Hello John, John, John . . ." I said in an increasingly raised and anxious voice. The line was dead.

I made a mental note to call John that night to chat about our joys and sorrows. I didn't give it another thought as I resumed my rush to Dr. Collin's O.R. to start and strip the leg veins of our second patient of the day.

In London, John told me that he had gone to Princeton to study electronic engineering so he could join his father at Westinghouse Electric. He married his high school sweetheart, and they were expecting twins when she was killed in a motor vehicle accident. Lost and feeling purposeless, he joined the U.S. Air Force. Given his educational background, he trained as an electronic warfare pilot in Pensacola, Florida. He learned to fly a Douglas EB 66 E-DL, an aircraft used in signals intelligence and electronic countermeasure operations near the Russian border. His squadron was deployed to Mildenhall Air Force Base in England during his late twenties.

When he was demobilized, he chose to attend medical school in London. Given our shared flying history, he told me countless stories about his time in the Air Force, life in the States, the warm, azure waters of the Gulf, and the alluring, exciting life in Florida.

He entered George Washington University's OBGYN Residency Program two years before Victoria and I began our residency in Boston in 1970. After marrying Margaret, a nurse anesthetist, "a delightful lady," he and Margaret had two lovely daughters born barely a year apart. Victoria and I visited them for a long weekend in Washington when their daughters were still in diapers. They seemed to be a happy family.

He joined a practice in Naples, a rapidly developing community on Florida's Gulf Coast. Victoria, our two-year-old daughter, and I visited them in 1975. During this visit, he took us to discover paradise on the barren Marco Island, navigating through mangroves to reach the world's most pristine seven miles of white sand beach, where we intended to picnic. I was awestruck by the endless, immaculate, peaceful expanse of sand. Then, he planted the seed for me to buy a house in Marco one day. Unknown to my wonderful, trusted friend John, my dream came true.

In the hubbub of being on call—operations, discharges, admissions, endless pages, and infinite tasks demanding attention, along with patients or nurses needing my full assiduousness—I overlooked my return call to John that night.

The next evening, I found a free moment and slipped into the medical records room, where I was guaranteed privacy and quiet. I rang John. To this day, I can still hear ring, ring—ring. Ring-ring, ring-ring, ring-ring, ring-ring, ring . . . come on, John, pick up the phone. I'm free to chat now, come on . . .

The line went dead.

He never picked up.

We never had that chat.

The busy and fast demands of surgical life consumed and subsumed me.

A few months later, I received a lengthy letter from Margaret. After living together for several years, she wanted a divorce. John, she wrote, threatened to kill himself. According to her letter, the marital stalemate persisted for several months until she initiated the divorce. John drove out of Naples, checked into a motel, and took an overdose.

I suddenly remembered what I was told early in the residency program to explain why the first three years of training were vertical and the last two to three years were pyramidal. During the initial years of the residency, one person drops out because it's too demanding. Then, during the following two years, one or two residents get divorced due to the long hours and neglect of their wives, resulting in fewer training spots during the last two senior years. I didn't quite believe it, but I was starting to see it because one of my colleagues was perpetually upset and spoke little except to express his anger and frustration about his wife and the acrimonious divorce he was going through.

Most of those around me were men of steel, determination, and ambition. They were the Brigham men. They seldom revealed the emotional aspects of their lives. Although it wasn't mentioned, rumors abounded about flings, romances, one-night stands, and some stable passions as a way to decompress their squeezed souls—men who yearned to feel special in someone else's arms.

I had been prepared earlier in life; from the age of four onward, I was forged at the anvil of my sadistic Prussian grandfather, learning ways to survive and push through at all costs to avoid the stigma and shame of failure. My training strained my relationship with Victoria. The daily worry and continual stress diminished my ability to reach out to the one I loved most—a strange phenomenon I didn't understand but detested.

No doubt she, too, experienced similar emotions from her arduous training. Fatigue left no room for my romance and fantasy, but I held on, knowing, or at least hoping, that life would improve and that the academic and financial rewards for both of us would justify the day's pain. I thought I understood both John and Margaret; nevertheless, I hated to see my good friend go down in flames in the isolation of pain. In my distress, I failed to mention the entire episode to Victoria.

My dear friend John—the electronic engineer, U.S. Air Force pilot, survivor of a North Sea crash, medical student, lover of English women, OBGYN, connoisseur of fine Stilton cheese and wines, and my teacher in crafting an exquisite Old Fashioned cocktail—the man who was the singular influence on my coming to Boston and Florida—was no more.

When Victoria and I visited him in Washington, D.C., he seemed to be his usual stoic self. We reminisced about our pub crawl through Scotland in his new VW. We planned, arranged, and met for another weekend after he joined the Naples practice. We also had plans to visit Florida, among many others after I completed my residency, but our busy careers displaced each trip. Tomorrow was always there, that eternal moment that never arrives.

Reverend John Donne stated in his Meditation XVII, written in the early seventeenth century, " . . . any man's death diminishes me because I am involved in mankind; and therefore, never send to know for whom the bell tolls; it tolls for thee."

Had I taken the time to listen to him when he rang me up that morning, despite the urgency of the cardiac case, would John be alive today?

I had let down a close friend.

John, I frequently visit you in my small cemetery of regrets. I can see your face and your wry smile. Your absence continues to be one of my greatest sorrows.

Around the Corner

by Charles Hanson Towne

Around the corner I have a friend,
In this great city that has no end.
Yet days go by, and weeks rush on,
And before I know it, a year is gone,
And I never see my old friend's face,
For life is a swift and terrible race.

He knows I like him just as well,
As in the days when I rang his bell.
And he rand mine. We were younger then,
And now we are busy, tired men:
Tired with playing a foolish game,
Tire with trying to make a name.

"Tomorrow," I say, "I will call Jim,
Just to show that I'm thinking of him."
But tomorrow comes—and tomorrow goes,
And the distance between us grows and grows.

Around the corner!—yet miles away . . .
"Here's a telegram, sir . . "
"Jim died today."
And that's what we get, and deserve in the end:
Around the corner, a vanished friend.

29

MAGGOTS & BLACK SNOW

An evil life is a kind of death.
—Ovid

The Brigham parking area was an unfenced lot of firm clay located beyond the last ward at the western end of The Pike's ground level. There was no attendant for the parking lot. The entrance to and from the hospital was through a heavy door. At night, the lot was poorly lit by a single lamp hung over the entrance door, its light gradually fading as one walked farther from the door to a distant car.

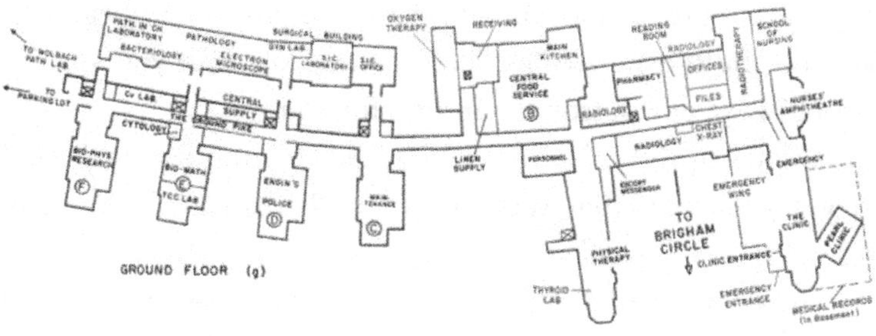

Access to and from the parking lot was via an unmanned boom barrier on Francis Street that rose when one swiped their ID card. The lot held about 100 cars parked closely together by their owners. If you didn't arrive before 6 a.m., you'd have to park on Francis Street. The walk to the E.R. took at least five minutes because it was located at the end of the long, seemingly endless Pike.

I was on an E.R. rotation. The weather report indicated that snow would blanket Boston, with forecasters predicting a potential accumulation of 20 to 30 inches of wet, heavy snow. This meant I should anticipate plenty of motor vehicle trauma, that I might only get a few catnaps during my night's workload, and that my car would be covered in snow and hard to locate; therefore, I might not make it home after this shift.

Even as a medical student, I enjoyed working in emergencies. An injured patient was a medical enigma that piqued my curiosity to solve. By assessing the situational awareness of who, what, where, and when the injury occurred, and by taking the patient's history and conducting an examination, including searching for clues that fit the patterns of injuries, I could usually arrive at a reasonable diagnosis, which, when it wasn't an acute, life-threatening emergency, could be confirmed with an X-ray.

On this six-week E.R. rotation, my shift started at 8 a.m. and lasted 24 hours. As soon as I came in, Nuala, the head nurse—an older, more jovial woman who was always upbeat and smiling—button-holed me. "Before you start, can you spare a minute? I've got a personal question for you."

"What's up?" I asked as she backed me into a cubicle and drew the curtain that was the door. "It's private," she said, adding, "Has it started snowing yet?"

It was not a confidential question, but I realized it was small talk, a nervous opening gambit for what she would share with me. She sat on the only chair in the cubicle while I stood perched against a gurney. "Tell me about it," I said.

"As I walk down The Pike from the parking lot to the E.R., halfway down, I get this terrible cramp," she pointed, "in my left leg." Her white nurse's stockings highlighted her lightly nicotine-stained fingers as she grasped her calf. "It feels like a squeezing pain. It has spread to my foot lately, making me stop and rest." She lowered her voice and looked around. Leaning forward, she almost whispered, "It's embarrassing. Friends walk past me, and I pretend I'm looking for my car keys."

I witnessed the confident expression of a head nurse transform into one of anxiety and worry—concern for what it meant health-wise and how it would impact her family, evoking Thoreau's line, "Most men live lives of quiet desperation." In her eyes, I detected the fear and uncertainty that illness brings, possibly even worries about financial instability. These are typical concerns that appear on the face of a patient confronted with unknown or distressing news.

"After a while, my charley horse goes away. It's strange, isn't it."

"Does it happen often?"

"The other day, I had to stop twice walking down The Pike to work. It doesn't bother me in the E.R. Could this be serious?"

"How long have you had this?"

She paused. As she searched her mind, I saw her thinking, "I'd say six or eight months."

"For how long have you smoked?"

"I started when I was in my late teens. It was fashionable, sexy," she chuckled. "Damn tough to stop. God knows I've tried. But my husband smokes, which makes it even more difficult."

Looking at her, I tried to lighten the mood during this informal consultation. "You won't tell anyone this, but I started smoking with my buddies when I was eleven, behind the garden shed. Made me sick as a dog." She laughed, her face lighting up. "So, I stopped by the time I was twelve," I admitted.

She smiled and then said, "You're funny."

She gave me consent to examine her as she lay on the gurney, kicked off her shoes, slipped off her white tights, pulled up her dress, and covered herself with a cotton sheet. At around forty, she was relatively thin. I could feel a bounding aortic pulse just below her belly button. I observed no scars on her abdomen. The pulses throughout her left leg were strong. On the right side, I could feel the femoral pulse, but I couldn't detect any pulses below that.

I squeezed her big toe capillaries, which caused the tissue to blanch. It takes time for the color to return after pressure. Her time was over three seconds, indicating insufficient blood flow in the artery of her right leg. There must be a narrowing or blockage. She swung around, straightened her hair and uniform, and folded the sheet.

"I believe you're experiencing a critically narrowed artery in the mid-thigh region—I'd say it's probably the mid-femoral artery, which is the most common. While walking around the E.R., you receive enough blood flow to your legs. However, when you walk briskly down our Pike, the demands on your calf muscles and feet increase the requirement for blood, oxygen, and glucose. The narrowed artery restricts your access to that additional blood when needed, leading to a charley horse. It's what you, no doubt, know as arterial insufficiency."

She nodded.

"Do you get any tightness in your chest?"

She shook her head.

"I wouldn't neglect it. This can worsen, so it's best to see a vascular surgeon. You know, Dr. Crane. He's an excellent vascular surgeon. You'll need an EKG to ensure there's no critical narrowing of your heart vessels, an angiogram of your leg vessels to confirm the diagnosis, find the area of narrowing, and then undergo an operation."

"What'll they do?"

"Depends. The most common procedure involves inserting a Gore-Tex Fem-Pop graft from the groin to just below the knee, thereby bypassing the narrowing."

"Why not see him?"

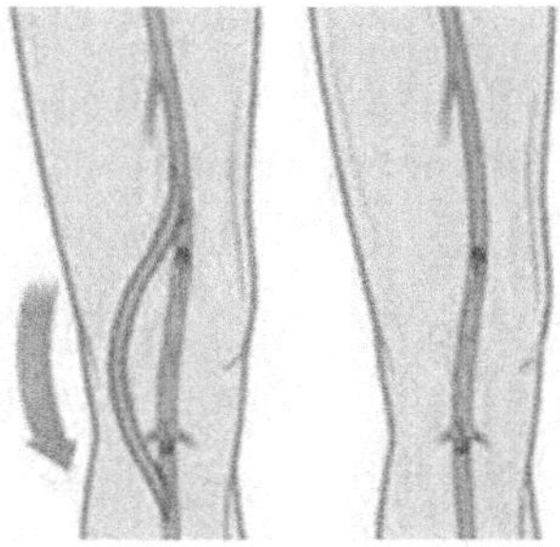

She nodded again, deep in thought. While I filled out a referral with a brief note of my history and findings, she slipped on her tights, straightened her dress, and put on her shoes. She pocketed my referral. Her head nurse's character returned to normal as she thanked me, leaving the cubicle with a hint of concern.

As it snowed lazily, with a few flakes here and there, surgical admissions to the E.R. decreased. I had a slow morning as clouds rolled in from the west. I lanced an extremely painful pilonidal abscess caused by an ingrown hair in the skin between the buttocks, and I loosely stitched up a cut from a kitchen knife. News of heavier snowfall arrived with the 3 p.m. shift change as the afternoon nurses began to arrive. Snow fell in waves in some areas of Boston, resulting in a heavy shower with some accumulation, while at other times, the snow was light, blowing in all directions and swirling in the wind.

By the middle of winter, Boston had already received around sixteen inches of wet precipitation, making the city appear dark and dirty. A few inches of snow had fallen each day, not enough to be considered a storm but sufficient to be an ongoing nuisance. The forecasters predicted heavier-than-usual snowfall for today.

I looked outside through the open E.R. door and the empty

receiving bays. Gray-white clouds hung low over the world while flurries of snow settled on and between the ambulances parked in the E.R. lot, gradually softening their sharp edges into rounded mounds. The biting cold, the squalls of snowfall, and the wind whipping up the loosely settled flakes painted the outside world a soft white.

In the distance, Brigham Circle and Huntington Avenue appeared bleak and gray, darkened by oppressively low skies. The monochromatic snow fell relentlessly onto yesterday's gray slush. Huddled, bundled figures leaned into blasts of freezing wind, hesitantly sliding with each step along the sidewalks. Citizens wore boots and heavy overcoats against the bitter cold, their scarves and hats transforming them into amorphous shapes as they moved. The passing traffic moved slowly, crunching along and squirting slush and slurry ice in all directions, striking passersby and parked cars. Traffic sounds were muffled, yet I could still hear the scraping of shovels on the sidewalks. Snowplows salting the roads lumbered by with their flashing yellow lights, beacons of more snow to come. It was a picture perfect scene of winter misery. As I stepped back into the E.R.'s warmth, it struck me that soon I would see old ladies with fractured hips slipping on icy sidewalks.

Homeless people began straggling in for a few hours of warmth, to thaw out, and perhaps to get a hot meal. Molly, a surgical E.R. nurse, said, "They come with chronic non-healing venous ulcers," adding, "One's compassion to admit them would put a tremendous strain on hospital beds. We keep them here to warm up and get them some coffee and a hot meal, but we don't house them except the few who have infections threatening frostbite or limb loss. After you've treated their sores, we apply a new Unna boot"—a compression bandage containing zinc oxide wrapped from the toes to the knee, leaving flexibility in the ankle.

As darkness fell over Boston, her prediction came true. A

trickle of older men bundled up to the hilt appeared with wet, soggy Unna boots. Some, like homeless Patrick, were regulars during such inclement weather. A few were poorly shaven, others had facial hair, and some reeked of alcohol, but all wore an assortment of woolen clothing that was damp from exposure to the elements. They were the underprivileged people living among us. They sat in an E.R. cubicle with their Unna-booted legs propped up, their wet wool clothing steaming in the warmth of the E.R.

Not having dealt with this problem before, Molly showed me how to remove Patrick's boots. Squatting next to me with scissors in hand, she said, "Start by cutting the gauze at the knee and work your way down towards the ankle to remove the semirigid mold around the calf."

As she did, we were overwhelmed by a musty pong from the mixture of macerated, wrinkled skin and the wet, compressive dressing. White maggots squirmed in various ulcers and fell, wriggling onto the pried-off dressing. Only the fresh smell of Molly's shampoo, which I actively inhaled as I leaned into her, prevented me from throwing up.

I cut off the remainder of the boot while she brought a basin filled with warm water and sponges. Once free of the semirigid molded gauze, I examined his swollen leg, removed the maggots with my forceps, and asked, "How long have you had this on?" His answer was hesitant: "Oh, about three weeks."

"You know, the gauze bandage is impregnated with zinc to speed the healing of your leg ulcers. You must return to our outpatient clinic for a new boot dressing every week until you are healed." There was no response.

After removing the Unna boot from both limbs, I stood up and stretched my back while Molly continued to squat on a stool in front of the patient's legs. She washed them with antiseptic Hibiclens in warm water. I admired her as she gently dried the legs and feet, carefully picking off dead layers of skin until fresh, healthy skin emerged. Then she applied a thin layer of medicated zinc ointment over Patrick's legs and feet. Molly could have been Mary Magdalene pouring fragrant ointment on Jesus' feet. Looking up at me, she spoke softly and showed me how to wrap a new boot diagonally, starting at the feet and crossing the ankle up the leg to cover the ulcers and compress the varicose veins. The trick was to wrap the limb so the patient could actively ambulate.

I admired the dedication of this young nurse, who couldn't have been older than her mid-twenties. As she rose, I could see the gratitude in the eyes of the older adult peering beneath shaggy, matted hair. Patrick sipped a steaming cup of coffee while we moved on to the next patient.

A lull in patient flow followed.

I checked out my bed in the E.R. resident's room adjacent to the E.R. Then I went to the kitchen to get some coffee. Molly must have had the same idea.

"Coffee? I'm just making a new pot."

"Sure."

"By the way, bringing us Dunkin Donuts is so nice of you. Saves the day when we're busy."

Unlike many of the nurses, Molly wasn't a smoker. As we stood around waiting for the coffee to stop dripping, she told me, in response to my question, that she was born at the Lying-In Hospital, that she was an only child, that her dad was high up in the Pacific Navy command and often at sea, so she lived with her mother in Chestnut Hill. She had gone to Radcliffe College, and seeing that the name didn't register with me, she added, "originally an all-girls college associated with Harvard."

"I tried to join the Girl Guides when I was a kid, but they wouldn't have me," I said, chuckling. She laughed, joining in the spirit of the banter.

"You must have traveled a bit with your dad," I said.

"Not really. New Hampshire up north in the winter to ski

and as far south as the Cape, where we have a house on Martha's Vineyard for the summer."

"Overseas?"

She shook her head. "I'd love to go to Italy or Ireland. They sound so pretty. Or somewhere exotic like Mexico."

By now, several patients with surgical issues were waiting. The first was a middle-aged man with a substantial girth who complained of back pain from shoveling the sidewalk. The X-rays revealed narrowed lumbar disk spaces and some osteophytes on the edges of the vertebral bodies. I prescribed muscle relaxants and painkillers and referred him to the orthopedic clinic.

Around 8 p.m., Molly approached me. "Would you see a young girl, Cindy? It's not a surgical case, but this is her sixth visit to the E.R. in the past 12 hours. Cindy is a teenager who keeps cutting her wrists, wanting to kill herself. I know she needs help. Would you speak to her?"

"Sure, put her in a cubicle."

"Hi. I hear you have some cuts that need cleaning. Can I see them?"

She was young and seemed in a dream, avoiding my eyes.

"Where are your parents?"

She shrugged. After a pause, she said in a distant voice, "They're always working."

She had ten superficial cuts over the veins of her left wrist, which I suspect were done with a blunt razor blade. They were clean. "You know, if you cut any deeper, you'll get the vein and perhaps even the artery, which will bleed and make an awful mess on your nice jeans," I said. She merely stared at her wrist and didn't speak.

"Is there a reason you're hurting yourself?"

She shrugged.

"What would you like me to do for you? You need counseling during this stressful period, and I want to help you."

Once more, she shrugged, then provocatively mentioned, as an afterthought, "They are never home. My Nana was always there for me when we lived in Michigan." She began to cry softly.

This was a psychological stress test for me, and I wasn't equipped to manage it. In many American families, both parents worked, thereby diminishing the energy and attention they could give to their children's emotional needs.

As a surgeon, I was trained to help people through action. However, with Cindy, I couldn't remove a mental illness from a troubled young girl. Her issue was far beyond my skill set and training. Cindy needed a psychiatrist, not a surgeon.

I picked up the phone and called the psychiatric resident. "I'm in the E.R. seeing a young girl with behavioral changes who is trying to commit suicide. She's been brought into the E.R. six times since this morning. I think you need to come in and see her," I said into the phone.

"Suicide is not an emergency," replied the passive voice.

"W-H-A-T? You listen here; she is trying to KILL herself and needs a shrink. If suicide is not an emergency, then what the fuck is an emergency in psychiatry?" I yelled. "You're on call, and you've got to come in and see her."

"It's snowing, so I can't come."

"The snow has tapered off. You are on call for emergencies," I repeated, "and you are responsible."

There was a pause before he said, "Let me see how bad it's snowing." He laid down the receiver. I could hear his footsteps as he walked to a window and back. "It's snowing here. Give her an appointment at the psych-resident's clinic Monday morning."

"She'll be dead. Have you heard me? DEAD, and your name will be all over it in the newspaper. You're on call. It's your duty, your hypocritical oath. If you don't come, I'll call your chairman."

"Go ahead."

"You, mother fucker, are a useless and outrageously irresponsible moron," I raged. He had hung up.

When called, the chairman entered and took the young girl from a surgical cubicle to a medical one. Two hours later, I saw them engaged in deep conversation.

I don't understand why the on-call psychiatry doctor didn't want to come in. It was his duty to do so. If extenuating circumstances prevented him from attending to this E.R. patient, he should have arranged for a colleague or even his supervisor to cover for him. I can't imagine being called to see a patient in the E.R. and refusing to come in. I'd be fired.

In surgery, we operated under a top-down command structure, while in medicine, the hierarchy was inverted. The intern's word was final. As a second-year resident, my directive to a psychiatric intern during an emergency carried the weight of an order, given his on-call status. This ongoing conflict in the chain of command sometimes resulted in situations where the least experienced medical professional, just one year out of medical school, faced off against the most skilled surgical resident, who had five to seven years of medical training. The patient found herself caught between these contrasting opinions.

By 9 p.m., traffic in the E.R. had significantly decreased as the worsening winter weather enveloped the community. An air of eerie stillness descended upon the emergency ward as cubicles emptied, patient visits to the E.R. dropped sharply, and the ambulance bay stood vacant. I could hear myself breathe while some nurses went off to dinner and others gathered around the nursing stations, enjoying a moment of peace, a coffee, and a smoke. Those who had remained past their shift's end to assist with the influx of E.R. patients chose to go home.

After a while, I became aware of increased activity in one of the larger E.R. rooms. Nurses hurried in, drawing the curtain behind them and speaking in hushed tones. I was called over to join the bustle. It took me a moment to realize that the confused patient was our Molly. She had stayed past her shift to help with the evening rush of patients.

"What happened, Molly? Tell me," the head nurse urged her quietly. Between bursts of sobs, Molly lay shivering and disjointedly whispered, "He held a knife against my throat." She wept some more. A nurse came in with a warm glass of apple juice. One moment, Molly was struggling to get up from the gurney, pushing away the blanket; the next, she flopped back and curled into a fetal position. "I opened my car . . . cleared the snow. That's when he came . . . I screamed for help" she sobbed some more, " . . . he covered my mouth and pushed me into the car." Her body shook again as she sobbed, waving her hands in front of her. "I tried to shout and kick him . . ." She thrashed her head from side to side on the pillow, " . . . his knife was cold against my neck . . ."

"I didn't know him." she burst out again, tears rolling down her angelic face, "he forced himself onto me." She grabbed the nurse's arm—a blanching squeeze, "I struggled, but he was heavy . . . no one came to help me. The car was covered with snow; it was dark. He was dark; he tore my clothes."

My medical colleague, Jean Ferguson, MD, the chief medical resident with training in sexual assault, joined me. She suggested that I examine the patient while she guided me using the E.R.'s sexual assault protocol for treatment and evidence collection. Molly calmed down and signed a consent form allowing us to examine her.

I recorded the circumstances of the event exactly as she had described them. While attempting to clear the heavy snow off her car, she was overwhelmed by an African American man about six feet tall and twenty to thirty years old. She was forced into the back seat of her car at knifepoint and raped. Following that, the assailant took off for the night.

According to Molly, she had completed her menses. She

would have to come back to get a pregnancy test. She didn't want her mother to be informed.

In the privacy of the surgical cubicle, I did a very gentle sexual exam, allowing her to guide our every step. Jean, Nuala, the head nurse, and an assistant were present. The head nurse wrote down my whispered findings: both labia were bruised and the introitus torn. Using an Ultraviolet Wood Lamp, I identified semen stains on her pubic hair and her undergarments. We took samples to test for various venereal infections, as well as the semen to document penetration and ejaculation. There was no evidence that there had been anal penetration, which Molly confirmed. When we finished, Molly started to cry once more because, as she said, "He violated me, and I could not defend myself. It all happened so fast after he surprised me, and he had a knife."

I suggested that the psychiatrist evaluate and treat her next. The head nurse went to get him.

Throughout my examination, I maintained my surgical composure. After finishing, I reached the men's room just in time to retch. I felt repulsed by the image of what poor Molly had endured. I called Victoria at the Children's Hospital to hear her voice and ensure she was safe. If she was off tonight, I asked her to have security escort her to her car.

A booth that operated 24/7 was located at the entrance to the parking lot.

PART II

1971-1972

Boston Children's Hospital, Harvard University

Junior Surgical Resident
PG-3

We are made to persist.
That's how we find out who we are.
—Tobias Wolff

30

AN AWESOME HOSPITAL

You are much stronger than your scars.
—*Anonymous*

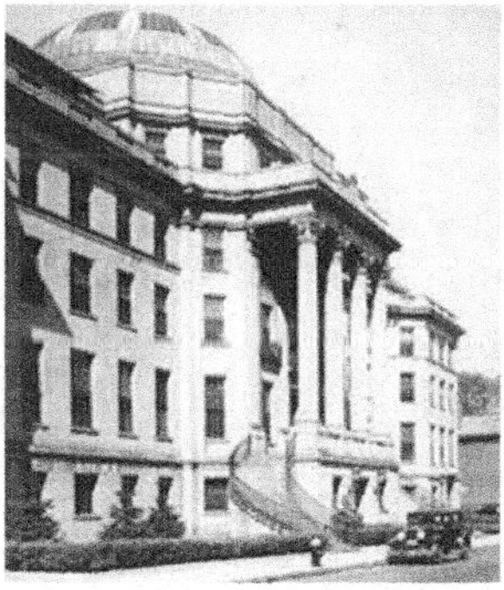

Boston Children's Hospital circa 1940

Until Every child is well.
~Boston Children's Hospital's tagline

Unlike the imposing façade of the Brigham, I saw no comparable view of the magnificent Children's Hospital's entrance, with its four Corinthian-style columns and sweeping staircase, as I typically entered the hospital through the conveniently located Emergency Room entrance on Longwood Avenue. It stood among residential and commercial buildings, including the Vanderbilt Hall of Residents across the street, where I had stayed about three years earlier while completing my surgical elective at Mass General. The original hospital was founded in 1869 in the South End of Boston, well before the Brigham was built, to serve the needs of poor children of Irish immigrants suffering from infectious diseases such as tuberculosis or traumatic injuries. Dr. Francis Brown, a Civil War surgeon and Harvard Medical School graduate, organized a group of fellow physicians and prominent civic leaders to establish one of the nation's earliest children's hospitals, a five-story brick townhouse. The small hospital's impact was felt almost immediately, and within a year, it was relocated to a new 60-bed facility on Huntington Avenue.

The Ladies' Aid Association provided essential supplies through community support, including food, clothing, linens, books, and toys. Adeline Blanchard Tyler, deaconess in the Episcopalian Church, was recruited to oversee daily operations. Sister Theresa and the Anglican Order of the Sisters of Saint Margaret succeeded her, managing nursing care until 1917, when they founded the Children's School of Nursing to ensure a steady supply of trained nurses familiar with pediatric issues. The hospital initiated a practical education program for medical students, many of whom attended Harvard Medical School. House officers were designated as "interns" to assist the surgical and medical staff.

Thirty years later, an even more significant and updated facility was needed to meet the demands of Boston's growing population. Hospital leadership recognized that a close partnership with Harvard Medical School would encourage discovery and drive major scientific advances.

By 1914, shortly after Harvard Medical School relocated to its current site on Longwood Avenue, Boston Children's Hospital moved next door. The partnership with Harvard and the establishment of a new nursing school helped the Children's Hospital emerge as a leader in exceptional research, medical education, and pediatric care and treatment.

And now, starting at the end of November, I will join my beloved Victoria at the Children's Hospital and spend 12 months operating on and caring for toddlers and infants. What a joy!

It would fulfill my earlier dream of working with children alongside Mr. Wilcox at Great Orman Street Children's Hospital in London.

The Children's Surgical Faculty in 1971

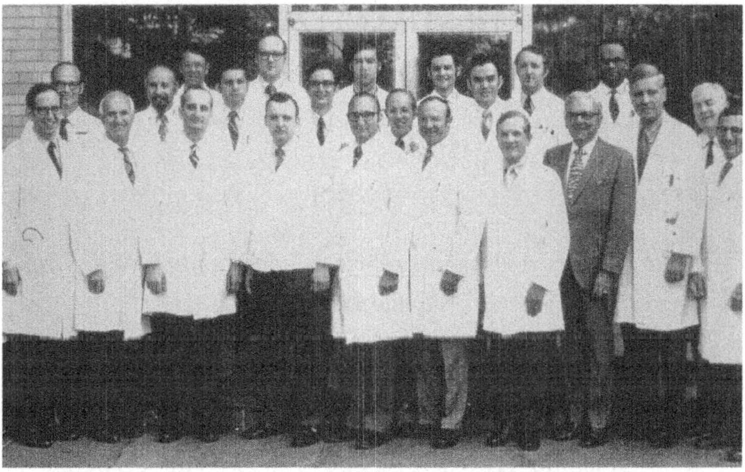

Left to Right

First Row: Ray Levy, Joseph Murray (Nobel Laureate), Judah Folkman (research chief), Willis Williams, Robert Filler (clinical chief), Kenneth Welch, Sam Schuster, Donald McCullum, John Gifford, Angelo Eraklis.

Second Row: Arvin Phillipart, Alan Perlmutter, resident, Mutaz Habal, Michael Mitchell, Michael Meguid, Garry Schwartz, Hillel Laks, Alberto Pena, Bill Crombie, John Daz, John Chamberlain.

31

THE MAGICIANS & THE TRAUMATIZED

A doctor is a person who gives people an opportunity for a healthy tomorrow.

—Anonymous

The surgeons who made up the faculty of Children's Hospital represented the Who's Who of pediatric surgery in Northeast America. They were clinicians with lifelong experience in operating on and caring for infants and children. Kenneth J. Welch edited the two-volume surgical textbook "Pediatric Surgery"; he was at the forefront of pediatric surgeons in the U.S., while his many associate editors were prominent surgeons and influential figures. His experienced colleagues at Children's Hospital contributed chapters in their areas of expertise, which is a hallmark of the American psyche, intensified by a surgeon's personality as a loner or someone who valued uniqueness. Occasionally, some came across as haughty.

To my surprise, not all senior faculty members were professors at Harvard Medical School, reflecting the old metaphor between "town and gown." The term originated in the Middle Ages when universities were cloistered, and students wore open-fronted black gowns to distinguish themselves from the town. It now describes the relationship between the non-academic physician population of a university town and its academic community.

At the Children's, we received a welcome overview upon arrival for our one-year rotation from Brigham and other Harvard programs, including Beth Israel Hospital and Deaconess. Drs. John Chamberlain and Angelo Eraklis headed the Emergency Ward, Outpatient Department, and Ambulatory Surgery. I would begin my rotation with my friends Mort Kahan, Howie Snyder, Hillel Laks, and a group of interns, including Dr. Richard Lynn.

There were two in-house general surgery services: the Gold team, headed by Kenneth J. Walsh, and the Blue team, led by Samuel Schuster. Additionally, the Urology Service was directed by the doyen of pediatric urology, Dr. Arnold Colodny, and supported by a younger colleague, Dr. Perlmutter. The Thoracic and Cardiac Services were connected through their combined chief, the legendary Dr. Robert Gross, the William E. Ladd Professor of Child Surgery at Harvard Medical School, Children's Hospital, and Peter Bent Brigham Hospital; a founder of both the American Board of Surgery and the American Board of Thoracic Surgery; and most enviably, a member of the prestigious National Academy of Sciences.

The Plastic and Reconstructive Service was led by Nobel Laureate Dr. John Murray, Dr. Donald McCallum, and Dr. John Gifford, who is the son-in-law of Dr. Moore.

Unique to the Children's Hospital, there were two chiefs of staff. Dr. Robert Filler served as the Clinical Chief of Staff for the training program. The Research Chief of Staff, Dr. Judah M. Folkman, Professor of Pediatric Surgery at Harvard Medical

School, emphasized the importance of academia, research, and development. Representing the audacity of innovation and daring, he suggested the courage to be curious and the necessity to think outside the box. This is where I first recognized that there are two tracks in professional surgery: clinical and research. I possess a strong appetite for curiosity. If I enter Dr. Moore's lab and eventually integrate research activities into my clinical surgical world, I will become a professor in time.

Dr. Folkman introduced himself to the assembled group at 8 a.m. on our first day following orientation. He quizzed the newly arrived residents from Brigham and the interns from the five Harvard hospitals. Besides our names, he wanted to know about our medical and surgical backgrounds, as well as our goals, interests, and hobbies. His curiosity about each of us was boundless. Among the group in the room, I was the only one who had included research in my career plans, which greatly intrigued him. He spoke generally about the philosophy of surgery, noted that at the Children's there wasn't a formal M&M session, and said he was available to meet with us if we had concerns beyond administrative issues.

He was far from the macho surgeon eager to cut. Rather, he was inquisitive and hesitant about providing definitive answers. He displayed hallmarks I later recognized as qualities of the surgeon-scientist type of thinker, focused on solving intriguing human problems instead of merely excising tissues—similar to Professor Carl Walter, with whom I performed a simple mastectomy while on the Ward Service at the Brigham. I appreciate this soft-spoken, unassuming surgeon who showed genuine interest in each of us. His reputation as a researcher and a gifted bedside teacher attracted students because he blended biology with clinical practice. I felt comfortable in the warm and inviting atmosphere he created.

He proceeded to orient us further.

We spent time on each of the two general surgical services

operating on patients with common, or what he referred to as, routine and recurring "bread and butter" cases. These cases encompassed a range of surgical illnesses, from hereditary diseases in newborns to a spectrum of congenital and acquired surgical conditions, as well as various types of trauma in children up to fourteen years of age. Each service had a senior and two junior residents who traditionally rotated through Brigham's training program. I continued working with Mort Kahan and Howard Snyder III as a second and third-year resident. Hillel Lacks and David Oates were our fourth-year residents, while Dr. Arvin Phillipart and another resident served as our seniors. Dr. Alden Harken was the chief resident of the Cardio-Thoracic Service. The schedule indicated that I was to start in the Emergency Room with Mort, Howie, and Hillel.

I subconsciously needed to care for the young, the neglected, and the vulnerable to soothe their pains and heal their wounds. I felt I hadn't received such love and nurturing from our mother for five years. Gulnar and I had been transported by our parents from our emotionally nurturing Egyptian grandparents and resource-rich surroundings in Cairo to our aging, war-weary maternal grandparents in ravaged Germany—grandparents who had lived through WWI, the Wall Street crash, with its inflation, the depression, and WWII.

My father went to England, which I accepted intellectually because, as a child, my sister and I would often play house in our condominium in Cairo. In our play, she was the stay-at-home mother who cared for her doll and my teddy bear, while I played the working father who left home, riding my scooter around our flat and returning to our make-believe house with imaginary food and money for the mother. This repeated role play subconsciously established in my mind the gender-defined positions in life. Translated: Fathers worked away from home, while mothers stayed home and cared for the children.

But my mother stayed with us for only a few weeks to help us "settle in" with our German grandparents, as we spoke no German. It mystified me why we were with them and had a new set of grandparents. Unlike my loving Egyptian grandparents, who hugged, kissed, and doted on me, these were cold, distant, and disciplinarian, unable to attend to our emotional needs. There was no explanation, limited amounts of bland food, no books, no toys, and no cousins to play with. It was an unpleasant, unending nightmare that I wished would soon end so we could join our Daddy in England. The weeks stretched into long, painful, and endless years.

Mother was a devotee of Johanna Haarer's child-rearing book *The German Mother and Her Child.* Haarer was the voice and influencer of the National Socialist German Workers' Party's philosophy in the early 1930s when my mother was an easily impressed teenager living in Hamburg. Haarer urged German mothers to ignore their toddlers' emotional needs, avoid expressing maternal love, and refrain from investing affection in their children to raise more hardened soldiers effectively. As a Nazi-promoting pulmonologist lacking any pediatric training, Haarer's widely circulated book recommended raising children with minimal contact and as few attachments as possible.

One night, my mother disappeared without saying goodbye, giving a kiss, or hugging me. She suddenly vanished from my life, leaving my sister and me in an emotional desert, as neither of my German grandparents, Oma nor Opa, were expressive or affectionate. Unable to understand or accept my mother's actions, her sudden departure created a deep rift between us with lifelong consequences. I became an angry, anxious, and confused person, desperately homesick. My sister grew distant from both of us, as she had been alienated. When my mother, in her eighties, sustained a stroke while visiting her daughter, instead of rehabilitation, Gulnar, struck by a vengeful mood, disposed of her via a sedation medication overdose. The ultimate payback. But was it the perfect undetectable murder?

Although I knew intellectually that I had a birth mother elsewhere to meet my emotional needs, Oma became my mother. It was Oma who sewed on my missing buttons, darned my socks, and loved me quietly, in the stillness infused with her daily involvement in my care, from making sure I did my homework and baking cakes and cookies for me, to the subtle vibes she transmitted that told me she loved me. I was raised seeking and receiving her love, approval, and acceptance, while the mother who walked away from me became a stranger I found difficult to accept.

I wasn't alone. Gulnar also missed our mother's maternal love—the nurturing and care we longed for during the critical stages of our infancy and childhood. The lack of that care contributed to significant adult personality disorders.

Many of the neonates, toddlers, and infants I encountered and treated during my time as a resident in the Gold and Blue Services had also been abandoned. Some had suffered domestic trauma and had consequently been taken away from their families, parents, or guardians. The Child Protection Program (CPP) at Boston Children's Hospital, established in 1970, addresses the issues of family violence and child maltreatment in conjunction with the Massachusetts Department of Children and Families (DCF). It was referred to as Children's Social Services.

As a result, the children were left alone in the Children's Hospital Blue and Gold wards. They didn't have visitors and lacked maternal love, nurturing, and care, which often brought tears to my eyes when I got home. I operated on these tiny human beings while my heart ached for them.

I loved being a children's doctor. The kids were frightened, anxious, and in pain when they came to the E.R. Despite this, I noticed that they remained curious about their surroundings. It brought back both fearful and joyful memories. I was scared when I was eleven and had my appendix taken out. I felt ebullient when I read a letter from my Mother to her parents describing my inquisitiveness: ". . . he sees everything, he hears everything, he smells everything; loves every animal . . . in short, he loves life and the world."

32

ONE E.R. & TWO MEGUIDS

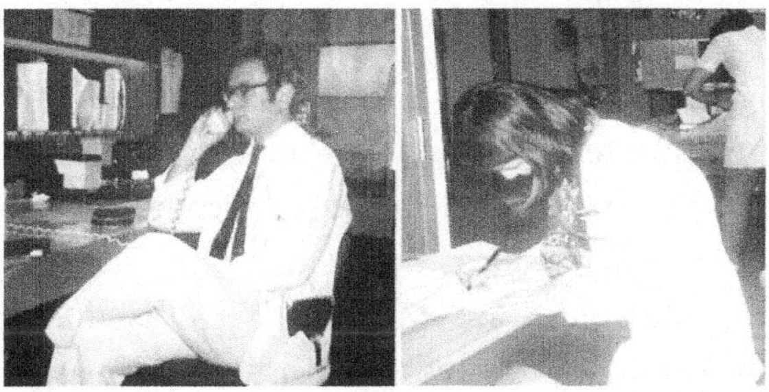

When my fingers can stroke at their leisure
Your head and your elastic
Back, and my hand gets drunk on the pleasure.
Of your body elastic.
—Charles Baudelaire

The first time Victoria floated into my view as an enchanting nineteen-year-old first-year medical student, she triggered explosions of passion reminiscent of Ode to Joy in my brain. I was mesmerized by her delicate porcelain English complexion, stunning figure, and understated joie de vivre. In that moment, I knew with crystalline clarity that this beauty would one day be my wife. After seven years of devoted engagement, during which we attended medical school, got married, honeymooned in Antigua, and became licensed physicians in England, we had now settled in Boston.

Finally, at Children's, we collaborated effectively. She managed the medical emergency services at one end of the E.R., while I handled the surgical ones at the other. We were a husband-and-wife team—the doctors Meguid, who operated the combined medical/surgical Emergency Room of the Children's Hospital Medical Center, one of Boston's most prestigious hospitals. Our move to America appeared to have been the right choice. What an extraordinary accomplishment. I no longer wished to quit or fantasized about returning to professional England.

Seeing my wife in the E.R. attending to sick children, directing nurses, teaching junior residents, and receiving the attention of her male attending evoked a complex mix of jealousy and eroticism within me. This scene filled me with immense pride and was incredibly sexy. While the staff viewed her through professional eyes, I saw her as my Botticelli's nude Venus, my Goya's Maja Desnuda, and my admirable partner and wife—the woman who wanted my babies!

I'd wake up a few minutes before our alarm went off just before 7 a.m. Victoria rose first as I stirred, anxiously hanging onto the fading winks of sleep, my body aching, reluctant to rise. Glancing through half-closed eyes, I observed her return to our bedroom after her bath as the dawn's delicate light crept through the window. Peeking at her through my eyelash curtain, I watched her wrap-around towel drop to her feet, exposing a lithe, fresh-smelling body. Her breasts trembled as she toweled her hair, the supple of her curved back and belly evoking fresh memories of her skin's taste, the feel of my touch and stroke, and the marble thighs that had encircled me the night before.

"Darling, the alarm has gone off. You'd better get going, or we'll be late." She said this to gently rouse me to action. I stirred as she put on her panties and sat next to me on the bed to put on her bra and pantyhose. I kissed her neck and inhaled the fragrance of her body as she slid the stocking onto each leg. "Do you know I love you dearly?"

She turned around and kissed me, replying softly, "I love you."

"How about a quickie," I whispered, "to start the day floating on air?"

"A quickie now? We'd be late, and anyway, I've had a bath and done my hair."

"A quickie or a passionate love for 20 minutes will do us good. But I'll settle for a quickie. That takes only three minutes . . . just the three most memorable minutes of our day, sweetheart, to reach a state of perfect happiness. You know I want you now," I pleaded, "to start the day in the best frame of mind," as I tugged at her clothes. "Three minutes? Or 20. Which?"

She looked at me questioningly. "Both. But I'm already dressed. Next time."

Ah. The proverbial next time. So pregnant with hope, promise, and lust. Better than the killer phrase "I've got a headache,' Goethe understood, "Only he who knows what longing is knows what I suffer."

I showered, shaved, and dressed. Victoria had prepared our breakfast in our kitchenette.

"You look so delicious, my darling. How did you sleep?" I asked.

Before I could answer or hug her, she asked, "Do I look all right?"

"Sexily stunning."

While I ate my scrambled eggs with toast, tea, and a second piece of toast with marmalade, knowing I wouldn't be having lunch, she finished her breakfast and got up. Through the bedroom door, I watched her routine of massaging her face, neck, and arms with cream and applying lipstick. She never wore perfume on a workday—a scent that evokes my ardor.

"Ready!"

We stepped into the crisp morning, inhaled the cool, fresh air, and listened to the uplifting dawn chorus, knowing we would be indoors for 36 hours. We drove to the hospital together, the rising sun reflecting in my rearview mirror, each of us lost in thoughts of our anticipated duties.

Having just completed my last rotation in Brigham's E.R., I was surprised to begin my next 12 months at Children's in the surgical E.R. But how better to assess a new resident's performance than by placing them in an urgent setting and observing how they function when facing unknown emergencies of varying magnitudes?

The rotation lasted 12 hours, starting at 8 a.m., while Howie covered the following 12 hours in the ER. Our third-year senior resident was Hillel Laks, with whom I had worked on Burley's Ward Service. He also covered the ER and was frequently my other 12-hour partner. I admired him immensely because he was a quiet worker, balancing Howie's friendly bellicosity while effectively getting his work done with a good measure of common sense. Born in South Africa, he emigrated to America via Israel. Was his status in the residency also that of a provisional resident like mine? The surgical interns were from Deaconess Hospital, the third of the Harvard teaching hospitals.

During the day, we covered the walk-in, non-urgent surgical clinic and Ambulatory Surgery cases. Once we gathered, Dr. John Chamberlain introduced himself. In his soft-spoken voice, he welcomed us, adding, "If you boys have any questions, my office is just around that corner," pointing some distance to his right. I estimated he was nearing traditional retirement age, as he looked frail despite his friendly demeanor.

As a house officer, I appreciated the surgical E.R. due to the diagnostic and therapeutic challenges presented by the patients, which tested my prioritization and organizational skills. Most of the time, I had to gather a history of their complaint, illness, or trauma from their parent or guardian to piece it together. This called upon everything I had learned surgically to help make a diagnosis and treat the child in the E.R., unless they needed to be admitted for surgery. Once more, the experience I gained when, as a medical student, I spent my free evenings examining patients in the University College Hospital Casualty Department instead of watching TV provided me with additional confidence.

As their "fireman," I tackled one crisis after another, addressing both physical and social issues. However, like all E.R.s, there were also mundane moments of quiet and boredom, as well as times of harrowing emergencies.

One day, a dreadful event occurred. Two sisters, ages four and five, were brought in, screaming and howling in pain, tears streaming down their angelic faces. Their grandmother had given them crayons to draw on paper, keeping them occupied. She had found them doodling in her precious Bible. As punishment for desecrating the Holy Book, she lifted them to the stove, and while they struggled and cried, she held their hands over a gas flame.

We treated their severe burns by lathering their fingers with ointment and applying light dressings, then admitted the still distraught and howling children to the Plastic and Reconstructive Service. It was a relief when the intramuscular pain medication began to take effect, causing the girls' sobbing to subside. The poor children were confused about being punished; such events were beyond their comprehension. Social services were called to assess the home environment. Deemed grossly neglectful, the children were removed from their families and consequently did not have parental visitors.

The surgical E.R. service was one of those rotations that fell into amorphous group activities, where I provided a service and was always busy, constantly giving of myself to others. This alone weighed heavily on my soul. I'd buy music records from the co-op to cheer myself up and give me something else to think about.

My musical repertoire extended from popular pop, country, and ballad singers of the time—the more romantic, the better—to the classics, ranging from piano and violin concertos to full-blown symphonic and choral pieces, including the latest songs from Andrew Lloyd Webber. I'd play these at home on my Fisher turntable while I relaxed and chilled out. Instead of meditation, which I had not yet discovered, I rejuvenated my spirits with music or poetry. In high school, while studying STEM classes, none of the boys in our macho clique would have admitted to liking poetry for fear of being labeled effeminate or a sissy, unaware that the poetry taught each Thursday by Miss Freemantle was like cosmic radiation, influencing us in ways we couldn't discern. At the time, poetry stemmed from our raging hormones and impulsive hurdles into adulthood. We didn't realize that poetry alleviated our fears, sadness, and worries while boosting our mood during stress, fatigue, and grief.

My day involved examining children, typically from the Roxbury African American community, with a presumptive diagnosis of "head injury." They were generally between three and six years old. The history was consistent: a bored child would jump up and down on the bed despite the supervising adult telling them to stop bouncing. Enjoyment drove them to continue, and they only stopped when they fell off the bed and bumped their head on the floor or a nearby dresser. The height of the fall was usually three to six feet.

Inevitably, the howling child, having been hit on the head for their disobedient behavior, was brought into the E.R. with a swollen scalp or a bleeding cut. In this working community, the supervising adult was not always the mother, making an E.R. visit even more crucial for the child's caregiver. A physical examination of the head, neck, and eyes was generally unremarkable. A child with a scalp cut would require stitching under local anesthesia.

I would talk to the frightened child just as Oma had spoken to and reassured me when I had a green stick fracture in my right forearm. I would explain everything I planned to do and what they could expect, even if an adult was with us. I would tell them that I understood why they were in pain, adjusting my language to suit their age and providing reasons for my intended actions to help them feel better. If it involved a surgical instrument, I would show it to them and explain how it worked and how I would use it carefully. Their curiosity outweighed their anxiety and fear, and their wide gaze indicated their engagement. Yet when I approached them or when the nurse held them, their curiosity was overshadowed by their fear and reluctance to undergo what I had explained.

The traumatic moment for the child always came when a needle had to be used to inject local anesthesia around a cut or when blood needed to be drawn. I vividly recall my terror, cries, and tears in grade school in Manchester at the sight of the small needle used for a polio vaccination. My fear exceeded the actual discomfort of a needle stick, and afterward, I felt embarrassed about all the fuss I had made. With this in mind, I continued talking to the children while using the smallest and thinnest needles to complete the task.

The head injury protocol involved a series of skull X-rays and measurements of the white blood cell count (WBC).

Imaging of the skull and brain was typically unremarkable, and the WBC functioned as a useful diagnostic indicator of trauma. Children with severe head injuries had a WBC that exceeded 10,500, significantly higher than that of those with minor injuries. The children were often discharged with a follow-up appointment, which was seldom kept.

Occasionally, a mother would bring back her child a couple of weeks later, wanting us to remove the sutures. "You said the stitches would dissolve."

I would remove them, thinking that the manufacturer deceptively marketed them as such because, frankly, they didn't dissolve. I had doubts when I placed them because they were made of a blue monofilament synthetic material that, to me, felt like nylon and reminded me of the drip-dry nylon shirts I wore as a medical student. Since time immemorial, sutures have consisted of plant fibers, horsehair, animal tendons, wool, silk, or catgut made from twisted sheep intestines. Catgut was found in Ancient Egyptian mummies and was still used during America's Civil War. However, this was America, and I was assured that this new material was superior to all previous suture materials, even the black silk that we traditionally used in London to close scalp or skin cuts—but which would have been exceedingly difficult to see in the kid's natural afro-textured hair.

We shared Victoria's assigned medical on-call room on the nights when we were on call together. I slept on the right side of the bed next to the phone, while she slept on the left. Exhausted, we fell asleep.

During the night, the phone rang.

"Hello..."

There was a gasp... Then the line went dead.

Nudging Victoria, I'd say, "I think it was for you."

It rang again. She leaned over to answer it. At Children's Hospital, we worked together as a professional team. She managed the medical emergency services at one end of the emergency room, while I handled the surgical emergencies at the other. We were a husband-and-wife duo—the doctors Meguid—operating the combined medical and surgical emergency room at Children's Hospital Medical Center, one of Boston's most prestigious hospitals affiliated with Harvard. Our decision to move to America seemed to be the right one. It was an extraordinary achievement, and I no longer wanted to quit or fantasize about returning to England.

The rumor circulated that she slept with a man in her room because the medical E.R. nurses were unaware of my surgical E.R. existence. On another occasion, the phone rang at 5:45 a.m. I answered it. A loud voice came over the receiver. "Dr. Meguid. Len Jones is scheduled for a hernia repair at eight. You wrote for Benadryl as part of his preoperative sedation but didn't write the dose. How much should we give?"

I was in a heavy phase of sleep psychosis, having fallen asleep after taking a call about another surgical patient barely 90 minutes before. It was almost like being in that awful jet lag I had experienced on my first night at the Brigham. I couldn't think clearly in my deep fog.

"What? Repeat the question," I muttered.

She did, rather loudly.

I still couldn't understand what the voice was asking. She repeated, "Dr. Meguid, what dose do you want to give?"

Victoria leaned over and said, "It's 1 mg per kilogram of the kid's body weight as a one-time dose."

"OK," came the reply as I fell back into the delectable depths of sleep, cruising until the harsh trill of my alarm. Once again, rumors suggested that I was having an affair with one of the pharmacists. But who? Most of them were men, and only a couple were women.

Whatever the rumors, waking up in the dreary on-call room and seeing Victoria first thing in the morning, before our day swung into action, was a moment of precious delight. We were alive, in good health, young, and had each other. What more could I wish for?

One day, to quell the rumors, I strolled over to the medical emergency room and introduced myself to the nurses and the secretary. They appeared pleasantly surprised to discover another Dr. Meguid—a surgeon.

Children from birth to six years old account for half of all trauma deaths, while this rate declines for those aged seven to seventeen. The leading cause of death in infants is asphyxia, while in toddlers, it is drowning and falls from heights, closely followed by blunt trauma. As children grow older, deaths are often caused by motor vehicle accidents.

I learned these statistics because one day, a five-year-old girl was tragically crushed to death when her mother backed up the car in the driveway, running over her daughter. Even on the operating room table, she appeared to be a beautiful child. Although I assisted in rushing her to the O.R. and the surgical team desperately tried to save her life, there was nothing my chief resident and the attending surgeon could do. I still see the tire marks across her back. As I returned to the E.R. in deep sorrow, I could not fathom the distress and pain of her parents.

This tragic accident brought me once again to my private cemetery. I built a chapel, which I entered to mourn, having witnessed the impact of childhood trauma that left a profound psychological scar. I prayed that the Almighty would grant special grace to these victims and forgiveness for the parents, and indeed the entire family, for the suffering they were enduring and would endure for the rest of their lives.

33

LONG SCARF SYNDROME

I am interested in finding and expressing a new form of life.
—Isadora Duncan

We were in the depths of winter, with enough snow on the hills around Boston to allow for skiing. Unlike the E.R. at the Brigham, where we saw a fair number of winter-related traumas, such as femoral fractures in older women with low bone densities, at Children's, this type of trauma wasn't frequently observed. Children tended to bounce off the icy sidewalks.

People bundled up and often wrapped scarves around their necks, not realizing that the loose end of a long-flowing scarf posed a well-known hazard. A twelve-year-old child was out sledding, and when she rode a ski tow to the top of the mountain, its winch caught the free end of her long scarf and dragged her into the machinery, smashing her face. Upon examination in the E.R., I found swelling and bruising of the tissue around her eye and eyelid, along with multiple lacerations on the right side of her face. The right side of the temporal arch was caved in, which gives the face its curvature between the eye and cheek.

X-ray examination revealed an open fragmentation of the right zygomatic arch. Several large muscles attach to it, allowing for efficient chewing. The zygomatic arch protects the right eye and forms a significant part of the facial contour, alongside other bones that make up the face. These bones were displaced and fractured into several pieces (a comminuted fracture), resulting in a skin breach and an open or compound fracture. Although she didn't lose consciousness, she complained of double vision, right facial pain, and numbness with loss of sensation in her teeth.

I alerted Dr. Habal, a skilled plastic and reconstructive fellow, because this young woman required an emergency operation to reconstruct her face. He and Dr. Murray, the Nobel Laureate and chief of that service, took her directly to the O.R. Once she was anesthetized and asleep, the surgeons irrigated the wound with poise, skill, and focus. They carefully explored the injuries and assessed the extent of the damage.

The floor of the right eyeball socket was fragmented. To keep the right eyeball in alignment and to prevent her from seeing double, the floor of the bony eye socket was reinforced with a silastic sheet. The fractures of the bones on the right side of her face that had fractured and sunken were realigned and wired together to reconstruct the shape of her face.

We wrote a brief account of this event, the ensuing injury, and, along with Drs. I co-authored Habal and Murray's manuscript titled "The Long Scarf Syndrome." Isadora Duncan, the renowned dancer, died by strangulation in 1927 when her enormous silk scarf got entangled in the rear wheel of an open sports car. The letter was published in the *New England Journal of Medicine*—my first publication in America. We posed the question of whether other physicians had seen similar injuries.

Brief Reports

The Long Scarf Syndrome—a Potentially Fatal and Preventable Hazard

Report of 11 Cases

Mutaz B. Habal, MD; Michael M. Meguid, MD; and Joseph E. Murray, MD

The long scarf syndrome refers to the entanglement of the scarf's free floating end into moving machinery. The death rate in 11 cases was an astonishingly high 45%. Prevention is simple and consists merely of removing or covering the scarf when worn near moving machinery.

THE long scarf syndrome was described in a letter[1] after we had cared for our first patient with this injury.[2] Since then, we have collected reports of 11 cases that meet our criteria, ie, the wearing of a long scarf, entanglement of its free end into moving machinery, and a resulting injury ranging from minor to fatal.

Clinical Material.—Of the 11 patients presented in the Table, nine were females between the ages of 10 and 30. As expected, all accidents occurred in the winter.

Four cases are reviewed in detail to demonstrate various mechanisms of injury.

Report of Cases

CASE 1.—An 15-year-old boy from Lexington, Mass, suffered total airway obstruction and respiratory arrest after his scarf became entangled in the engine of his snowmobile. The scarf was loosened and his mother revived him by mouth-to-mouth resuscitation. The boy recovered and was seen by his ophthalmologist for retrobulbar hemorrhages with retinal damage. Spontaneous recovery without visual damage occurred.

CASE 2.—A young mother in her early 20s from Rochester, Minn, was hauled out of her seat while riding a ski lift when her scarf became wrapped around an oncoming chair. She died of strangulation as she was carried down the chair lift, suspended by the scarf.

CASE 3.—A teenager in San Diego, Calif, sustained severe facial lacerations and bruises when her scarf became entangled in the rotating wheel of her boyfriend's stationary motorcycle as she leaned over to inspect the running machinery. Fortunately there was no airway obstruction, but treatment for facial injuries was required.

CASE 4.—A 16-year-old girl from Fort Wainwright, Alaska, was knocked to the ground and dragged under a safety gate that failed to operate when her scarf became entangled in the rope tow at a ski slope. She passed through the gate and was dragged by her scarf into the moving machinery. She suffered only facial lacerations and bruises requiring surgical treatment.

Advertisement for a new life insurance company as it appeared in the October 1971 issue of Esquire.

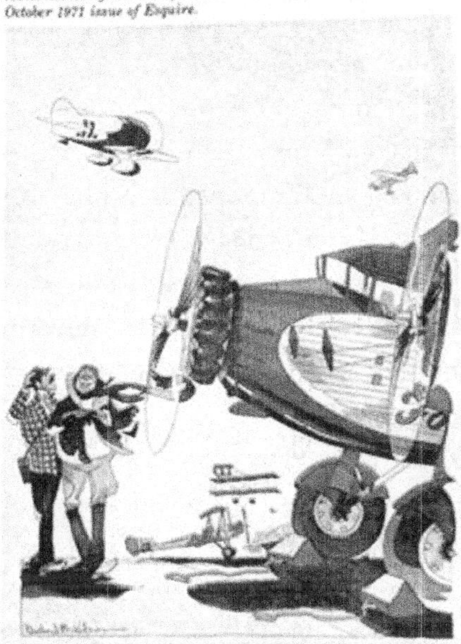

"My insurance company? New England Life, of course. Why?"

From the Department of Surgery, Peter Bent Brigham Hospital, Children's Hospital Medical Center, and Harvard Medical School, Boston.
Reprint requests to 721 Huntington Ave, Boston, Mass 02115 (Dr. Habal).

JAMA, Sept 11, 1972 • Vol 221, No 11

The Long Scarf Syndrome—Habal et al 126

His creativity, energy, and positive attitude drew me to Mutaz Habal as a successful mentor, surgeon, scientist, and friend, particularly as he embraced the academic surgeons' saying, "publish or perish." In response to our letter, we received over twenty case reports of similar injuries in children and young adults. We examined each case and identified eleven instances where a long scarf had pulled the wearer into machinery, causing facial injuries, and in five patients, leading to suffocation. We authored another brief report published in the widely read JAMA—the Journal of the American Medical Association. It was also noted as a cautionary tale in "Reader's Digest." This case paved the way for Dr. Habal, who went on to become the Director of the Tampa Bay Craniofacial Center, Research Professor at the University of Florida, and Editor-in-Chief of the prestigious Journal of Craniofacial Surgery. After retiring, Mutaz and I remained colleagues, friends, and even geographic neighbors.

Dr. Moore's entreaties and expectations of his residents were that each should publish two papers per year. Mutaz encouraged and demonstrated how to pursue this goal despite my busy surgical learning and skill application. In both published reports, our co-author was Dr. Joseph E. Murray, Nobel Laureate, who in 1952 performed the first successful kidney transplant at Brigham, opening the new field of transplant surgery.

I wasn't sure Dr. Moore was aware of my publications. To keep him informed, I sent a reprint of each of the published papers. I was delighted to learn I was still a contender for a senior residency spot in the Brigham training program. This news encouraged me to continue working hard. This interaction taught me that providing juniors with positive feedback was a strong motivational force to keep them engaged and happy. Strangely enough, he didn't reference the paper or my co-authors.

Dr. Moore had worked closely with Dr. Murray, having his laboratory perform all the immunological work that contributed to Dr. Murray's fame, leading to his first kidney transplant. The Nobel committee didn't extend the fame to Dr. Moore. When Mutaz and I chatted and the information came out that they had worked closely on the immunological problems, I wondered if the Chief of Chiefs felt left out and hurt by the injustice done by the Swedes? After Dr. Murray had a heart attack, he retrained as a plastic surgeon. Thereafter, Dr. Murray informed me that he played tennis every morning to stay fit.

HARVARD MEDICAL SCHOOL
DEPARTMENT OF SURGERY

FRANCIS D. MOORE, M.D.
Moseley Professor of Surgery

Peter Bent Brigham Hospital
721 Huntington Avenue
Boston, Massachusetts 02115
Telephone 617 - 566-6226

September 20, 1971

Dr. Michael Meguid
The Children's Hospital Medical Center
300 Longwood Avenue
Boston, Massachusetts 02115

Dear Mike:

Thank you very much for your letter and for the article about the long flowing scarfs.

That certainly is a hazard and I can remember when our children were small, taking special precautions to avoid such things.

As to your senior residency. Your work has been excellent and we regard you as highly desirable for that position.

We are making our planning sessions now and will be in touch with you soon.

I will ask Dr. Vineyard to bear in mind your desire for more urologic training as part of your rotational scheme.

All best wishes.

Very truly yours,

Francis D. Moore, M.D.

FDM:imh

34

QWERTY DISASTER

The quick brown fox jumps over the lazy dog.
—The Boston Journal

"I can't type these manuscripts for you," Victoria declared. After all, she was still a resident at the same hospital, just like I was, and she came home just as tired as I did. I understood her position well.

"But I found a three-week typing course at the local high school starting next week. I've signed you up for it," she said triumphantly, adding, "You'll learn to type, which will stand you in good stead for the rest of your life."

"You're kidding! I'll be a surgeon and have a secretary to do all my manuscripts," was my reply.

"That's a few years away, so you might as well learn it now."

The following Thursday, I excused myself from evening rounds and drove our VW to the high school. I didn't know what to expect. As soon as I walked into the classroom, I was overwhelmed. On every desk was a typewriter—some sixty desks and sixty typewriters. Awesome. I'd never seen such affluence before, certainly not at our high school in Cairo or

England. I realized that most American youngsters were allowed to learn to type while in high school. This was totally out of this world!

When we lived in Egypt, Mother had her own "sewing room." It was better suited for a typing salon. I grew up familiar with my mother's portable Olivetti. After breakfast, she'd retreat to her salon with a steaming cup of Nescafé and close the door. The door to her salon had a large, frosted glass pane. Gulnar and I could see her shadowy figure sitting by the machine, typing away, as we played in the nearby living room under the casual watch of the servant. We could hear the clicking sound as she typed, one letter after another in German—some three hundred and fifty of them over time—to her parents in Wedel near Hamburg, complaining about the isolation of her life in Egypt. She described how she was "holding herself apart from the primitive life in Egypt," as her letters referred to it, while in her mind, she was dwelling in the 1930s world of her remembered Germany.

She was isolated because she refused to learn Arabic, describing the Arabic language in one of her numerous letters to Oma, her mother, as "an ancient language invented by some donkey," conveniently forgetting that her Egyptian husband—my father—was a professor of Arabic and Pedagogy at Cairo University, a wordsmith who dedicated his academic life to reading and writing children's textbooks in Arabic and propagating the use of Modern Standard Arabic.

Unwilling to learn the language, she couldn't converse with my Egyptian family members—led by my grandfather, Sheikh Amin, my grandmother, Sit Nazifa, and Daddy's ten siblings. She also refused to learn about Muslim culture, the society in which she lived that defined daily life in Egypt. She looked down on the Egyptian family, whom I loved dearly. Every Friday, my Egyptian family—my grandparents, Daddy's siblings, and the partners of those who were married, including Afaf, an uncle's out-of-wedlock daughter who was accepted into the family—would gather for a communal lunch at Sheikh Amin's home in the Arabic quarter of Cairo. Mother consistently refused to join Baba, Gulnar, and me as we left our flat to be with them. She didn't like "the noisy family gathering, their heavy, greasy food, their stinking toilets, their gray towels, and their lack of English," as she described in her letters to her parents in Germany.

On the first day of my typing class, the high school classroom was crowded with people milling about. Since I arrived close to 5 p.m., I found an empty desk near the back of the room, surrounded by chatting young girls. The only other man in the room was the instructor, a balding man with a toothbrush mustache, standing about five feet one or two inches tall with a ramrod-straight back. He wore a black shirt and trousers tucked into shining knee-high leather boots. He slapped his boots with his ruler, creating a loud, clacking noise that silenced the room, and introduced himself in a rather strange accent—a mixture of Italian and Austrian German. He may have considered himself the high school typing coach, but I viewed him as an escaped SS Blackshirt, which captured the fear he effectively instilled in me, and probably in the other students as well.

He rambled on about our training manual, which lay beside the typewriters, the care of our typewriter, which already had a blank sheet, and on and on. I realized I wasn't following him because fatigue and hunger distracted me after working 36 hours. Not only was I starving, but I was also dehydrated and hadn't had enough sleep.

"Open your manuals and type the first sentence to familiarize yourselves with your machine," he said. It read, "The quick brown fox jumps over the lazy dog."

Amazing! This sentence contains all 26 letters of the

Modern English Alphabet. How ingenious! Who would have thought of it?

Since I didn't know the layout of the keys, it took me a while to finish the sentence. We spent nearly half an hour typing various phrases from the manual as my enthusiasm for this class waned. The teacher moved around the room among the young girls, who glanced over their shoulders at the unusual figure among them. Suddenly, he barked, "Now, we'll have a one-minute speed test. When I say go, copy the text on page twelve." I flipped to the necessary page in the manual.

"Go," came the command with gusto as he cracked his ruler against his boots. His zeal matched that of my former school track and field coach at the start of the 100-yard dash.

The clatter was deafening as 59 women sat upright, hands hovering over keyboards, and typed away. I diligently started to type. A loud crack marked the end of the minute as a hush settled in the room. "Now, take a word count."

The coach smartly walked among the desks, listening to the counts.

"OK." Another crack from his ruler as all eyes focused on him, "The average word count is 52."

Crack.

"We aim to increase that to one hundred words per minute in the next three weeks!"

I was shaken. I'd typed twelve words using two fingers in the allotted minute, and each one was misspelled. Apart from feeling inadequate, I knew I had been conned. This wasn't a beginner's course. Twelve words compared to fifty-two made me think this was an advanced course, not one for beginners. I felt out of place here.

As he instructed us about homework, I felt my fingers were meant for better purposes. I slipped out of the classroom, a humiliated, tired, and defeated man determined to keep begging and cajoling secretaries to type my medical papers.

35

TINY TOTS

You're in Great Hands
—Surgical Aphorism

On a late Friday afternoon, a two-year-old girl was brought in by her parents. Nancy appeared irritable, lethargic, and refused to eat. Upon examination, she had a high fever, an elevated white cell count, and a rapid pulse, likely due to a combination of dehydration and an inflammatory process in her abdomen. Her symptoms worsened throughout the day. She had a history of blood in her stool and episodic abdominal pain. Continuing my examination, I observed that her abdomen was distended and tender, consistent with an acute abdomen.

Using two fingers to examine her abdomen, I felt a mass on the right side, and a gentle rectal exam with my well-lubricated, gloved pinky revealed some blood. Despite my cautious exam, it must have induced some discomfort and pain, as she started crying again.

My diagnosis, based on her history of episodic abdominal pain with bloody stool and the presence of a right lower quadrant mass, was that intussusception most likely caused her acute abdomen. This condition involves the telescoping of the terminal ileum or small bowel into the large colon, obstructing the passage of fluids and food, and strangulating the blood vessels into which it has telescoped. Typically, the end of the small bowel, the lead point of telescoping into the colon, presents with enlarged lymph nodes resulting from a viral infection. However, her high temperature concerned me, so a perforated appendix causing an abscess was also part of my differential diagnosis.

My discovery of an acute abdomen automatically brought Dr. Judah Folkman, Chief of Surgical Research, to the emergency room. He lived in a high-rise next to the hospital and came faithfully whenever the nurses informed him that the emergency room resident had a child with a suspected acute abdomen.

Dr. Folkman listened to the summary of my findings and differential diagnosis before examining the toddler. Agreeing with my assessment, he began to chat, saying that I must have been trained in England because I had made a diagnosis first based on my physical exam instead of relying on an X-ray, adding, "There is no way to make a diagnosis of appendicitis except by physically examining a patient." Pausing and looking at me, he said, "Not many of our American-trained residents do as thorough, careful, and comprehensive a physical exam as you are trained to do. They often overlook diagnostic findings. I'm impressed."

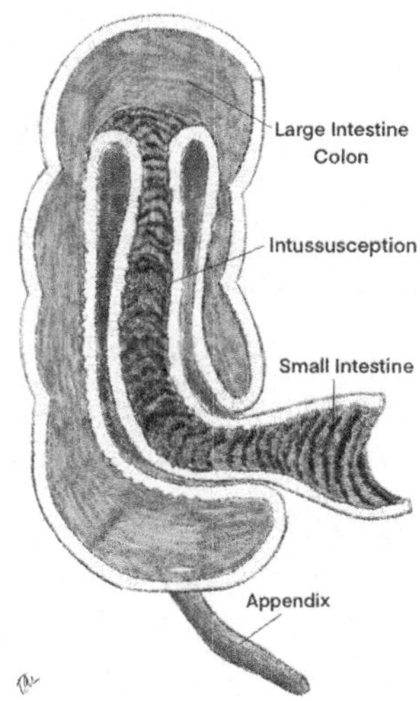

I reveled in the compliment. He couldn't have known the many hours of joy I experienced at University College Hospital E.R. in London, examining abdomens as a student. He discovered that I was interested in research and was a provisional resident in Dr. Moore's program. Perhaps I had found another mentor at the Children's who would support me for a senior residency.

To rule out an intussusception, we ordered an emergency X-ray of her abdomen was taken after securing an intravenous catheter, through which we began hydrating the patient and administering antibiotics. If the X-ray indicated an intussusception, the gentle pressure of a barium enema would gradually push back the telescoped small bowel, straightening the gut and correcting the condition. However, the X-ray of this very sick toddler didn't show any signs of intussusception. We agreed she probably had a perforated appendix with an abscess. I informed Tim Canty, the chief resident, and Dr. Robert Filler, the Chief of Clinical Surgery, who had just completed an operation and would be coming down shortly.

A past event triggered Dr. Folkman's quick arrival in the E.R. Some time ago, a little girl had been seen in the E.R. with abdominal pain, and the difficult clinical diagnosis of appendicitis wasn't made in that pre-CT scan era. In the absence of an appendicitis diagnosis, she was sent home. Her parents returned with their daughter when her condition worsened, and she was admitted and underwent an emergency operation to remove the perforated appendix.

The error caused a scandal, and some whispered about the possibility of a lawsuit. The parents were extremely distressed because the diagnosis had been missed. They rightly argued that an infected gut leaking material from a perforation could spread to the fallopian tubes and result in sterility in adulthood. Whether a lawsuit was filed for negligence remained a rumor. To prevent such an event from happening again, Dr.

Folkman decided to examine every child diagnosed with an acute abdomen personally.

Tim came down from the O.R. to examine her. With a fever of 102°F, a mass, and X-ray findings indicating small bowel obstruction, we had to operate. Since the E.R. was quiet and had no surgical patients waiting, I accompanied Stephaney to the O.R. to assist in the operation. Tim and Dr. Filler operated, and I assisted by holding retractors, wondering how many kids two years and younger had undergone surgery for perforated appendices, as it wasn't common.

We made a small horizontal incision right over the mass. Upon entering the abdomen, we discovered an abscess. The cause wasn't a perforated appendix; instead, we encountered a mass made up of loops of small bowel matted together by inflammatory tissue, which resulted in the bowel obstruction caused by a perforated Meckel's diverticulum.

That diagnosis reminded me of a mnemonic rule of two that I had learned during my anatomy days in medical school. The diverticulum occurs in about 2% of the population as an outpouching of the small bowel. It is approximately two inches long, located about two feet from the ileocecal valve, where the small bowel enters the large bowel, and is most commonly found in two-year-old toddlers. In about two-thirds of patients, the Meckel's diverticulum contains gastric tissue similar to that found in the stomach, making it prone to a perforated gastric ulcer.

We removed a short segment of the small bowel surrounding the diverticulum pouch. To achieve this, we utilized Dr. Filler's new non-crushing German clamps, positioning them an inch above and below the diverticulum to prevent digestive juices from leaking into the abdomen. By using the non-crush clamps on either side of the small bowel, we could sew the two ends without trimming any crushed tissue, thereby re-establishing gastrointestinal continuity. The patient recovered well and was eventually sent home.

I was immensely impressed by these clamps.

What a great invention!

A surgeon must have been tired of squashing bowel tissue and trimming the mashed ends before he could sew fresh, uncrushed gut together. He probably studied the mechanics of squeezing human tissue and, together with an engineer, invented a bowel clamp that didn't mash the delicate tissues.

Hallelujah!

That was surgical progress!

Dr. Robert Filler, a generous man I held in high regard, could afford to buy a precision-made German clamp for bowel surgery. In line with New England frugality, the rest of the staff used relatively old, worn hospital instruments that displayed significant wear and tear. Instruments were refurbished in the hospital tool shop, after which they were recycled, resterilized, and repacked into an operative kit for use in subsequent surgeries.

Finally, when a surgeon decided they had outlived their usefulness, they deliberately dropped onto the floor from the sterile operative field. In an emphatic statement to the circulating nurse, they would exclaim that they were useless and should be discarded. They were generally consigned to the animal lab for further service.

The day when DHL delivered Dr. Robert Filler's precious new clamps from Germany, I happened to be assisting him on their inaugural application to resect a loop of diseased small bowel in a nine-year-old. The rumor had rapidly spread through the changing room and the surgeon's lounge that Bob Filler had the latest surgical instruments and was stupendous! In the presence of curious colleagues who had moseyed into his operating room and in a somewhat festive atmosphere specifically for demonstration, Bob Filler, who had a big, boisterous personality, showed off the beauty and virtues of this new precision technology by applying the two clamps to the diseased bowel, some inches apart. He then resected the diseased bowel in between, expounding with a professorial air, "Gentlemen, they did not crush the tissue within their jaws. I do not have to trim the crushed tissue to get freshly bleeding ends before anastomosing each end together." Looking around at the now-gathered crowd of colleagues, he crowed, "The new clamps merely stem blood vessels and stymy gut content from leaking out into the abdominal cavity, allowing rapid anastomoses of the new cut ends of the small bowel to re-establish gastrointestinal continuity and integrity."

With a celebratory air, a parade of colleagues gathered to congratulate Dr. Filler in a euphoric love fest of swoons, ums, and aahs! While Dr. Filler basked in the praise and limelight of his moment of glory, eyeing everyone surrounding the operating room table, I stood on the opposite side of the patient, waiting for Dr. Filler to give me the green light to start closing the abdomen. It occurred to me that I could use at least one of these overly expensive personal clamps to approximate and not crush the foreskin above the penile glands when I next performed a circumcision in the E.R. clinic. They were perfect for this.

During our Labor Day meeting with Dr. Moore at Marion near the Cape, he indicated that residents should publish two monthly non-case reports for their surgical maturation process. With this in mind, I spent my evenings and weekends working on manuscripts that were essentially surgically oriented and descriptive, based on intriguing patients I encountered. I then compared and contrasted my experience with a literature review in the field. I asked the staff of the medical record room to pull all the cases of Meckel's diverticulum in children two years of age and under who had been operated on at the Children's Hospital during the previous two decades.

I found 770 cases on my record room shelf!

"Are you guys crazy? Seven hundred and seventy cases in kids under two years of age? This can't be! This is not a common finding in humans, let alone in kids."

"That diagnostic code is like a wastepaper basket. All Meckel's diverticulum cases and any other undefined abdominal cases are coded under that number. You'll find cases that aren't Meckel's," came the reply.

And they were right.

In the end, I found 60 infants who had undergone surgery for complications related to Meckel's diverticulum. Just over half of them were less than one year old. Common clinical manifestations included lethargy, irritability, loss of appetite, fever, abdominal tenderness, and the passage of blood in the stool. Infants whose diverticulum was discovered incidentally during the operation were excluded from the study population. Of the 60 patients, 32 had gastric mucosa with rectal bleeding, while the others had perforation or intestinal obstruction due to inflammation.

I submitted the data to the prestigious *Journal of Surgery, Obstetrics, and Gynecology*. The editor accepted the manuscript, and it was subsequently published.

COMPLICATIONS OF MECKEL'S DIVERTICULUM IN INFANTS

Michael Meguid, M.D., Timothy Canty, M.D., *and*
Angelo J. Eraklis, M.D., F.A.C.S., *Boston, Massachusetts*

The authors of my medical ethics book should only include those who contributed directly and significantly to the work. Dr. Eraklis, a junior professor in charge of the E.R., learned of my manuscript and requested a copy. His response indicated that he should be the first author. This was the action of an unspeakable scoundrel. I was indignant that someone who had neither seen the child in the E.R. nor been involved in the pre- or post-operative care of the patient, who had not participated in the operation, nor conducted any of the time-consuming data collection, analysis, background research, or written many drafts of the paper would pressure his junior not only to add his name but to insist on being the first author! For a head of the Outpatient Department to claim authorship on my paper seemed to me to be immoral. Just because medicine is not an exact science, it doesn't mean it should favor quackery.

The science of morals, encompassing the science of human duty—including the science of law and the rules of conduct that distinguish right from wrong, good from evil—has been firmly established in our moral codes since 1690, which is four hundred years older than the concept of ethics.

Even as the head of the Outpatient Department, even if he had trained me, which he hadn't, it would have been unethical and akin to Cronus the Titan in Greek mythology, "eating his children as they were born to maintain power and prestige." No one threatened him or his job because he never invested in the process. He should have felt embarrassed and ashamed. Credit should go only to those actively involved in the work's concept, research, and writing. Anything else is a betrayal of science—fraudulence and scientific dishonesty. And I viewed him as a surgeon and as a human being.

I had spent hours collecting data, interpreting it through simple statistics, and writing a paper. I did not have any coercion. Yet I wondered what the payback would be and how it might hinder my advancement. The key question for a colleague who wishes to be gratuitously added to a paper should be: If your colleagues meet you in the street, hospital, or bar and ask about the paper, can you honestly describe the data and outcome, or will you embarrass yourself?

I wrote him a letter, politely pointing out that I had been

involved in the case and had spent more than 100 hours in the medical record room going through 770 charts, collecting data during the evenings when I should have been home with my wife. I had written several drafts, which Tim Canty had read, and his lack of standing in the enterprise didn't warrant being a first author or even being on my paper. Finally, I asked him whether "surgical training was so competitive that it eats its children?" Eraklis backed down on being first but still insisted on authorship by virtue of being head of the department. As a resident, there wasn't much I could do about it other than not publish the data. I added his name resentfully and reluctantly. From this experience, I learned that in the future, I'd acknowledge an unwanted name rather than compromise my moral beliefs, however unpragmatic this may be.

The curse of "publish or perish" hangs over every academic, as promotion often depends on publishing. Fascinated by this case and having invested much intellectual energy in the topic, I wrote two more papers as the first author. First, I collaborated with the radiologist Dr. Wilkinson and the rest of the team on a paper entitled "The Futility of Barium Sulfate in Diagnosis of Bleeding Meckel's Diverticulum." The second was "Barium Studies in Meckel's Diverticulum." Both manuscripts were submitted to The Archives of Surgery and were subsequently published.

Tim used a slice of the data after he had discussed his project with me and, with my agreement, wrote a more focused manuscript. He shared it with me, and I made the necessary corrections. He then submitted his manuscript to the *Journal of Pediatric Surgery*.

Another advantage of publishing a data set in multiple surgical journals is that a broader audience of surgeons across various fields can learn from our mistakes. Hopefully, this information will help prevent them from making similar errors.

Since I received Dr. Moore's encouraging letter, I have been convinced of the "publish or perish" philosophy, and I published my work. By this point in my early career, I had published thirteen surgical papers, primarily cited in PubMed. This online database contains most citations from previously printed publications and is managed by the National Library of Medicine. This was sure to impress Dr. Moore when we next had our annual evaluation.

36

PERFECTING THE CROWN JEWELS

He who wishes to be a surgeon should go to war.
—Hippocrates

Part of the second-year resident's E.R. duties involved running the circumcision clinic. Howie, Hillel, and I scheduled six to seven kids each week for the one-morning-a-week clinic to perform the procedure. The young patients were primarily African American boys between six and fourteen years old from the Roxbury neighborhood. Most of the patients suffered from phimosis, which is the inability to retract the foreskin covering the head or glans of the penis. Upon examination, the phimosis appeared as a tight ring of foreskin around the tip of the penis, nearly blocking the opening of the urethra. This made urinating difficult and frequently led to bladder infections due to the accumulated contagion, or what we called "driftwood," under the nonretractable foreskin. Older patients often experience a painful condition called paraphimosis. In this case, the foreskin becomes stuck behind the head of the penis and cannot be pulled back down into a normal position. Circumcision effectively treated both conditions.

Once the patient was anesthetized, Howie and I took turns operating while the other served as the assistant as we worked through the operative list. I took a brief history and examined the patient. They were understandably frightened. Howie and I spoke to them to reassure them about the operation and address their questions.

On the first day, Hillel demonstrated to us how the operation was performed. It was a relatively simple procedure where we excised the superfluous skin so that the penile glans was liberated. Under the standard surgical training rubric of "see one, do one, and teach one," the procedure of doing a circumcision was mastered within an hour, with each circumcision taking about 20 minutes to perform.

For our dynamic minds, these operations felt repetitive and dull, leading us to question: How many different ways can we perform this operation, and how can we accelerate it by inventing safe variations on a theme (referred to as "independent research" and frowned on profoundly)?

Dr. Robert Filler's highly prized personal non-crush clamp was the most aesthetically pleasing approach. I was inspired to use this marvelous, innovative application for circumcisions during this operation, where I stood idly by as Dr. Filler's first assistant, waiting to close the abdomen.

After a significant amount of stealthy cajoling and persuasion directed at Judy, the instrument nurse in the O.R. who seemed to be the personal custodian of Dr. Filler's non-crush GI clamps, along with my vow to keep this potentially treacherous act secret, she—who was always hoping to snag a surgeon, if not for a potential husband, then at least for an initial date—handed me one sterile, non-crush clamp in a secretive act of possible treason.

I tucked the clamp, sterilized and packed it beneath my white coat over my scrubs. When it was safe, I felt it through the sterile wrapping, tracing it out with reverence and a sense of triumph. It was an exhilarating moment! It felt like magic, light stainless steel with two interlocking rows of delicate, precision-made teeth designed to hold but not squeeze the tissue in their jaws, locking with just one magical ratchet click. It is truly a marvel of high-quality surgical engineering. All instruments should be such a pleasure to work with—the Ferrari or Lamborghini, the Mercedes-Benz, the Cadillac of surgical instruments, worthy of use on a penis as much as on other vital structures in the body. I was certain this new application for circumcision would enter the annals, if not the Hall of Fame of Surgical Progress and Great Surgeons. What a marvelous instrument, as aesthetically pleasing as listening to Beethoven's 9th Symphony, sipping a single malt whisky, or slowly melting the finest dark chocolate in one's mouth. This was the joy of operating.

I made my way down several floors to the outpatient operating room for my upcoming circumcision of an eight-year-old. This O.R. was far removed from regular operating room traffic and safe from the prying eyes of other surgeons, especially Dr. Filler.

The three residents, Howie, Hillel, and I scrubbed, and the patient was anesthetized. I donned a sterile gown and gloves while the circulating nurse cleaned the penis and the surrounding pubic area and draped the operative field with sterile towels. I was enthusiastic to proceed, filled with exhilarated joy and unrestrained enthusiasm for the fame with which, as the first to write this surgical history, this procedure would be associated with my name. I was as excited as Magellan must have been in finding the westward passage. At that moment, a biblical passage about angels blowing their trumpets flashed through my head.

I drew up the foreskin over the glans and applied the magic

clamp, locking its jaws with one gentle click about the foreskin. With a scalpel, I swiftly and neatly cut off the redundant skin above the clamp, elegantly slicing it along it in one gliding motion. It was a moment of exquisite bliss. And while I was lost in divine reverie, my innervation worthy of a Nobel prize no less, the operating room door opened, and Dr. Filler stood in the doorway in his street clothes.

His expression showed absolute disbelief and horror as he watched what I was doing with his sacred GI non-crush clamp. Mortified and speechless for one brief moment, he was overtaken by panic and agitation at my apparent sacrilegious use of his prized possession. He rushed toward the sterile operative field in his street clothes like a crazed man, disregarding the sterility of the operating room, whimpering, "Give me my clamp . . . give me my clamp! You can't use my clamp on a penis. They are my new bowel clamps; you'll ruin them!"

Ruin them?

Really?

How could I ruin a stainless steel clamp on the delicate foreskin versus a thick bowel?

And with that, he snatched his instrument out of my hand.

Having retrieved his precious Fabergé-like jewel, he held the blood-stained clamp in the palm of his bare hand, tenderly examining it.

"Where did you get these? Who gave them to you?"

"I don't know. I just found them in the instrument kit."

"Where is the other one?"

"What other one?'

"They come in pairs; they are mine; no one else is to use them," he whined.

I found just one and applied it gently with a single click, like you do. They are wonderful—the ideal instrument for a circumcision." Teasing him, I said, "Can I use them again?"

"No," he bellowed, hiding the instrument behind his back.

"Are you crazy? They are my bowel clamps, and you'll spoil them! They cost me $500 each." With that, he ran out, pocketing his clamp like a little boy who had discovered that another kid was using his beloved toy. As he rushed out, the saying that came to mind was, "The only difference between men and boys is the price of their toys."

37

THE HOLY GRAIL

The aim is to operate only when necessary but not to delay an essential operation.
—Moshe Schein

The whiteboard dominated our operational world at the Children's Hospital O.R. In the morning, the chief of anesthesia, with absolute authority and certainty, documented each case awaiting operation, noting the patient's name, surgeon, surgical service, start time, and the operating room where the case was to be performed. Missing was the name of the gas provider, whether an anesthesiologist or nurse anesthetist, who would put a vulnerable child to sleep. We often thought that withholding the name was a power play—no extraneous pressure on a no-name to get going. As we joked, "A surgeon loves to operate; an anesthesiologist is reluctant to give anesthetics." This idiom often held a kernel of truth, as putting a patient to sleep is an uncontrolled physiological experiment, because the outcome cannot be predicted. Nevertheless, "the board" had the surgeon by his short curlies. The Chief of Anesthesiology jealously guarded the whiteboard—no one touched it or added a case without his approval. As with all organizational endeavors, the schedule was only valid at the start of the day or until the chief left for lunch or used the bathroom. Then its vulnerability was exposed to puffed-up, egotistic surgeons who wanted to operate on an urgent in-house case here or a presumed emergency there, not as an add-on to operate late into the day. One could almost see the small child stomping his feet during a temper tantrum, crying, "I must operate right now!" Knowing an O.R. supervisor nurse well helped the surgeon get his way.

Surgeon: "I have a strangulated hernia that must be operated on right away."

Anesthesiologist: "Can it wait?"

Surgeon: "Absolutely not."

Anesthesiologist: "How long?"

Surgeon: "Only forty-five minutes."

Anesthesiologist: "Use room six. Their case is scheduled to start in thirty minutes. Let Dr. Jones know you'll be bumping him and using his room." This is a common courtesy.

"Hello, Dr. Jones?"

"Yes?"

"I'm starting an emergency in your room."

"No, no, no, you can't use my room." The surgeon hangs up.

Despite this chaos, all scheduled cases were completed by the end of the day. Some surgeons were satisfied, while others expressed their frustrations about the drawbacks of this human horse race.

Observing the give-and-take of such behavior, I resolved that in my surgical future, I would be the first to start operating in a room at 7:30 a.m. I would stay in that room, performing one case after another, even during lunchtime. I recognized that once I left my room, those who ran the board sensed that I had a crack in my schedule and would sneak a case into my room. I often thought lightheartedly: "If necessary, I'll have a porta-potty placed in the corner of my O.R. room so the nurses and I don't have to leave my O.R."

38

AUSPICIOUS SURPRISE

It is the supreme art of the teacher to awaken joy in creative expression and knowledge.
—Albert Einstein

When I moved from the E.R. to the Blue Service, the senior resident who was intended to lead the service was a man with wild, bloodshot eyes from prolonged sleep deprivation, excessive coffee, heightened nervousness, and fear. In his frantic, existential mood, turmoil surrounded him. He was non-functional.

Uncle Sam wanted him. He felt distraught because he didn't want to go to Vietnam. He awaited a call from his father with the crucial news that never came—no absolution. All other options for deferment had been exhausted. Vietnam awaited him despite the U.S. military's drawdown in anticipation of a Paris Peace Accord.

He sat at the nursing station in an agitated mental state. He neither greeted Mort nor me when we arrived to begin our in-house rotation. In his miserable confusion of self-absorbed nonsense, he was unable to provide us with information about the status of the patients in the service he was about to abandon.

Surrounded by incubators, crying babies, infants, toddlers, and busy nurses, a general chaos that felt unfamiliar to us prevailed. If Burley had been my George Washington, the departing senior resident resembled Pigpen from Charles Schulz's popular cartoon, Peanuts. He finally left the service, a pitiful sight, like a squealing pig on its way to the abattoir, grumbling as he walked out the door.

Mort and I wandered through the neonatal intensive care unit, or NICU, and the wards in his absence, searching for our patients. We found critically ill newborns and preemies in incubators, toddlers in cribs, children in small ICU beds, and young adults in hospital beds. Some were awaiting surgery, while others were post-operative and recovering. Meanwhile, some faced ongoing sepsis and required constant attention from multiple services, including pulmonary, infectious disease, and gastrointestinal departments, as they existed on the knife-edge of life. In managing septic patients, the surgical residents provided minute-to-minute and daily care, and so did Mort and I. We were on the wards 24/7, including during holidays and weekends, alongside some incredibly devoted, well-informed, and educated nurses. They played a crucial role in teaching us the delicate nature of caring for sick children.

In our search for patients, a nurse would grab us. "If you're on the Blue or Gold service, this is one of your patients. And in your absence, I've been taking care of it," she would say, briefing us about them and asking us to renew or amend medical orders after examining our new responsibilities.

Among the dedicated nurses was Ann Saxbe, the wife of fellow resident Bart Saxbe. Bart is the son of Republican diplomat and politician William Bart Saxbe, who served as a U.S. Senator from Ohio and as Attorney General for Presidents Richard M. Nixon and Gerald R. Ford.

Ann was recognized as conscientious, dedicated, knowledgeable, and efficient. The unfortunate story is that Bart informed her of his decision to divorce her during the birth of their daughter, Katherine. According to Ann, he was leaving her for a young dermatologist. Her alimony wasn't enough, forcing her to work at the Children's Hospital to make ends meet despite having a newborn. Despite her sad circumstances, Ann Saxbe maintained a positive and friendly demeanor. She was the go-to nurse whenever I had a medical issue with a baby. Ann was always searching for a babysitter for Katherine. Our daughter, Bonnie, was born two months after Katherine, and Victoria occasionally encountered Ann during her ward rounds with surgical patients who had medical issues.

The squealing pig's departure caused a dilemma. A replacement senior resident was urgently needed, and no obvious backup existed. Senior faculty racked their brains to find someone to replace the departing soldier. A senior resident, a mere cog in the medical wheel, was needed for Dr. Kenneth Walsh's Gold service and Dr. Samuel Schuster's Blue team to serve for the next six months to finish the academic year. Neither Dr. Moore at the Brigham nor Dr. Austen at Mass General could provide a senior trainee to fill the departing warrior's shoes at a moment's notice.

During the first 48 hours of the lengthy void of uncomfortable uncertainty, rumors swirled about potential candidates. Proposed candidates were suggested, but none were known. In this dire situation, no objections could be considered. Two days passed before a possible candidate was judiciously floated, in a whispered rumor that seemed to gain a grain of credence: Dr. Gross, chief of the Cardiac Service, proposed the absurd, unmentionable improbability of a Mexican physician.

The nurses were in disbelief. "Did I hear you correctly?" "Yes, a Mexican," they whispered. It was said with an uneasy feeling. "Really? Who? You must be joking," they muttered skeptically during coffee breaks and lunch, shaking their heads in disbelief. "Can you imagine a Mexican in this prestigious environment? Where did they find him? Did he cross the southern border illegally?" I found the murmurs uncomfortable because I, too, was a foreigner.

In reality, he was a Research Fellow in Dr. Gross's laboratory. Thus, I imagined an educated man, a surgeon of some standing. Nevertheless, his nationality was the source of astonishment rather than his credentials.

I thought people at Harvard were open-minded, cultured, and sophisticated. I disliked classifying people, vividly recalling my childhood in post-war Germany during the early 1950s when my sister and I faced taunts because we came from Egypt. As kids, we were surrounded by a surge of newcomers, internally displaced Germans, and so-called dubious "East Germans," fleeing west from the Red Menace. We greeted them with suspicion and apprehension, even as they became neighbors.

This whispered candidate had the courage to leave his country and travel to a foreign nation to conduct research for Dr. Gross. He was bold and brave to step into a maelstrom of prejudice and volunteer to help, whether at the Children's Hospital or the residency program. No one considered how this mysterious Mexican might feel about his reception.

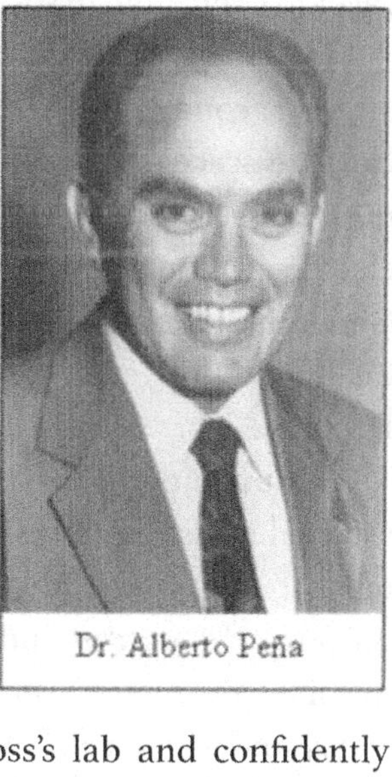

Dr. Alberto Peña

The prejudiced uncertainty vanished when Dr. Alberto Peña, tall, handsome, and soft-spoken, emerged from the depths of Dr. Gross's lab and confidently strode onto the ward. Our new Senior Resident, defying all stereotypical definitions of a Mexican, was a kind person with an open and curious smile. What I liked most about him was his thoughtfulness and profound wisdom.

Dr. Peña was a qualified pediatric surgeon. He trained in general surgery and pediatrics at the Military Hospital of Mexico City. He served as Chief of Surgery at the National Institute of Pediatrics and as a Professor of Surgery at the Autonomous University of Mexico, where he managed a wide range of routine and complex operative cases, mirroring the large population of Mexico City—a deceptively young heavyweight well beyond the resident stage!

His presence as a resident was as unlikely as Victoria and I, two doctors from England, running the E.R. at Harvard's prestigious Children's Hospital. In the annals of Children's Hospital, these two events were a Sputnik moment, no matter how small, but they were memorable milestones. They reflect the benefits of America's generosity and the strength of its policy of welcoming international scholars seeking higher education, eager to contribute to society and pursue the American dream.

Tragically, Dr. Peña's son, Gustavo, was born with biliary atresia, a condition where the bile ducts inside and outside the liver are scarred and blocked. There is no cure, and the prognosis is about three to four years. Alberto and his family traveled to Boston seeking clinical help from physicians at the Children's Hospital. Dr. Gross operated on Gustavo, extending his life by five years, while Alberto worked as a researcher in Dr. Gross' lab.

His trademark was his camera bag. He took photos of the unusual gross physical signs and pathology he encountered in our patients, which inspired me to get a camera for the same purpose. I've used it and its subsequent upgrades throughout my life. My motto eventually became, "Have a camera and slides, and will travel."

Alberto brought calm, order, and confidence to the chaotic

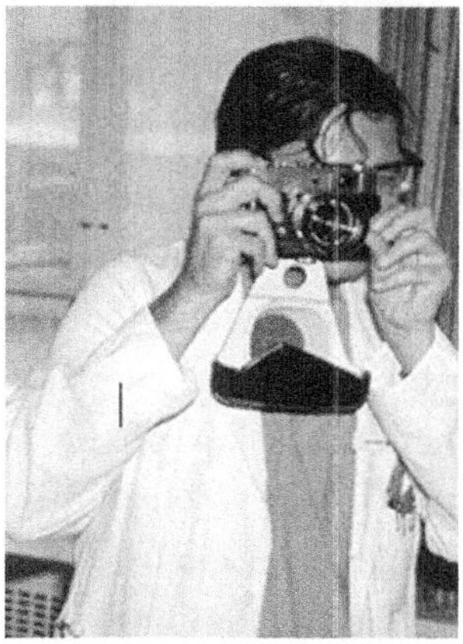

Dr. Meguid with camera

atmosphere of uncertainty and insecurity that prevailed in the wards after the departure of the previous senior resident. Although he was older than most senior residents, his appearance belied his age: the surgical attendings, Drs. Walsh, Schuster, and Filler, initially treated him like a resident. They supervised him during surgeries, occasionally allowing him to perform parts of operations while they anxiously observed his every intra-abdominal move, his instrument use, and his suture technique—his approach to every standard operative procedure.

Alberto, Richard Lynn, and I crowded around the operating table, where an infant lay the length of my forearm. In this small space, as the second assistant, I saw more of Richard's masked face than the details of the operative field. I'd reach into the wound to mop up blood, ensuring the operative field remained dry to allow Alberto to see the organs or tissues he was operating on.

Only surgical instruments are used in pediatric surgery due to the downsized organs and small operative field. In contrast, we insert our hands and use instruments to accomplish our tasks during adult operations. As Dr. Peña operated, he demonstrated to the supervising American attending surgeons, who were more his peers than mentors and, in many ways, less experienced, that he understood anatomy, grasped the pathology, and was agile and comfortable with the appropriate surgical instruments, needles, and sutures. They observed how he gently worked on delicate tissues with meticulous care and technical skill, minimizing blood loss.

Holding a retractor was frustrating. I wanted to operate. Instead, I had to make do with watching and memorizing every step of his intra-abdominal moves as he performed operations more suitable to my level of training. My disappointment was based on my original decision to select this rotation because I was led to believe that at the Children's, residents were encouraged to operate. It was I who wanted to hold the scalpel to incise the skin of the abdomen, I who wanted to part the wound edges, to carefully feel the intra-abdominal organs and note their miniature structures, their warmth in my hands, and the bowel familiarly slithering on the back of my hand. I wanted the experience of applying the clamps, cutting the small or large bowel, excising the disease, reconnecting it, and healing the child. I knew the abdomen, and I wanted to return to it, even if only under Alberto's watchful guidance. I could now relate to the acting chief resident's orthopedics complaint: "Dr. Primo should leave operations to us young guys."

39

STATURE & DIGNITY

Egotism is the anesthetic nature that allows us to deaden the pain of being a fool.

—Michel de Montaigne

Alberto was to assist Dr. Schuster, the attending physician, in performing surgery on a five-year-old girl who had congenitally duplicated collecting systems draining into the bladder from a kidney—the operation aimed to remove the ectopic ureter.

Dr. Schuster's faint German accent reminded me of my autocratic Prussian grandfather. Even before the operation began, while the little girl was asleep and covered, a tug-of-war ensued between him and the six-foot-tall Alberto over the height of the operating table. For Alberto, the comfortable height was too high for the attending, who objected and preferred the table set at a comfortable height that was too low for Alberto. The struggle continued as the anesthesiologist constantly adjusted the table based on their requests. Finally, Alberto tactfully suggested that Dr. Schuster could stand on several stable 5-inch stepping stools to gain additional height.

The mere suggestion pushed his short man buttons! He went ballistic, and his response was far from friendly to Alberto's practical proposal. He wouldn't be told to stand on a stepping stool; his manly height was a sensitive issue! As they openly squabbled, the clash of personalities escalated the tension in the room even before a drop of blood was spilled. I stood back, waiting and watching how this ego tussle would be resolved while the anesthetized child lay on the table, and the meter for the cost of the anesthesia was ticking.

Like a dutiful mother trying to resolve a squabble between two kids, the circulating nurse rushed in with two interlocking platform stools for the attending surgeon. He rebuffed her, pushing them aside with his foot. The table would be set at an intermediate height, satisfying neither the operator nor the assistant. I thought this was a poor compromise, and he was stubborn, sulking, and willful, just like my oppressive Prussian Opa.

Dr. Schuster stood to the right of the operating room table, preparing to operate on his patient. However, in a fundamental error—perhaps to atone for his guttural, unbecoming behavior—he hesitated when the scrub nurse passed the knife into the operative field and Alberto took it to open the child's belly. Alberto confidently and steadily proceeded with the operation. Dr. Schuster grew anxious, agitated, and uneasy, uttering disconnected words and attempting to grasp the scalpel to take over the procedure himself. He searched fiercely for opportunities to wrench it from Alberto's hand. Alberto repelled his intrusive hand by deflecting it with his right elbow as he continued with the surgery. I could tell that Alberto had performed this operation many times before and was very comfortable continuing to work.

Dr. Schuster's disturbance became more vocal, and he babbled about irrelevant drivel, lamenting his wife's insistence on having their pictures arranged symmetrically on their wall, referring to her as "irritating." It raised my blood pressure and tension further, creating an operative environment of crepuscular gloom. Next, he escalated the tension by angrily criticizing Alberto's every move in the abdomen, thereby fostering a hostile work environment, as described in today's terminology. I was becoming increasingly annoyed. I preferred peace and quiet while assisting and operating because tranquility allowed me to concentrate and memorize the steps of each procedure.

Alberto was not distracted; instead, he remained calm and continued to operate confidently. He took great care with the tissues while I gently dabbed the blood to maintain a clear operative field. When Alberto carefully removed a small adhesion from the left kidney, he unintentionally caused a tiny, isolated tear in the splenic capsule, from which a drop of blood emerged, creating the impression of slight bleeding.

"Look what you've done," shouted Dr. Schuster accusingly, looking up at Alberto. "Now we'll have to remove the spleen, increasing the danger of post-splenectomy sepsis in this child." Translated: You idiot, you don't know what you're doing because I would never have done that. Give me the knife; I want to operate.

The capsular tear was minor. In a series of five papers and an abstract from a recent meeting presentation on minor splenic trauma, the philosophy of preserving this organ following a splenic capsular tear and bleed has evolved due to the availability of Gelfoam, a white, pliable, water-insoluble product containing anti-bleeding factors. A small piece of Gelfoam is placed onto the capsule, covered with a sponge, and pressure is applied. The bleeding eventually stops, preserving the spleen and avoiding the need for its removal, which is essential for developing immunity, particularly in preventing pneumonia in infants, children, and young adults. Gelfoam has been a surgical game changer for inadvertent splenic injury. I spoke up spontaneously to save the day and reduce the anger and tension. "Why not save the spleen? Isolated splenic tears heal spontaneously with Gelfoam."

A fuming, purple-faced Dr. Schuster turned to me and used me as a lightning rod for his frustration and anger and snarled, "You know nothing about splenic trauma. Get out of my O.R."

Splenic trauma? You are an old, miserable, ignorant fool. It's a capsular tear, NOT splenic trauma!

He repeated, "Get out."

You are evicting me from the O.R.?

How dare you! I'm up all night caring for your patients, and you humiliate me by throwing me out of the O.R.—the very reason I'm here?

The O.R. was my personal Mecca, the Church of the Holy Sepulcher, the Grand Shrine, and the Mahabodhi Temple—the sum of all divine places. The O.R. was my rightful place!

Nothing would keep me out of the O.R.

I had crossed the Atlantic to be in an O.R.

I was enraged at the injustice, and I refused to leave.

He turned on me once more, "Go!"

I stepped back and, in my fury, inadvertently broke all sterility protocols by first tearing off my gloves, gown, and mask. I then spat out, "Kiss my ass!" barely avoiding adding, "You fucking moron," as I stormed out of the O.R., seething with anger and humiliation.

Still dressed in my scrubs and fueled by visceral outrage, I marched into the library. I printed five abstracts from the surgical literature on the paradigm shift concerning splenic salvage. Incensed, I sought out Dr. Folkman to lodge my complaint about the hostile work environment. "It's a travesty of justice," I added. "Dr. Schuster abused his power, but I'm sorry for having cursed him. It was an expression of my frustration. I'm flitting away from my assigned 16 weeks of general surgery training by having to assist the likes of Schuster."

I wanted to operate!

Continuing my polemic, "He isn't up to date with the surgical literature since there has been a watershed development about splenic salvage based on the degree of injury," I explained, still agitated. However, I was concerned that my offense might lead him to write a damaging comment in his evaluation of me, jeopardizing my promising prospects of being promoted to a categorical senior resident at the Brigham.

Dr. Folkman, a fair-minded surgeon-scientist, listened to my complaint about his colleague's behavior and lack of knowledge regarding current surgical literature, as well as my spontaneous outburst. "I was an idiot," I contritely confessed as I calmed down.

Expressing empathy, he briefly read the five abstracts as I stood beside him.

He nodded. "You are right," he said. "Looks like applying a sponge with some homeostatic powder and gentle pressure can stop the splenic capsule tear from bleeding, preserve the spleen, prevent a splenectomy, and maintain the young patient's immune status. It's good to know."

Then, looking at me once more, he asked, "Do you know if a splenectomy was done?" I shrugged my shoulders. He continued, "Some surgeons practice at the level they were trained years ago, and their frequency of reading the surgical literature decreases with age, along with a narrowing of general information as specialists become experts in one field."

I had cooled down and tried to assess which side of the fence he would be on.

"So? Why get so upset about being asked to leave the O.R.?"

I explained that the O.R. was my temple, my home, and how a senior surgeon at the Brigham had defined me as a "born surgeon."

"OK." He added, "Don't worry about your evaluation—I write them. Avoid working with Dr. Schuster from now on. You are assigned to the Cardiothoracic Service for 12 weeks. Not all of that time will be spent on the heart, lungs, and chest. Dr. Gross handles many abdominal cases and doesn't always have an assistant. Join him. He has vast experience, and he'd love to have juniors on these operations."

As I left, having licked my wounds, I made it a point to assist Dr. Gross whenever I could. The old surgical adage came to mind: "Residents keep abreast with surgical developments by reading research papers, young professors by reading the NY Times, and old farts by flicking through Readers Digest."

I hurried to the OR, where Dr. Gross was about to begin a splenectomy on an infant.

"Scrub," was all he said.

By the time I finished and walked into the OR to assist him, he was placing the last stitch in the abdominal fascia to close the abdomen. The circulator waved me off as we both realized I was too late. She smiled to reinforce what was known: that Dr. Gross was a fast operator, and I laughed, feeling foolish, especially since Dr. Gross looked up and winked at me. We had raced to see who could scrub or operate faster. But he was a quick surgeon, not because he hurried, but because he saved time by avoiding wasted motions. I liked that, and I could operate quickly too, as I knew the anatomy intimately and didn't waste movements. Later in my residency, I met other surgeons of the same kind, with whom I operated, and where operating became a joy.

I remained in the O.R. with Dr. Gross in case I could be of assistance.

Fortunately, I learned a useful trick. Dr. Gross had left a red rubber catheter inserted through the abdominal closure into the abdominal cavity before finally closing the abdomen. His scrub nurse injected the infant's 24-hour intravenous fluid requirement through it, after which she quickly removed the catheter while he tightened the last stitch.

This infant wouldn't need an intravenous catheter for the

next day as it recovered from the operation. I filed this clever trick away, intending to use it one day.

I caught up with Dr. Folkman in the radiology department, where he was examining a chest X-ray.

"Dr. Gross had completed the splenectomy by the time I had scrubbed," I said.

"Stick with him. He has many other cases for which he requires an assistant."

He then turned to the chest X-ray on the screen and asked me inquisitively, "Have you ever wondered why pulmonary metastases, the so-called cannonball metastasis, grow to the same size and then stop? Look at these." He pointed at the lung mets. "They've all reached about two centimeters in size."

"I believe they reach a size where the nutrients can no longer support their growth. After all, the Peyton Rous sarcoma cancerous cells live on glucose and metastasize to the lungs, as Rous showed in his 1935 experiments, subsequently stopping at the same critical size."

"Yeah. But I think they stop growing when they reach the limit of blood vessel growth," he said.

"That's interesting . . ."

He added, "Aren't you scheduled to do research in Dr. Moore's lab?"

I nodded.

"We should discuss an alternative opportunity for conducting research and, if necessary, a position to complete your fourth and fifth years of surgical training."

I registered his comments. Were these engaging baits?

He then turned back to view the chest X-ray with the cannonball mets, lost in thought.

Dr. Folkman proposed that cancer cells or tumors can recruit new blood vessels by producing a protein that stimulates vascular growth, a process known as angiogenesis. Once the new blood vessels connect to the tumor, the cancer cells

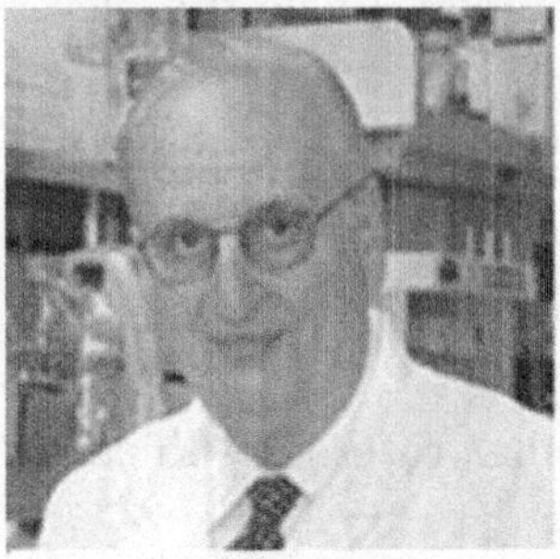

Dr. Judah Folkman

access the general circulation and obtain glucose and other nutrients to colonize distant organs, thus spreading the cancer. "That's why these cancer mets are only 2 cm in size until their protein spouts and attracts new blood vessels. Isn't that exciting?"

To test his hypothesis, he injected several cancer cells into the cornea, which is the clear part at the front of the eye that typically lacks blood vessels, of rabbits. He expected to see blood vessels beginning to emerge from the side of the cornea in a direct line toward the cancer cells. They did. Once the vessels reached the tiny tumors, the cancers grew vigorously and then metastasized, or spread, throughout the body.

This was exciting. I loved the inquisitiveness that is a part of human nature.

I found a fellow soulmate driven by curiosity—an intellectual who took for granted that operative surgery had to be mastered but recognized that surgery was merely a means to an end in treating a patient. Surgeons like Elliott Cutler, Dwight E. Harken, Robert E. Gross, Francis D. Moore, Joseph Murray, and now Judah Folkman possessed the boldness to question why and how a matter accepted as a given in human physiology occurred. This was the thrill and great joy of being a surgeon scientist—an individual with the vision and imagination to see beyond the horizon. These men wouldn't have condemned the use of a GI non-crush clamp on the delicate foreskin of young kids.

There was opposition to his research proposal at the Children's Hospital. Once again, a visionary surgeon brimming with enthusiasm rushed forward with his experiment, ahead of the administrators and naysayers who put the brakes on his work

—the brakes and balances of animal research. They objected to his lack of formal approval for the project. Was this a remnant and a repeat of the situation Dr. Gross had become entangled in when he proceeded to tie off the first Patent Ductus Arteriosus in a child while a senior resident at the Children's Hospital in 1938? I was reminded of Arthur Schopenhauer's saying, "Talent hits a target no one else can hit. Genius hits a target no one else can see."

The pushback against Dr. Folkman's lab studies came from those who were skeptical because he hadn't proven his theory or identified and isolated the 'tumor angiogenesis factor.' As a result, his project was halted.

One cannot stop an idea simply because it can be executed elsewhere. To continue his work, he relocated the rabbit colony to the guest bathroom in his high-rise flat next to the hospital. It was not uncommon to see residents rushing out of the hospital to care for the rabbits. Dr. Folkman observed blood vessels beginning to sprout from the limbus of the cornea in a direct line toward the cancer cells, as he had predicted. Once they reached the tiny cluster of cells, the cancers grew explosively. He and his team eventually isolated two small molecules —an angiogenic factor and an antiangiogenic factor. The former stimulated the growth of new blood vessels, while the latter inhibited their growth. Their Nobel-worthy discovery opened an entirely new field of cancer therapy. Could one starve a tumor's growth by cutting off its blood supply? Unfortunately, Dr. Folkman passed away at 75 in 2008, but he had made his mark in life.

Alberto Peña was another surgeon driven by curiosity. He once told me, "Michael, when there is more than one operation for the same surgical problem, then the surgical problem isn't understood." I agreed with him, but I didn't understand what thought process had prompted him to share this conviction.

Eventually, I would learn that Alberto focused his surgical

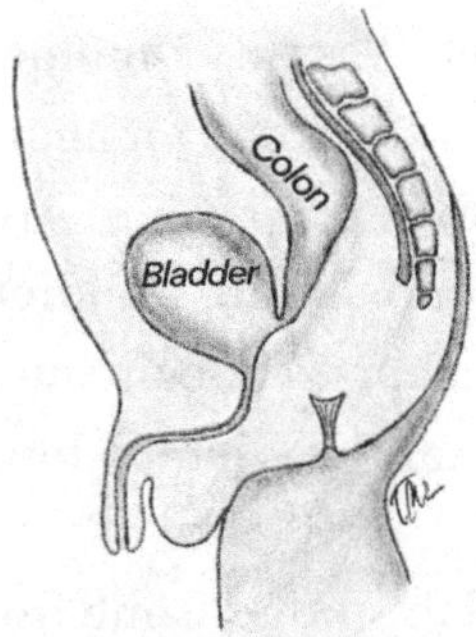

curiosity and skills on a common issue of rectal and anal malformations. During the early stages of embryonic development, the human hindgut, or lower colon, forms a shared channel with the urogenital tract known as the cloaca. A few weeks later, a septum forms that divides the common channel into two openings: the urogenital opening in front of the rectoanal canal. The urogenital opening develops into the bladder, urethra, and vagina in females. In males, it forms the bladder, prostate, and urethra. The colon grows downward to create the rectal canal, which connects with an upward-migrating skin puckering of the anus.

When the membrane in the cloaca fails to separate, the rectal canal connects not to the anus but to the vagina or bladder. The infant is born with an imperforate anus and other anatomical malformations.

To study this problem in detail so that he could develop a surgical remedy, he mentioned an opportunity to study imperforate anus in piglets at a local farm. With the farmer's permission, he was given the piglets born with rectoanal malformation. Studying these, Alberto devised an elegant operation that untangled the anatomical problem using these piglets that were going to be sacrificed by the farmer.

He approached the problem by surgically opening the area right between the buttocks like a book, rather than addressing the anatomical abnormalities through the front of the abdomen. Known as the "Peña pull-through procedure," this has become the standard treatment worldwide, bringing him recognition and fame. His operation definitively corrects the rectoanal malformation.

Like any immigrant to this country before achieving fame and fortune, Alberto faced the dilemma of either returning to Mexico or staying in the States after finishing his work. He visited me while I was working at the City of Hope Medical Center in Duarte, California, to seek my advice.

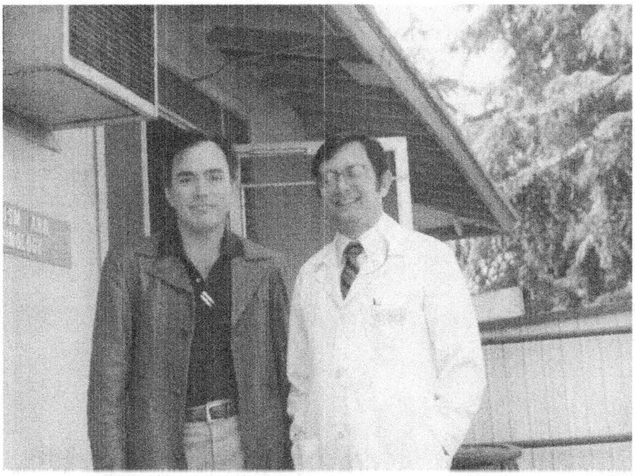

Dr. Alberto Peña visiting the author in 1978 at the City of Hope National Medical Center, Duarte, California

As he saw it, the future of his children was at stake. They would grow up disconnected from their rich Mexican heritage. I felt honored that my former senior resident sought my advice. Yet, we were both outsiders who, through our hard work and research, advanced the surgical field and improved the community's health. I told him that his eventual wealth would allow him and his family to travel to Mexico every weekend. In keeping with the Surgical Resident's Survival Guide, we supported each other and became lifelong colleagues and friends.

Similarly, fifty-two years later, Dr. Richard Lynn and I met again at the Clinical Congress of the American College held in Boston in 2023. He was now an Emeritus Professor and 2nd Vice-President of the American College of Surgeons. Over dinner, we exchanged war stories from our joint residencies, recalled the long nights we spent together salvaging sick kids, laughed at the Schuster farce once more, and expressed our admiration for Alberto Peña, recognizing his monumental contribution to pediatric surgery, as well as our awe for Dr. Folkman. Each of them provided both positive and negative lessons to our individual lives. Richard and I are practically neighbors since we both live in Florida.

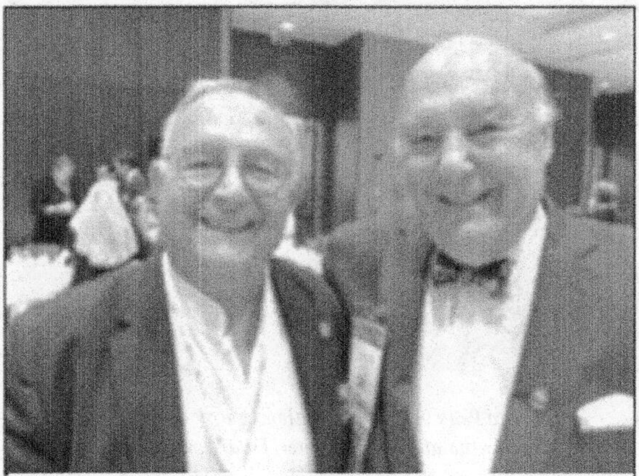

Dr. Richard Lynn & Author

40

BETTER THAN GOOD SEX

Anybody who believes the way to a man's heart is through his stomach flunked geography.
—Robert Byrne

I observed Alberto being assessed as a surgeon worthy of becoming a senior resident for ten days of pure frustration, while I was relegated to holding a retractor and not even given a chance to close the abdominal incisions. Once the senior attendings approved Alberto's competence, they allowed him to supervise the juniors, manage the surgical services, and operate independently on routine cases. Once again, I could cut while he guided and taught me.

Hallelujah!

In pediatric surgery, as in general surgery, many common conditions affect adults and children. Routine operations are familiar to all members of the operative team, including Alberto, the scrub nurse, the circulating nurse, and the anesthesiologist. During these procedures, a series of repeatable techniques is performed in the same sequence each time a specific operation is conducted. When everything goes smoothly, the operation resembles a perfectly choreographed ballet performed on and around the anesthetized child's body.

I loved these bread-and-butter cases. As I operated on them, I distinguished myself for my sensitivity and intelligent adaptations; despite this, the scrub nurse worked seamlessly with me, anticipating my upcoming steps and providing the exact instrument or suture I would use. The whole operation progressed quietly and in an orderly manner. It was an enjoyable work routine because it increased safety, reduced the length of the operation and anesthesia time, improved the quality of my work, and allowed me to predict how long a case would take, enabling me to schedule my next one. As a result, my skills grew, and I left the O.R. feeling accomplished and elated. It reminded me of the simple mastectomy I performed early on at the Brigham while I was on the Ward Service with Dr. Walters.

Alberto had a sharp sense of perception, an almost uncanny awareness of surgical disease and the depths of life itself. His love for children and their care, as well as his passion for operating, matched his enthusiasm for teaching his juniors. He inspired me with his calm and steady manner. He seized every opportunity to teach during operations and ward rounds, exemplifying the true essence of apprenticeship, a hallmark of surgical residency. Rounds with him on the Blue and Gold services, particularly concerning those few children who existed on the knife-edge of life due to their unstable conditions, were conducted at a reassuringly deliberate pace, engaging with the patient or their nurse while ensuring that we learned along the way.

As I got to know Alberto better, I discovered that his other trademark was his sense of humor. How fortunate I was that we developed an affinity for each other and stayed in touch throughout our careers.

When Alberto was on call, Richard and I worked alongside

him. In many of the operations, he assisted me with the common procedures that had become ingrained in my surgical DNA. My skills and proficiency grew, and I became a confident expert in handling human tissue and correcting diseases, structural abnormalities, and uncomplicated congenital issues in children. The instruments became familiar and comfortable tools. The fact that I could extend my hand to receive the suture or instrument I needed accelerated the operation, as I could maintain the golden thread of my concentration and visual focus on the depth of the wound without needing to look up at the scrub nurse or negotiate with her about what I required. This method avoided the wait for it to be found and handed to me, enabling me to refocus my eyes on the wound's visual depth to execute the next part of the operation safely.

Throughout my surgical training, I performed many recurrent operations. My operation logbook indicates that I was the surgeon in approximately three daily operations during my 16-week period on the Blue and Gold General Surgical Service, totaling nearly 80 operations. This count does not include cases where I served as the operating surgeon during my rotations in Plastics or Cardiothoracic Surgery. I took pride in my general surgical experience because operating is what made me happy.

As Dr. Gross said, operate often. For the general surgical record, this included thirty hernia repairs, sixteen appendectomies, twelve abdominal operations to correct a testicle that had become stuck during its descent, ten abdominal procedures for cancer, where I removed either the small or large bowel, and one operation to close a colostomy. Additionally, I performed single cases such as a tracheostomy to place a breathing tube in the windpipe, a gastrostomy to insert a feeding tube into the stomach or jejunum, the removal of an enlarged spleen due to Hodgkin's lymphoma, a kidney resection, removal of a benign breast mass, a vascular operation in trauma, a cholecystectomy for cancer, and a lung wedge resection. I was the first resident to assist in inserting a central venous catheter for total parenteral nutrition in an infant. The catheter was inserted in the operating room—we now insert TPN catheters at the bedside.

Alberto assisted and taught me in most of these cases. Therefore, I was learning to become proficient in operating, discussing issues with nurses, parents, and patients, and, above all, in humility, because any of these operations, at any stage, could have had complications.

There will always be operations that are not routine. In such cases, I must rely on surgical principles and adapt to other procedures. I believe that the many months I spent learning anatomy in England helped me feel comfortable with the organs I was operating on, their relationships, and the knowledge necessary to avoid pitfalls. Additionally, part of my record-keeping included the requirements set by the American Board of Surgery before my board certification examination. I had to submit a record of the types and numbers of different operations I had performed to demonstrate mastery of advanced surgical knowledge and skills. These would eventually be assessed through written and oral examinations.

Luck was on my side. The overall volume was heavy, so I was fortunate to perform some operations above the usual experience level of a resident. One such case in pediatrics involved a six-month-old infant boy presenting with projectile vomiting. The latter is pathognomonic, a telltale sign in infant males with hypertrophy or increased sphincter muscle thickness, which allows food to pass from the stomach to the small intestines. The hypertrophy blocks food in the stomach until it is overfilled, causing the child to vomit forcefully. The history alone of projectile vomiting in the absence of stooling provides the diagnosis of pyloric stenosis.

This was regarded as a Chief Resident's case of significant

magnitude. I had witnessed Tim Canty perform one, so when the next four infant boys were admitted with a diagnosis of pyloric stenosis, Tim was busy operating on other patients. I was free, available, and willing. With Alberto's assistance, I opened the upper abdomen by making a small subcostal incision to enter

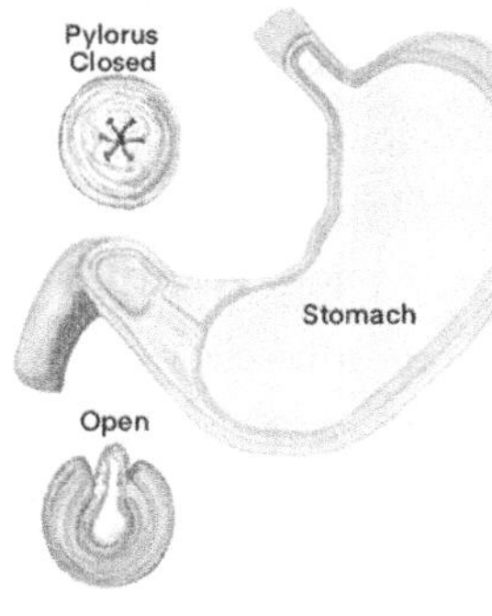

the upper abdominal cavity and locate the pylorus, which resembles a white olive. I created a small incision through the avascular muscular layers of the olive until I encountered the relatively bloodier mucosal lining of the stomach. I bluntly yet gently separated the musculature with a hemostat until the mucosa protruded, ensuring that the obstruction was relieved. Satisfied, I placed the expanded olive and stomach back into the abdomen, then closed the wound layer by layer. The infant began eating voraciously without vomiting, indicating the success of the operation. To my satisfaction, he, like the others, recovered quickly.

A handful of pediatric patients who needed plastic and reconstructive surgery were mixed in with the general surgical patients. In addition to Dr. Murray, the other physicians included Dr. McCullum, Dr. Gifford, and Dr. Moore's son-in-law, who is a maxillofacial dentist. The post-graduate fellow on the service was Dr. Mutaz Habal, my Lebanese friend. I was the resident who assisted in caring for their patients.

Donald McCullum had a private office outside the hospital where he saw patients; we would admit them. He preferred to operate on his patients, with Dr. Habal assisting him. I wasn't required to participate because Dr. McCullum was one of the nonacademic surgeons who didn't believe that residents could safely operate on his private patients. However, he expected us to care for them postoperatively. He didn't address me once during the six weeks I covered the Plastic and Reconstructive Service.

One day, during rounds, we stood by a patient's bedside after Dr. McCullum had performed surgery to repair a cleft palate and cleft lip on a child. Dr. Habal asked him to clarify his post-operative orders, as the nursing instructions indicated that the harelip suture should be gently cleaned and mineral oil lightly applied to the wound with a Q-tip every day. Addressing Dr. Habal, he said, "I want my wounds covered. Don't remove the dressing on my patient's face. To prevent it from becoming infected, I'll remove it myself next week when I know the incision has healed." Somewhat confused by the mixed instructions and eager to impress Dr. McCullum, Dr. Habal mentioned that a recent scientific paper showed that lip wounds seal over within six hours; even when human feces were dabbed on the wound, they didn't get infected, so they could be left open without a dressing.

Dr. McCullum's face reddened, then deepened to purple with rage. "If you put feces on my patient's wound, I'll rub shit all over your face!" He then stormed out of the ward. Mutaz and I stifled our laughter, then burst out laughing, unable to contain ourselves.

Dr. McCullum was an old-timer who disliked residents sharing advances in knowledge with him. Years later, when Mutaz and I met, we recalled the humorous event.

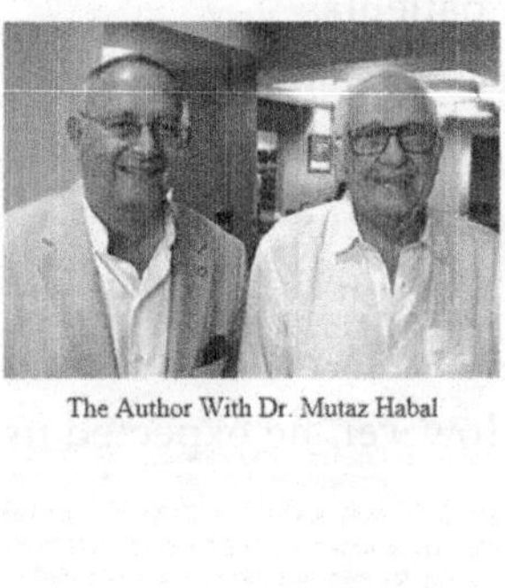
The Author With Dr. Mutaz Habal

Drs. Murray and Habal performed numerous surgeries on children, and I assisted them. Two were little girls with burned palms and hands. We debrided the skin, and I was taught how to handle the thin skin. As with all surgical procedures we were taught as residents, this technique would become useful at some point in our future careers.

I also assisted in surgeries for sixteen children with syndactyly, a condition characterized by webbing between two or more fingers. While webbing is present in utero, it usually disappears as the fingers develop. However, in some cases, it persists and is identified after birth. Syndactyly is the most common abnormality among newborns; approximately 10 to 40 percent of children with this condition inherit it from a parent.

However, Harry was the most fascinating patient on this rotation. He was a remarkable and handsome seven-year-old with a positive outlook on life and a broad smile that brightened the world around him. I enjoyed taking care of him because his curiosity about everything happening in the ward was even more remarkable. After all, he was born with the congenital absence of a nose, nasal passages, and sinuses—a condition termed Bosma arhinia microphthalmia syndrome.

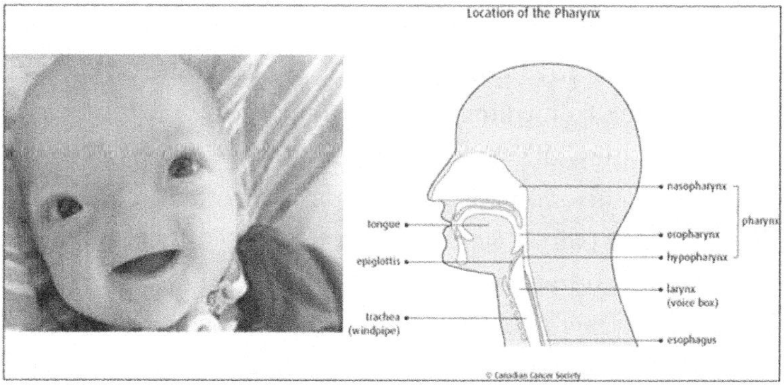

I can't imagine living without the smell receptors in the mucous membrane of the nose, which are finger-like extensions of the brain poking through the cribriform plate at the top of the nose and transmitting impulses to the olfactory nerves. How I'd miss the scent emitted from Victoria's skin, the fragrance of her body, and the lingering aroma after we made love, which was better than any pizza I've had. Like a dog that knows his neighborhood, I possess a mental map of her extraordinary body, thanks to my acute sense of smell.

Poor Harry.

His extremely rare genetic disorder affects one in 197 million births. Fewer than 100 patients worldwide have been reported in the past century. In addition to a complete absence of the nose, the syndrome includes eye defects and a lack of sexual maturation. Harry's main problem is that he cannot eat and breathe simultaneously. Dr. Gifford cares for him with great compassion and tenderness.

The day arrived when Dr. Gifford and I took Harry to the O.R. After he was anesthetized, I steadied Harry's head. At the same time, Dr. Gifford utilized an old-fashioned handheld carpenter's drill to create a passageway from the exterior through his facial bone into Harry's pharynx. We inserted a wide silastic tube through the newly created nasal passage into the nasopharynx, having lined the passage with several strips of skin for grafting. For a while, we monitored Harry with his nasopharyngeal tube during rounds. The tube was eventually removed after confirming that the skin grafts had taken and were now lining the nasal passageway. One day, Dr. Gifford brought in a custom-made external nasal prosthesis attached to the frame of a pair of glasses. When Harry put them on, there were cheers, and an even broader smile appeared on Harry's face when he saw himself in the mirror. He looked very handsome. Shortly thereafter, he was discharged. A team of medical and surgical subspecialists continued to follow him into adulthood. Psychosocial support was also provided for the entire family.

41

AGONY OF THE GOLD & THE BLUE

He who has a WHY to live can bear almost any HOW.
—Friedrich Nietzsche

The senior residents, Drs. Alberto Peña, Tim Canty, Junior Residents, Mort, and I, along with our fantastic interns, including Richard Lynn, covered both the Gold and Blue Services for a period of 16 weeks. The services grew busy as summer approached and school vacations began. On average, we had twenty to thirty patients in each service who were sick. Fortunately, most children recovered well after the operations that cured them. However, a small number of patients were chronically ill and lived on the wards, cared for by dedicated nurses and residents.

Similar to the routine at the Brigham, after early morning rounds, one resident would go to the O.R. to assist with the day's elective cases. These included routine maladies in children, such as inguinal and umbilical hernias, undescended testicles, exploratory laparotomies for various gastrointestinal diseases, including Hodgkin lymphoma—a type of cancer that develops in the lymph system; colostomy closures; inserting gastrostomy feeding tubes; tracheostomies; and breast biopsies. I loved every moment in the O.R.

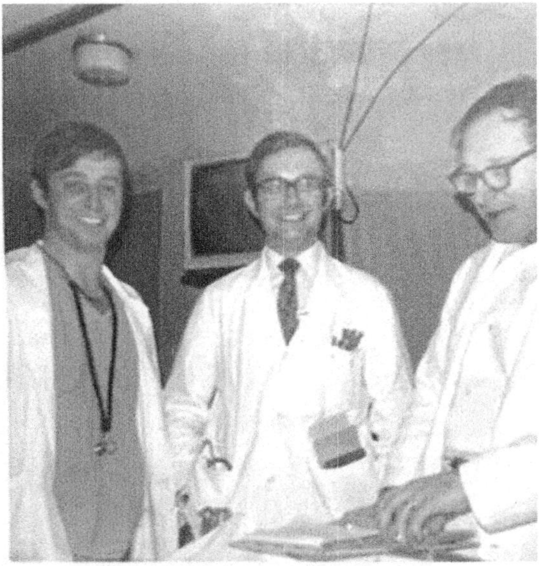

Drs. Canty, Meguid, and Kahan

In one of my evaluations, it was noted that I "initiated aggressiveness in the O.R." While this might sound terrible, in surgical language, it meant that I advanced the operation by acting swiftly and confidently, allowing myself to be taught and guided by my seniors at any time on any day. This assessment pleased me because, from the beginning of my interest in surgery, I knew I had a lot to learn and that I had been given a once-in-a-lifetime opportunity to gain this vast fund of knowledge and operative skills at Harvard. Such a comment also supported the assessment that I was "very comfortable in the O.R. and with handling instruments."

The operation was only one aspect of treating a patient. Additionally, it involved learning and applying the best pre- and post-operative care to manage the patient. As we were repeatedly told at Brigham, "You'll have a lifetime to operate, but one chance to learn the appropriate perioperative care of your patient." I found that saying hard to believe as a young man, but I have come to find it true with advancing age.

The residents who are not working that day would stay in the ward to care for yesterday's patients, perform scan work, attend emergency operations, and prepare new admissions for the following day's operative list. The days were so busy that I developed the habit of skipping lunch, which allowed me to complete all my surgical activities.

Evening rounds began after the day's cases were finished. We gathered in the X-ray department to review our patients' X-rays, then went to the recovery room to check on our post-op patients. After that, we proceeded to the wards for rounds.

Compared to working with Alberto, rounds with Tim were quick, even though several seriously ill children had complex illnesses that required no further surgery at the time, but could experience life-threatening flare-ups at any moment. Despite their complicated medical situations, Tim breezed past the children, giving Mort and me the impression that he expected the junior staff to handle their non-operative issues. Meanwhile, he was only interested if a patient required surgical intervention.

As juniors, we cared for these very sick youngsters whenever we were not in the operating room. We needed thoughtful feedback from our seniors during rounds about the care we provided them throughout the day while the rest of the team was operating. I wanted to confirm that managing patients without senior residents was appropriate, as I felt less secure in my knowledge and experience with these children. Had I cared for them properly? Like Mort, I needed that affirmation.

Among them were children with congenital bowel or lung diseases who, when they had a sudden acute incident such as uncontrolled GI bleeding or an acute breathing problem, abruptly became very unstable, like a volcano that could unexpectedly erupt.

The resident who had been in the operating room would stay overnight, caring for the patients he had operated on or assisted during the day. He'd also operate on any lingering emergencies that may have accumulated or those that arose during the night, managing these complex patients while praying he could get some sleep. The other dragged himself home, presumably following the numerous commandments in the Surgical Resident's Survival Guide, and then collapsed in bed.

These stable, chronically ill children, who were post-operative and possibly required further surgery, were prisoners of their precarious lives. To survive, they lived in the hospital. An abrupt change in their existential equilibrium could trigger a sudden emergency necessitating an urgent operation that might save them. Discharging them would be like toying with their already unstable lives. They existed on the cusp of medical and surgical knowledge, as neither discipline provided definitive treatments or additional elective therapies to cure them or resolve their operative or nonoperative dilemmas. Lying in bed under our care, they teetered between life and death, held together by compassion and our soul-felt cry "to keep them as well as possible," while I hoped that a sudden emergency wouldn't occur on my watch.

However, flare-ups did occur, typically in the late evening when much of the staff had gone home and the residents were already exhausted from the day's work. The chronically ill child suddenly became acutely sick, and it was our responsibility, both medically and ethically, to treat the child as conservatively and appropriately as possible, hoping our management of the flare-up would prevent another trip to the O.R.

When such an emergency occurred, I wasn't alone. As Dr. Moore had stated, "Don't be a lone wolf." The nurses were always present, but I demanded that ancillary services, such as X-ray technologists, radiologists, blood bank services, or other personnel, be available and responsive to my calls to salvage a child's life. And they were.

We utilized every means we had learned or recently read about in scientific journals to treat them without taking them to the O.R. During such events, we used all available supplies without concern for how much we were consuming or what the costs might be, including blood, blood products, catheters, and medications. This encompassed drugs, even if their efficacy for a disorder was marginal. Our mindset was to overcome the exacerbation. We didn't rest until we regained control, and the patient was once again stable, despite our awareness that we were not curing the patient but merely extending their existence.

Was I doing the right thing by prolonging their dying process? There was no staff member to discuss this with regarding the issue of doing "something" for the patient without actually doing "something" for the patient. I feared being labeled ineffective if I voiced my concerns. Indeed, I didn't want any child to die, let alone on my watch, although their continued presence with us sometimes seemed painful or almost inhumane.

We understood the biochemistry of their diseases and the absence of the gene believed to cause these unfortunate children's illnesses. However, we did not yet have the remedy. We could not replace their gut or remove the diseased organ and substitute it with a healthy one.

Although Dr. Joseph Murray transplanted a healthy kidney into a genetically identical twin in 1954, the transplantation of healthy intestines, a pancreas, or lungs to replace severely diseased ones remained a dream. It was still not clinically feasible even in the early 1970s.

Our immense efforts and investment of time and resources

to keep these chronically ill children alive were a hope for purchasing time during which a medical miracle drug or advancement in transplantation techniques would be discovered. All the while, Mort, Richard, and I lived in the purgatory of chronic worry.

Such acute exacerbations of their disease take a significant emotional toll on me, and undoubtedly on Mort and Richard as well. I could not shake off the weight of it when I returned home, feeling physically and mentally drained after spending the previous night fighting for a child's life following a full day of intense surgery. It was a debilitating exhaustion, a crisis that plunged me into deep depression and sadness, to the point of feeling like a human failure.

No chaplain for doctors.

No priest to console.

No psychiatrist to explore our frailties.

Intellectually, I grasped Martin Heidegger's philosophical argument that ". . . death is an inextricable part of life. But the fear of death leads us to seek medical help to save us from dying." Nevertheless, I felt that the death of any patient under my care diminished me. As John Donne stated, "We humans are connected; no man is an island." This was my fervent belief, and I had not yet come to terms with any loss.

There was another, more subtle anxiety from my childhood that subconsciously invaded my mind. As a child in war-devastated Germany in 1948, I was of similar age to these very sick patients whose lives were precarious and whose futures were uncertain. My mother had vanished for several years for reasons I didn't understand, and my beloved Oma would sing Johannes Brahms's lullaby at night when she put me to bed. Its last two lines ended, "Tomorrow morn if God wills, you'll awake once again."

It neither soothed nor comforted me; it had the opposite effect. The thought of not waking up again or dying in the darkness terrified me, as I was already in an alien world, apprehensive and frightened. Moreover, Oma's lullaby did not alleviate my feelings of helplessness. This anxiety irrationally arose like a fog while I was taking care of these kids.

Tim breezing by the children during rounds was hardly reassuring. Please linger and tell me that what I did for them was right; it became my silent prayer during rounds. Yet the fact that we moved right along should have reassured me that my care for the child had been adequate. Once I reached 45 Marion Street, I'd sit in our armchair, unable to shed my frustration and accumulated anger, and weep uncontrollably. I felt lost—a moral telos crisis—a lack of justified medical purpose.

I felt like a failed human being who couldn't help the patients I desperately wanted to save. This monumental cost led me to emotionally shut down, resulting in emotional blunting and detachment. It drained away all thoughts of love, making intimacy impossible and causing emotional distancing as a form of self-preservation.

Victoria, too, must have been in an emotionally challenging situation dealing with her pediatric patients and their related turmoil. She was not in a position to hear my fears or offer sympathy and comfort, nor was I capable of doing the same for her.

I wanted to curl up in a fetal position and sleep during such times. I wished I could drink; after all, wouldn't a bottle provide comfort with each glass? Instead, over time, I found solace and consolation in novels, art, poetry, and music from various genres, which offered relief and a mood boost during periods of suffering and grief.

Perhaps Mort experienced a similar emotional reaction when he got home. Maybe he had an empathetic or expressive wife who wasn't in the same profession. Perhaps he possessed a stronger sense of internal security, supported by his religious beliefs. He might have had a cat that curled up on his lap, bringing him calm, perspective, or serenity. Or perhaps he drowned his sorrows for failing a child.

We worked closely together for most of our junior residency years, but that did not translate into knowing each other beyond a mutual trust. Whenever one appeared to relieve the other, the other would vanish. All I knew was that at the end of my 36-hour shifts, he would be there to take over the children's care. I always regretted that this working bond never developed into a lasting friendship.

Later in life, when Mort and I met, among the topics we shared, rather sadly yet honestly, was that during the physical and emotional stress of working at Children's, neither of us was willing to let a child die appropriately on our watch. It was not due to a lack of compassion, but rather from fear of reprimand. Instead, the child had to survive until the other partner arrived in the morning and took over the responsibility.

With time and maturity, I came to understand that curling up into a ball or wrapping my arms around myself to nurture and heal my wounded self wouldn't have been as silly as it seems. A small child still resided within me, holding the memory of the fear of dying, and I needed reassurance after the emotional trauma of caring for my vulnerable charges. It was okay to weep without fully understanding why. It would have been compassionate for me to recognize that I wasn't Superman, despite being a Brighamite.

Throughout my general surgery rotations—eight weeks on the Gold Service and eight weeks on the Blue Service—I performed 102 operations. We were constantly trained in operating skills and in pre- and post-operative care but were never taught to help patients die. Nor were we instructed to reveal our emotional vulnerability or taught empathy, compassion, understanding, or love regarding a patient's suffering. No! In this mecca of surgery, it was understood among the resident staff that we never say or even think, "We give up."

Despite the lack of salvation for a child, during our conservative treatment, the patient would eventually fall off the knife's edge yet again, leading to another bout of surgical intervention. These repeated emergency operations were not routine and had to be performed as individualized undertakings, depending on the variable pathology and conditions encountered during the procedure. How many times did the attendings, the men the residents revered, sweep their gaze past my eyes as we stood before a child's open belly and think aloud, "What should we do now?"

The various ways that attending surgeons managed such operative crises depended on the totality of their surgical skills and the expertise they had gained throughout their training and subsequent lifetime of operative experiences.

Emergency operations had a vaguely formulated pre-operative strategy and faced an uncertain chance of success. Once inside the belly, the procedure we performed depended on the type of lesion encountered. The operation placed stress on the body of a child already teetering on the edge of survival. It was conducted as a last resort, perhaps in response to and with the consent of a pleading mother to "do something," or a surgeon's nagging conscience, or a wisp of hope for a surgical triumph—just perhaps, perhaps to enhance the child's condition or from a simple unwillingness to accept the fact that the end was in sight.

I rarely saw such acute-on-chronic conditions during my travels to less affluent countries. They didn't have the resources to try to save these children. Instead, their pragmatic approach was one of helplessness and prayer until death occurred. It was a tension I observed repeatedly throughout my life, watching sick patients in these countries being cared for by educated physicians trained in England, Canada, or the US, who now had insufficient resources. In contrast, others around them recognized that death came at God's will.

42

WILL DEATH COME TONIGHT?

So good evening and good night,
With roses bedight,
With lilies spread,
Snuggle up in your nest.
Tomorrow morn, if God wills,
You'll awake once again.
Tomorrow morn, if God wills,
You'll awake once again.
—Johannes Brahms
"Lullaby" 1864

With my childhood invading my subconscious, fear of their death haunted me as I cared for three specific children. They never had parental visits or any visitors, as, in some cases, their families lived far from Boston. In contrast, others had been removed from the family environment by Children's Social Services. In their isolation, they were long-term residents with chronic illnesses who teetered precariously on the brink of life. Was there a cure just around the corner? I prayed for them every day.

Six-year-old Adam was one of them. During the initial emergency operation on a Saturday morning for uncontrolled rectal bleeding, Adam was found to have hereditary hemorrhagic telangiectasia, an inherited disorder characterized by soft arteriovenous malformations (AVMs) that form throbbing, live vascular tumors under the lining of the bowel mucosal lumen.

Telangiectasias are clusters of small blood vessels with irregular connections between arterioles and venules, creating worm-like vascular tumors in multiple areas. They disrupt blood flow and oxygenation of the colonic mucosa, unpredictably eroding the delicate mucosa and causing bleeding into the gut.

Most of Adam's tumors were isolated to specific portions of the large bowel. In other children, they tend to form multiple skip lesions in the length of the gut, raising the quandary as to how much of the bowel should be cut out, especially since the next bleed was unpredictable.

We resected a segment of the large bowel that contained what we believed to be the most AVM tumors, including the bleeding one. The massive blood loss stopped. After reconnecting the bowel, the abdomen was closed, and Adam was moved to the recovery room. I wrote orders to transfer him back to the ward when he was stable. We felt we had truly treated him during a late Saturday morning breakfast.

But as I ate, I realized that since it is an inherited, congenital disease, it is possible that after we resect such a mass, other tumors could develop. Angiotensin stimulates the formation of new arteriovenous malformations (AVMs). Thus, removing parts of the gut wasn't the definitive answer. The solution would be to treat the AVM tumors with clotting agents. But which ones? In the 1970s, we lacked the techniques to deliver a clot or clotting factors directly to a bleeding mass. Adam already had smaller tumors present. So, I revised my impression that we may have performed a definitive operation. Adam could experience another massive and fatal bleed.

Adam was stable for most of Saturday afternoon. I was surprised that he had no visitors. I sensed his loneliness, sitting up in his bed by himself in a strange hospital environment, bewildered by pain, nasogastric tubes, IVs, and an oxygen mask, uncertain about what would happen to him next.

I recalled the bleak time I woke up after my appendectomy at 2 a.m. when we lived in Cairo. It was dark, and I felt disoriented, miserable from pain, and nauseated by the ether anesthesia that still saturated the tissues of my tongue and mouth, blurring my vision. Neither of my parents visited for what felt like a long, long time. Mother eventually arrived late in the morning after driving my father to the airport for his flight overseas. I didn't see him again for six months. Once more, I was without him. Wasn't his absence from my infant life, when I so desperately needed him as I grew, a sufficient period without bonding with his son, I without a father? My poor Dad. He, too, grew up having to rely on his wits alone in Cairo's streets without the reassuring presence of a father at that age, and seeing Adam brought back such dark memories of my lonely recovery.

By evening, at the start of the night nursing shift at 11 p.m., Adam remained stable, giving me a false impression that he was doing well. After my late evening rounds, I went to my on-call room, thinking I could finally rest my aching body.

In the early hours of Sunday morning, the nurse called me, "We found a pool of blood in Adam's bed. Bright red blood has started to come in spurts out of Adam's rectum."

She didn't need to say anything more. I immediately made my way to the ward. The sweet odor accompanying rectal blood loss preceded my arrival at his bedside and confirmed the news even before I saw him. Adam looked fearful, ghostly pale, with a rapid pulse, low blood pressure, and diminished urine output —all signs of ongoing life-threatening blood loss. Why these bleeding events seemed to occur almost exclusively at night mystified me.

While the ward was in semi-darkness and we hoped the other children were sleeping, we drew the curtain around Adam's bed and turned on all the lights so we could work. We spoke in hushed tones, fearing we might wake the nearby children. As we labored over him, his agitated face transformed from fear to terror. I hoped we could get him through this episode of bleeding.

Over several hours, I administered numerous blood transfusions to Adam, a flood of platelets, along with a variety of costly specific clotting factors and saline fluids, in a race against his ongoing bleeding to assist with clotting. I hoped these conservative treatments would prevent another operation.

The nurses changed Adam's sheets and cleaned him off after each ongoing spurt of bright red rectal blood. The area surrounding his bed was a mess—a plethora of empty IV bottles, small transfusion bags, and syringes as we busily dealt with the emergency. Despite our valiant efforts, the bleeding continued in rushes, interspersed with periods of no bleeding when I thought the hemorrhaging had finally stopped. But it was merely wishful thinking, for barely an hour later, another trickle of blood would precede an evacuation of bright red blood mixed with gelatinous clots, odorous farts, and a precipitous fall in his blood pressure.

I was losing control of the situation and fearful that with several AVMs in the gut lining bleeding, Adam would require another operation. I alerted Alberto, who contacted Dr. Gross.

Both joined me at the bedside, appearing sleepy, to assess the clinical situation for themselves. Adam was slipping from our grasp, becoming progressively more unstable.

We moved him from his bed to the O.R. In this emergency, the anesthetic team administered more fluids into his veins in an attempt to keep up, or even get ahead, of Adam's blood loss and maintain his blood volume. We changed into O.R. clothes and scrubbed, while the nurses quickly gowned and gloved us. When Adam was asleep, Dr. Gross reopened the abdomen, assisted by the team gathered around the operating room table.

We searched for the bowel length of the bleeding submucosal mass in enlarged, fragile AVMs. We identified several possibilities, any of which could have been the culprit. One issue was that the anesthetic drugs lowered blood pressure and obscured the AVM that was the likely source of bleeding.

Searching further, we found one in the left sigmoid colon and convinced ourselves, with some trepidation and doubt, that this AVM tumor appeared to be a source of Adam's blood loss. Despite observing darker blood, it would require resection resembling a blackish paste with a few specks of fresh, reddish blood in the transverse colon. We reasoned that the findings in the transverse colon were likely due to backwash from the left colon.

Dr. Gross performed a sigmoid colectomy—removing his sigmoid colon. A seasoned and experienced surgeon, known for his speed, moved rapidly in electric silence. Alberto and I clamped and tied off vessels, mopped blood in the field, and assisted him as we worked in the small hours of the night. Toward the end of the procedure, I felt the old, fearful sensation of my infant days, remembering Brahms' lullaby and thinking, "Will Adam wake up again? Will he survive?"

After the sigmoid colon was removed, the transverse colon was freed from its attachments to allow for the anastomosis, or joining, of the two ends of the remaining colon. The bleeding seemed to have stopped, and the anesthesia team sighed in relief, as they had managed to stay ahead of the child's blood volume and stabilize his condition. The Foley catheter I had inserted earlier was draining a good volume of urine. These were the reports we heard from the anesthetic team at the head of the table as we closed the abdomen. Dawn was creeping over Boston as we degloved and disrobed, feeling we had achieved our aim.

Once in the recovery room, Alberto, the nurses, and I hooked up the child, who had an anesthetic tube through his mouth leading to his lung, to the various monitors and life-support equipment. We established Adam's baseline condition as he awoke and gradually rejoined us in the land of the living.

With Adam stable, Alberto and I headed to the men's room. Standing side by side before the urinals, we gradually felt the tension abate as we relieved ourselves. "There's nothing better than a good piss," I said, facing the wall and emptying my bladder. He chuckled.

"Have you ever wondered if your prostate gets larger or your bladder smaller as you grow older?" he said, facing me and eliciting a smile on my tired face.

We stripped our bloodied O.R. clothes and realized that we had spent four hours during the night with Adam.

"Breakfast?"

Before we could change into our daytime clothes, our pagers squawked simultaneously. The nurses reported that the rectal bleeding had resumed. As if it were a bad movie, we were again in the O.R. reopening Adam's abdomen. We stared at the large bowel, trying to figure out where the bleeding source was, as I fought off fatigue. Evidence now suggests the right large bowel. The blackish-brown blood challenged us as we pondered, hearing the questions from anesthesia as to what we were going to do. Indeed, what should we do to save Adam? I felt a gnawing emptiness grow inside my stomach.

A total colectomy seemed to be the lifesaving solution. Dr. Gross performed this quickly and efficiently in a state of quiet desperation and doubt. Once again, the bleeding ceased. We surgeons had skated on fragile ice and, out of sheer frustration and based on probability, removed the rest of the large bowel to stay ahead of the blood loss and save Adam's life as the sun shone over Boston. We left Adam with an ileostomy, fashioning and exteriorizing the end of the small bowel into a nipple—a Brooks ileostomy, to which a bag was attached, and another four to five hours had passed.

Each section of the bowel has a specific function in the digestion and absorption of food and water, as well as in the interaction of its bacteria with the colon's microbiome. The microbiome supports the immune system, aiding Adam's physical growth and intellectual development. Blindly removing the entire bowel saved a life but may have ultimately left the patient a G.I. cripple.

Adam was stable as we began our new day of scheduled activities. We were drained. Our bones felt like they weighed a ton within our skin. Like the ward, the O.R. resembled a battle scene, with discarded paraphernalia and the remnants of the necessary kits to rescue and save a life.

Some 50 years later, we would ask our interventional radiologists, who are very skilled, to insert a catheter via the aorta into the superior mesenteric artery, which supplies blood to the arteries of the colon, and inject a contrast medium to locate the bleeding site. We expect to see the contrast blush as AVMs leak into the colon, indicating which part of the gut should be excised. The days of blind colonic excisions are a thing of the past. Today, this problem is targeted.

Jacquie was a radiant child, a lively and engaging five-year-old full of curiosity and trust. In a moment when no one was watching, she had taken a drink of caustic, corrosive Drano that burned her throat, esophagus, and the fundus of her stomach. I inserted a feeding tube into her jejunum, the beginning of her small bowel. The nurses fed her homogenized food through this tube to help her gain weight and grow.

Like the two infant girls whose hands had been burned by a God-fearing grandmother, Jacquie was also removed from her home, siblings, and parents by Children's Social Services. Under the pretext of protecting her from an abusive environment, Jacquie was deprived of family visits and left alone as a form of safety. (As I write this, parental visits are permitted with supervision by a social worker or personnel from Social Services.)

Jacquie stood in her crib, smiled constantly, and waved her arms and hands, eager to touch every nurse and resident who passed by, yelling, "Hello, hello." She yearned for a human touch.

Jacquie faced many challenges: she was an African American child, neglected, and severely injured. Yet, despite these misfortunes, she always smiled and remained friendly, calling out to those who passed her in the ward. Jacquie was under our care but was also treated by the medicine residents, one of whom was Victoria. When we were home and relaxed, we dreamed of adopting her to give her a fair chance in life. However, the reality was harsher. For many reasons, she and others like her were considered unadoptable due to systemic restrictions.

Annabel was an eight-year-old red-headed beauty whose name reminded me of Edgar Allan Poe's poem "Annabel Lee." She had advanced cystic fibrosis, an inherited disease that damages the lungs, digestive tract, and other organs. It causes abnormally thick and sticky mucus, affecting the production of sweat and digestive juices in the pancreas, other organs, and the airways of the lungs.

In the absence of visitors, Annabel had no mother to soothe her fears, provide emotional support, or kiss her goodnight. She faced the world alone. Reclining in her bed with her eyes wide open, she watched everything around her, dependent on a ventilator and a tracheostomy.

To ensure that this critical tube remained in her windpipe, her hands were secured to the bed frame for fear that she might pull it out in a panic during a stressful episode when she couldn't get enough oxygen to breathe. A similar tracheostomy tube was kept in a Ziplock bag and pinned above her bed for safety. If the tracheostomy became dislodged or was accidentally removed, a new sterile one was readily available to save her life.

Annabel's lung mucus accumulated, resulting in repeated, severe lung infections. The tissue surrounding the alveoli, or air sacs, had become damaged, thickened, and scarred. As the lungs scar and stiffen, breathing becomes increasingly difficult, and insufficient oxygen enters the bloodstream.

I visited her before rounds to see and chat with her, even though she couldn't reply because of her tracheostomy. Her face lit up, and for a brief moment, I felt I was connecting with this beautiful, angelic child. When she was in good spirits and her left hand was free, she'd disconnect from the respirator, place a finger over the opening of the tracheostomy tube, and attempt to speak to me with her innocent, saintly voice. She could only utter a few words before she went into paroxysms of coughing, and her face became alarmingly red. Distressed, her eyes searched for a nurse who would spring over, suction out the thick mucus in her tracheostomy, grant her the gift of breath, and then reconnect her to her respirator. I stroked her forehead as the nurse secured her arm to the bed frame. How could I feel such love for this virtuous little girl? Was it her innocence or my feeling of helplessness to cure her of the disease that would cut short her faultless life?

As I departed, her bright eyes followed me, filled with fear and apprehension, as she wondered what I would do next. Her eyes conveyed confusion and resentment toward the world for her suffering, not understanding what was happening in her body. Despite my soothing, reassuring words, she never smiled, remaining too afraid and distrustful of the universe.

Occasionally, a scarred alveolus would burst, causing the air from the ventilator to collect beneath her skin, tracking up her neck and head, which led to subcutaneous crepitus. This crackling and crunching noise could be felt when pressure was applied to her skin. The thick mucus in her lungs prevented her breath from escaping her trachea. Annabel's face would swell with subcutaneous air, doubling in size as the ventilator forced air into her lungs . . . air that could not escape.

The subcutaneous emphysema and its accompanying crepitus extended down her neck onto her chest wall, creating a barrel-shaped appearance. She repeatedly bucked against the tracheostomy and respirator as she experienced paroxysms of attempted coughing to clear the plugs of mucus. With each cough, her frail body lifted off the bed; her eyes bulged even more, her veins stood out, her face grew redder, and sweat gathered on her brow, flying off with each cough. In terror, she would grab my hand and squeeze my fingers until they turned pale. Her helpless gaze frightened me.

With my hands captured in hers, preventing me from sucking out her tracheostomy, I'd urgently yell for the nurses. They'd come running and disconnect Annabel from the respirator, squirt fluid down her tracheostomy once more, snake a catheter down her tracheostomy and trachea, and suck out the softened goop.

Dollops of goop.

Breathing easier, she flopped back, exhausted, closed her eyes, now nearly buried in her swollen, air-filled face, and relaxed her grip on my hand. I stayed by her side, monitoring Annabel's breath sounds. I ordered a portable chest X-ray and prepared to insert a chest tube through her ribs to relieve a pneumothorax and further ease her breathing. Her X-ray revealed that she had a 10% pneumothorax, meaning 10% trapped, unusable air between her lungs and chest wall, which was insufficient for me to insert a chest tube. My suggestion to my seniors to remove the air via a needle inserted through her chest wall and attached to a vacuum tube was dismissed. But I knew that in an imminent emergency, I would do exactly that because I wanted her to live.

My pulse, blood pressure, and sweating would rise and fall in tandem with hers. In her isolation, unable to speak due to the tracheostomy, her fear and anger toward the doctors and the world were understandably justified. Annabel was a powerless victim of her disease, while I felt like an impotent physician without a cure.

One morning, I noticed that a different patient occupied her bed. During the night, an emergency had arisen; she must have looked around for me to help bail her out, as had occurred numerous times when I was on call at night. But that time, I wasn't there. I wish I'd been able to say goodbye.

Today, I'm aware that scientists have successfully used gene editing (called CRISPR, for Clustered Regularly Interspaced Short Palindromic Repeats) to delete genes associated with the fatal disease Sickle Cell and perhaps eventually Cystic Fibrosis. However, CRISPR was a scientific development that came too late to save Annabel.

We residents were soldiers on the front lines. Tense and ready to act, we suppressed fear, helplessness, and guilt for failing our patients. Despite sleepless nights and fatigue, we worked as effectively as possible on their behalf. I would later learn that the toxic mix of flashbacks, childhood post-traumatic stress disorder, and occasional suicidal thoughts was common among persistently sleep-deprived, chronically fatigued residents. We eventually became competent, compassionate physicians. Along the way, some of us would stop at our private cemetery, praying for forgiveness for our human failings. But at the time, we were Brigham residents who, when asked to jump, only replied, "How high?"

Annabel Lee
by Edgar Allan Poe

It was many and many a year ago,
In a kingdom by the sea,
That a maiden there lived whom you may know
By the name of Annabel Lee;
And this maiden she lived with no other thought.
Than to love and be loved by me.

I was a child and *she* was a child,
In this kingdom by the sea,
But we loved with a love that was more than love—
I and my Annabel Lee—
With a love that the wingèd seraphs of Heaven
Coveted her and me.

And this was the reason that, long ago,
In this kingdom by the sea,
A wind blew out of a cloud, chilling
My beautiful Annabel Lee;
So that her highborn kinsmen came
And bore her away from me,
To shut her up in a sepulcher
In this kingdom by the sea.

The angels, not half so happy in Heaven,
Went envying her and me—
Yes! That was the reason

That the wind came out of the cloud by night,
Chilling and killing my Annabel Lee.

But our love it was stronger by far than the love.
Of those who were older than we—
Of many far wiser than we—
And neither the angels in Heaven above
Nor the demons down under the sea
Can ever dissever my soul from the soul
Of the beautiful Annabel Lee;

For the moon never beams, without bringing me dreams.
Of the beautiful Annabel Lee;
And the stars never rise, but I feel the bright eyes
Of the beautiful Annabel Lee;
And so, all the night-tide, I lie down by the side.
Of my darling—my darling—my life and my bride,
In her sepulcher there by the sea—
In her tomb by the sounding sea.

43

SAVING BABY IAN'S LIFE

Nutrition for those who cannot eat or cannot eat enough
—Stanley Dudrick

Dr. Folkman caught up with me in the ward. "Dr. Filler and I will be starting on a case with a rare condition, called chronic intestinal pseudo-obstruction. We'll need some help."

"I'm free. What is it?" I asked.

"Chronic intestinal pseudo-obstruction," he repeated. Seeing that I didn't register the diagnosis, he continued. "He's a two-month-old who has failure to thrive from this rare disorder in which the intestinal nerves and muscles don't work together, preventing food and fluid from moving down the gut from the stomach, leading to malnutrition since he isn't absorbing enough nutrition."

While we changed, he continued my education. "About three years ago, a team of researchers at Penn led by Stan Dudrick demonstrated that they could provide all the necessary nutrients intravenously, known as Total Parenteral Nutrition (TPN), which helps infants grow and develop. I know you're interested in metabolism, and this is a good case for you."

"What are we going to do?" I asked inquisitively.

"Insert a central venous catheter to give him TPN."

"Oh. And we're going to do this in the O.R.?" I asked.

"I have a copy of the paper in my office. The author, Stan Dudrick, did some incredible work to feed infants and pups with his TPN. It might interest you!" he said as I followed him into the brightly lit operating room.

We joined Dr. Filler and a team of nurses who were assisting baby Ian, who had a securely placed peripheral IV in his hand. The baby lay on the O.R. table, swaddled in blankets, with only his head, neck, and shoulders exposed as anesthesia checked for the endotracheal tube. I was still confused about why so much fuss was being made over inserting a central catheter that would ultimately end up in the superior vena cava, leading to the heart. I had placed several of these in the ward and couldn't comprehend all the heightened concern. What was I missing?

While Dr. Folkman and I scrubbed, Dr. Filler tilted the table to a head-up angle of about 45 degrees. A nurse shaved the right side of the baby's head. Dr. Filler, already gowned and gloved, applied an antiseptic to the side of the head, ear, neck, and chest, while the nurses covered and draped the baby. A sterile towel covered the left side of the head, and anesthesia stood on that side, ventilating our patient—baby Ian.

The adults, Drs. Filler, Folkman, and I crowded, body to body, around the right side of Ian's head while the scrub nurse, with her instrument table, stood at the top end of the O.R. table—all huddled about baby Ian. Both Drs. Filler and Folkman spoke over my head, strategizing how to proceed. Finally, Dr. Filler took a skin marker pen and made a small mark on baby Ian's scalp behind and a few inches above his right ear.

"Give him the knife," Dr. Filler said to the scrub nurse. I took it and hesitated, unsure of what I was supposed to do.

"Make a 5 mm cut in the scalp. Don't go too deep."

I did. Then Dr. Filler took over the operation, and while I observed, he created a subcutaneous tunnel that extended from the incision site down behind Ian's ear. At each stage, both attending surgeons discussed and confirmed the actions taken and the next steps.

Dr. Folkman turned the baby's head sideways and held it there so that the right sternocleidomastoid muscle, the major neck muscle connecting the skull to the sternum, remained straight. Lying beneath the muscle is the central vein, which leads to the superior vena cava and the right side of the heart. With Baby Ian's head in that position, Dr. Filler took a syringe filled with saline, attached it to a long hollow needle, placed it through the subcutaneous tunnel, and, after consulting with the anesthesia team, thrust the needle into the internal jugular vein. In the intensity and quiet of the moment, we could almost hear the needle pop through the wall. Drawing back on the syringe handle, he withdrew some blood. The tension in the room eased, and he passed a silastic tube, no wider than 1.5 mm, through the hollow needle. Having previously measured the distance from the skin incision to the approximate position of the heart's right atrium, Dr. Filler advanced the sterile tubing filled with saline into the desired position. An X-ray of the baby confirmed that the catheter was in an acceptable position in the superior vena cava at the junction with the right atrium. A lot of head nodding followed, indicating that the procedure had gone well.

Dr. Filler then dressed the venotomy site on the scalp, securing the catheter to prevent it from being displaced by baby Ian's movements once he was awake.

Until now, I was unaware of why the procedure needed to be performed in the operating room and why precautions were taken with the long subcutaneous tunnel and the Total Parenteral Nutrition fluid flowing through the catheter. My curiosity and ignorance were clarified when I picked up the paper from Dr. Folkman's office. Ian was the first baby to receive Total Parenteral Nutrition, and I was among those who placed the catheter in the first case at Children's. Little did I know how nourishing patients would become a significant aspect of my surgical life.

About 100 children are born with chronic intestinal pseudo-obstruction in the U.S. each year. This illness is a lifelong condition that can be managed with proper medical care. While I wasn't impressed with this operative case, Dr. Folkman's paper provided all the answers.

Long-term total parenteral nutrition with growth, development, and positive nitrogen balance

STANLEY J. DUDRICK, M.D.
DOUGLAS W. WILMORE, M.D.
HARRY M. VARS, PH.D.
JONATHAN E. RHOADS, M.D.
PHILADELPHIA, PA.
From the Department of Surgery and the Harrison Department of Surgical Research, School of Medicine, University of Pennsylvania

Sick, malnourished babies typically require at least 80 to 100 calories per kilogram daily and over 2 grams of protein per kilogram each day. This is administered as TPN, which includes glucose, protein, essential fats, calcium, other minerals, and all vitamins in minimal amounts appropriate for their age, dissolved in saline. This solution is compounded in the pharmacy to ensure stability and sterility. It is hyperosmolar and must be delivered via a pump into the central venous system to mix with the blood flow, preventing thrombus formation.

TPN did not exist until 1968. Dr. Stanley Dudrick's research was groundbreaking. The evidence indicated that Beagle pups given TPN for 72 to 255 days grew into healthy dogs, comparable to a control group fed dog chow.

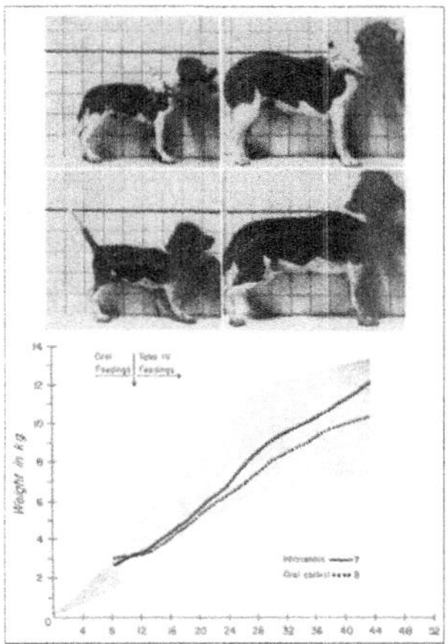

For patients who cannot eat, will not eat, or are unable to eat enough, nutrition in TPN aids growth, increases body weight, and prevents further weight loss during chronic illness.

This was initially demonstrated in animals, newborns, and acutely ill or chronically sick patients. This resulted from several years of research conducted by fellow surgical researchers. This significant medical advance emerged from scientific, technological, philosophical, and practical progress in basic science and clinical medicine achieved by countless researchers and clinical scientists over several decades.

I am deeply grateful to Dr. Folkman for enhancing my education. After reading Dr. Dudrick's paper about this groundbreaking research and its benefits to our patient population, I became convinced that he and his team deserved the Nobel Prize in Medicine. Furthermore, I believe surgeons inclined to do so should engage in clinical or basic research during their training.

I could hardly have predicted that surgical nutrition support for patients would become a focus of my life. In this capacity, I traveled the world lecturing, often alongside Dr. Stan Dudrick, who was my co-lecturer. We collaborated on writing book chapters and remained close friends until his untimely passing. His absence was a great sorrow, as we had many enjoyable adventures after our scheduled talks.

44

CHALLENGING CUTS

The longing for ignoble things;
The strife for triumph more than truth;
The hardening of the heart that brings
Irreverence for the dreams of youth;
—Henry Wadsworth Longfellow

Victoria and I finally got a break and traveled to the nation's vibrant capital. We returned from our sunny Washington, D.C. getaway feeling refreshed and more in tune with each other, optimistic about living in Boston and continuing my surgical training. The urge to return to London had lessened, although the pleasant memory of life on the Isle of Wight lingered like the aftertaste of Cadbury's Fruit & Nut chocolate.

What lay ahead of me was unexpected.

For the next three months, I was assigned to assist with the care and treatment of premature babies and infants under one year of age who lived in incubators. They suffered from congenital heart deformities that developed before birth—a topic we never studied in anatomy or embryology during medical school. Dr. Bert Litwin was passionate about correcting these abnormalities, hoping to follow in the trailblazing footsteps of Dr. Gross by making a profound contribution.

Approximately 40,000 babies are born with congenital heart defects each year in the United States. These anomalies can vary from a small hole between the heart's chambers to absent or severe deformities of the aorta or pulmonary artery, affecting the flow of oxygenated blood through the heart and into the rest of the body. These defects have unique names, such as tetralogy of Fallot, congenital pulmonary stenosis, and vascular anomalies. Regardless of the specific heart issue, they result in fragile, very sick newborns who require constant and careful medical attention. About a quarter of these babies need surgery within their first year of life to survive.

More delicate than china dolls, their symptoms include abnormal heart rhythms, such as atrial fibrillation, heart failure, and blue-tinted skin. Therefore, we referred to them as blue babies who suffered from shortness of breath and an inability to feed or develop normally. Because they were premature, they were on respirators and received medications to lower their blood pressure and control their heart rates. We fed them through feeding tubes inserted in their stomachs to help them grow to a size where surgery would be possible. The babies who needed surgery ended up on the Cardiac Service in the infamous NICU, or neonatal ICU, where we, the residents and highly skilled nurses, ensured their survival until Dr. Litwin could operate on them.

This field was on the extreme periphery of my surgical interests, as I didn't intend to become a neonatal cardiac surgeon. Intellectually, I read about and understood congenital abnormalities. I empathized with the humanity of the situation and the anguish of the parents, knowing their baby would die if such abnormalities were not corrected.

As a medical student at University College London, I

enjoyed studying embryology because it made grasping anatomy easier. How a four-chamber heart developed from a simple blood vessel fascinated me. However, I wasn't interested in how embryological abnormalities of the heart and major vessels occurred.

Mort Kahan and I occasionally assisted in caring for Dr. Litwin's patients. We were at the forefront of surgery, and admirably, Dr. Litwin was dedicated and determined to operate on their hearts and major vessels to repair them. He aimed to save lives that might otherwise be lost.

Even less engaging were the operations themselves, which lasted two to three hours, during which Dr. Litwin closed a small hole in the heart or created a 2- to 3-millimeter aortic-pulmonary shunt—a passage between the aorta and the pulmonary artery—to improve the oxygenation of body tissues. These procedures were performed in a hyperbaric oxygen chamber, where the ambient air pressure was increased to three times normal pressure to significantly enhance and saturate the oxygen in the infant's lungs, brain, and tissues before the heart was stopped. The beating heart was temporarily halted because there was no heart-lung bypass machine available for such tiny patients.

The chamber was located in the sub-basement of the Children's Hospital. It resembled a submarine, crammed with all the necessary paraphernalia and personnel: an anesthetized infant with an anesthesiologist, a scrub nurse with her instruments, a circulating nurse, Dr. Litwin with his technician, and an assistant like Mort or me. Due to the crowded space, when it was my turn to assist, my view of the surgical procedure was limited. I stood clear of the operative field, with my arm extended toward the baby, holding a retractor so Dr. Litwin could see and operate. There was neither teaching nor operating for the residents. The fun part, if one can use such a description, was that as the oxygen pressure increased, the

pitch of our voices rose so that we sounded like Alvin and the Chipmunks.

I took care of these delicate patients post-operatively, whether they were in incubators, beds enclosed with heavy plastic to maintain high oxygen levels and a moist steam environment, or open beds in this special ICU. I counted my blessings that the emphasis on pre- and post-operative care had been instilled in me at the Brigham, where the saying was: you'll hone your operative skills throughout life, but now is the time to learn your patient's care. These infants and young patients demanded obsessive attention to every detail of physiological care, testing the limits and then some of my 24 hours of wakefulness, drive, and determination to ensure these patients survived, recovered, and were discharged. The nurses caring for them were like walking superwomen who knew much more than I did. If I left knowing a fraction of their knowledge in caring for these fragile babies, I'd consider myself lucky. Throughout this experience, I worked closely with a patient's nurse. Each nurse typically cared for one or two patients at a time. Despite my relative ignorance, I looked up to them and drew on their experience to enhance my management of the fragile kids.

Dr. Litwin, with my assistance, operated on baby Francisca, who weighed just over 4 kg, or 8.8 lbs. Francisca had a hole in the septum, or wall, between the left and right atria. This hole was closed by sewing a patch of artificial material, such as Teflon. She required 16 ml of IV fluids per hour, or about two cups of liquid, post-operatively. A few hours after the operation, Francisca's nurse called me. "Baby Fran is fussing about, and her oxygen saturation is decreasing."

I examined the patient but couldn't reasonably determine the problem. I ordered a chest X-ray, thinking that perhaps the patch Dr. Litwin sewed over the hole was leaking—or worse, it had ruptured. I informed Alberto, my senior resident, that day;

he, too, couldn't identify the issue. We checked the X-ray. To our horror, we saw that the infant was in severe pulmonary edema. I miscalculated the amount of intravenous fluid baby Fran needed. I mistakenly gave her 20 mls or two and a half cups per hour. The mere 4 ml difference was drowning her. By providing some diuretics, she expelled the extra fluid, and no residual damage was done.

Surrounded by such fragile babies, any of whom could deteriorate at any moment for any reason, the deafening chorus of beeping machines made it challenging to remain alert, awake, and combat fatigue. For this reason, the on-call rooms were just a step away across the corridor. After an 18-hour surgical day in the operating room and wards, I would make evening rounds, typically around midnight, with each nurse reporting to me the latest status of every baby, infant, or child in the ICU, which was a large, open room filled with incubators, cribs, and infant beds.

Feeling punch-drunk, I became vulnerable to the potential dangers of making an incorrect decision around 2 a.m. I'd succumb to phenomenal fatigue. Lying fully clothed on my bed, I'd be instantly asleep. Just 2 or 3 hours of deep sleep refreshed me sufficiently to resume my duty. One night, while I was fast asleep, the door of my on-call room was flung open. In the glare of the light, a nurse stood in the doorway and yelled, "Michael arrested!" Then she disappeared. In an instant, I was in the ICU, ripping open the plastic over Michael's humidified, oxygenated bed. I thumped his chest with my fist to shock his heart. The eyes of terrified seven-year-old Michael opened and stared at me in horror as I was about to give his chest another blow. The nurse grabbed my sleeve and yelled, "Over here. This Michael!" I joined a cluster of nurses and helped resuscitate an infant, Michael. After writing a note in infant Michael's chart, I apologized to the first Michael for waking him up so abruptly. He stared at me in horror and mistrust.

Neither Dr. Litwin nor his associate ever stepped into the ICU. They trusted the nurses more than the residents to care for their patients at 5 a.m. I would do ICU rounds again, draw blood, get X-rays, run EKG strips, and read them. Each morning, Dr. Litwin's associate would page me at 6 a.m. Instead of asking for a progress report about a patient, he would demand to speak to their nurse. Even though I had spent most of my day, evening, and night caring for his patient, he was never willing to talk to me.

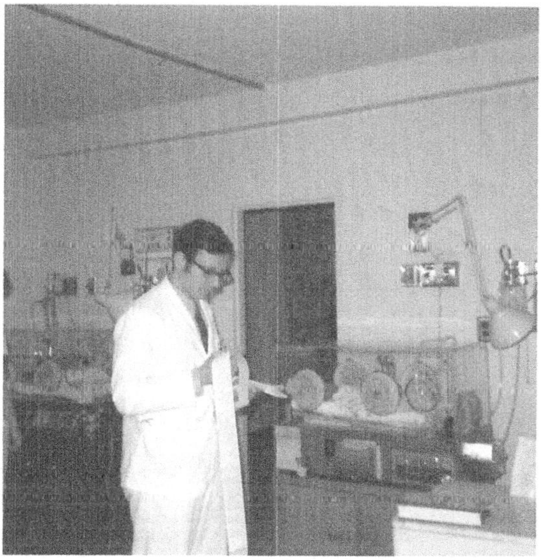

After being ignored several times, I decided to disregard his call. Eventually, he understood the message. He entered the ICU just after 6 a.m. and spoke only to the nurse. It felt entirely impersonal.

Finally, when he appeared, I would get a shower and breakfast, not knowing when I would next have food or the chance to see Victoria and regain my sanity. In three months, he showed no improvement in his discourteous behavior. Dr. Litwin's technician didn't want to talk to the residents. He assumed that we had dedicated our extraordinary efforts to caring for Dr. Litwin's patients.

My final rotation at the Children's Hospital was on the Thoracic Service. The senior resident was Alden Harken, the son of Dwight Harken, a cardiac pioneer in the history of surgery, like Dr. Gross.

Alden was a lively, cheerful, and fun-loving person, as well as an exceptional teacher. We became lifelong friends, and I was pleased to work with him. Secretly, I hoped that if I had a son, he too might become a surgeon and feel as proud of me as Alden was of his father. However, I recognized the immense pressure on a son who chose to follow in his successful father's footsteps.

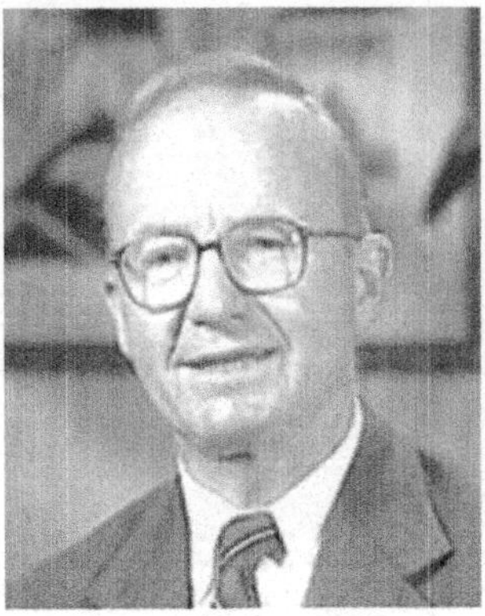

Dr. Alden Harken

Together with Alden, we operated on eleven-year-old Paul with pectus excavatum or concave chest, a condition in which his sternum or breastbone is sunken into his chest, giving the appearance of the chest center having been scooped out. This condition is caused by the cartilage at the end of the ribs growing excessively faster than the ribs, resulting in an out-of-proportion growth rate compared to the sternum. Like all patients with pectus excavatum, the sternum presses against the heart, large vessels, and lungs. Paul suffered from shortness of breath, fatigue, irregular heartbeats, and embarrassment from the unusual appearance of his chest. My buddy, Howie Snyder, assisted us with this operation. Once the patient was asleep, I made a horizontal incision below the breast, extending it from side to side. Howie removed the perichondrium, a dense, fibrous layer surrounding the cartilage similar to the periosteum that surrounds bone. We worked as two teams, with Howie on the patient's right side and me on the left. I started adjacent to the sternal angle and worked toward the xiphoid—from the first to the seventh rib, allowing the sternum to move forward into a normal position. We could see the heartbeat, large vessels pulsating, and the pink edges of the lungs expanding and deflating. Then, we fixed the breastbone into a more normal convex position with surgical metal hardware supports. These were removed after 12 months, when the chest wall had returned to its normal convex position and was no longer pressing on the heart. The operation was stressful because Howie chatted constantly. His distracting gibberish drove me crazy.

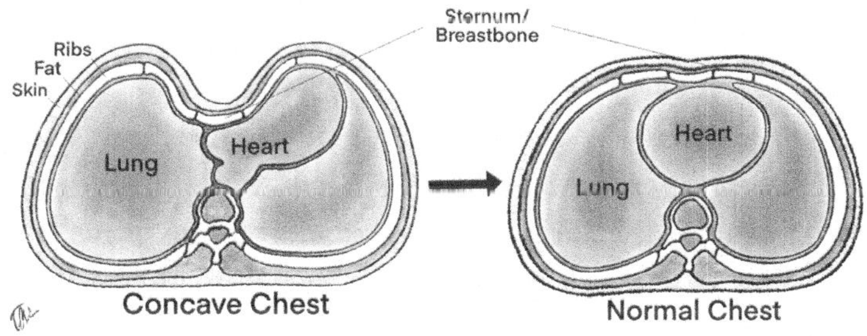

I preferred a silent, operational environment where I'd only speak when necessary and could genuinely make a difference in the operation. With Howie, it felt like verbal diarrhea. I told him to rest his voice, and when he continued yapping, I finally said, "Please shut up so we don't make mistakes."

He did. I wondered what the payback would be.

While the silent Mort and I were buddies for most of our rotations during the two years of junior residency training, Howard McCormick Snyder III, affectionately known as Howie, was my buddy on only a few rotations. Thoracic surgery was one of them.

I first met Howie during the infamous ortho rotation when he was serving on the Urology Service. Our on-call rooms were next to each other. He often woke up a few minutes before my 5 a.m. alarm went off. Each morning, I'd find him in our shared bathroom—similar to a Swedish sauna due to the thick mist billowing from Howie's long shower, which fogged up the room and caused condensation on the mirror above the multi-sink counter. On the counter lay his Dopp kit with his shaving gear, frameless spectacles, and a small transistor radio blaring Howard Cosell's sports commentary delivered in a blustery, clipped, rapid, and grinding voice that seemed alien and outlandish compared to the soothing BBC's Queen's English I was used to at such an early hour. The noisy assault was Howard Cosell's fast speech. I wondered whether Cosell's cadence influenced Howie's loud, clipped, staccato voice and rapid speech delivery.

With an increased and continuous noise level, my sleep's tranquility evaporated into the mist, while my anxiety and stress heightened, making me feel irritable and on edge. I was frustrated that Howie repeatedly and unknowingly disrupted the delicate hours of dawn when my brain was sorting and storing away the previous night's thoughts and dreams, all while preparing and prioritizing the activities of the coming workday. He was unaware that it impacted those with whom he shared a bathroom.

Howie operated at a higher decibel level and exhibited more activity than the other residents in the program, both in speech and movement. His loudness was so pronounced that I began to worry he might be partially deaf, as it appeared he was unaware of the volume of his voice.

As it was, when Howie was in the shower, he couldn't possibly hear Cosell's loud, high-speed, clipped sports commentary. I would turn down the volume based on the principle that if one wanted to listen to a program, they should come and hear it.

When Howie finished his shower, he'd yell, "Hey Mike, did you turn down the volume?"

"Yep. You can't possibly hear it. Come here and listen to it. Otherwise, it's irritating noise pollution. And my God, it's so early in the morning."

Howie stepped out, wrapped in a white towel that exposed his hairy simian chest. He wore wet shower shoes and squinted as he searched for his glasses.

The first time I met Howie, he introduced himself without any prompting. He told me he was named after his daddy and grandpa, explaining the "third" after his name, which he emphasized with gusto. He continued to rattle off his past and expected future without further encouragement.

I'm from Georgia. I attended a military school. The significance of this quintessential American institution eluded me at the time. Continuing, he mentioned that he wanted to become a pediatric surgeon "because children fascinate me." The men in his family had fought in the Revolutionary War, also known as the American War of Independence, in 1775, which secured American independence from Great Britain. After residency, he aspired to own a white mansion in Georgia with tall columns at the front, and he desired to marry a Southern belle, much like Scarlett O'Hara in Gone with the Wind.

His lineage and life plan truly impressed me, especially as a newcomer to America. My horizon stretched only to July 1, 1972, when my clinical commitment with Dr. Moore came to an end. However, I aimed to extend it by a year or two to continue my research in his lab. What a peculiar way, in an unusual place, to introduce oneself! It was a time of uncertainty and new beginnings, a feeling that would become familiar during my extensive training.

Howie was a conscientious buddy with the gift of gab—the ability to converse confidently and loudly in a way that made people want to listen and believe. We relied on each other and worked seamlessly as a team during the cardiothoracic surgery rotation. In those early, challenging days, Howie taught me the detailed method of presenting a patient at the bedside. He believed this thorough approach was crucial for effective patient care. When we collaborated, we frequently exchanged information about the patients we shared across various services, keeping each other updated. Since I had missed the orientation session held before I arrived, I didn't know at the time that he'd be my buddy on and off during the next two years.

During the three months on the Thoracic Service, Alden assisted in the operation of six children with pectus excavatum. Throughout this time, he contributed guidance and spoke only to teach and direct the procedure. I found comfort in the calm, reflective atmosphere he projected during the operation.

Although Alden was very generous in taking me through the cases and allowing me to operate, I wasn't enthusiastic about this procedure. Was it that dealing with ribs reminded me of my time on the Ortho Service, or was I starting to miss operating on the abdomen? In retrospect, I believe it was the latter.

During my extensive training, I learned that we were being prepared for an academic surgical career. As stated in the Surgical Credos, "Be helpful to fellow residents who will become your colleagues and friends for life." It was important for us to assist one another.

A few years later, Alden became a professor of thoracic surgery at the University of Colorado, Denver. He was one of the individuals who invited me to join the highly selective, limited-membership Surgical Biology Club II (SB II) of the American College of Surgeons, of which he was a member.

45

DR. ROBERT E. GROSS

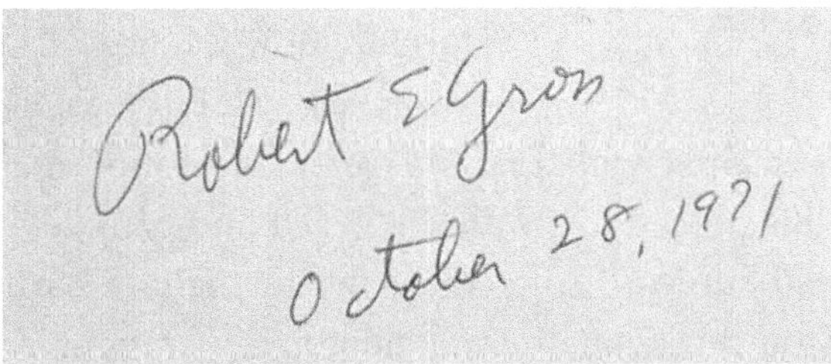

If an operation is hard, then you are not doing it correctly.
—Robert Gross

A pair of white leather lace-up shoes appeared in my O.R. locker, a personal gift from Dr. Robert E. Gross, who was not only the William E. Ladd Professor of Child Surgery at Harvard Medical School and the Children's Hospital but also the Chief of all the Surgical Services at the Children's. I was to wear the white leather lace-ups on his Cardiac Surgery and Thoracic Service with my white pants and coat. I was informed that Dr. Gross expected me to keep them squeaky clean and never allow dried blood on them. Additionally, I was warned that he lived with one of the nurses on his operating room team, Elsie, and that any remarks made during an operation were akin to addressing Dr. Gross himself. Fortunately, we operated silently and only spoke to convey transactional messages.

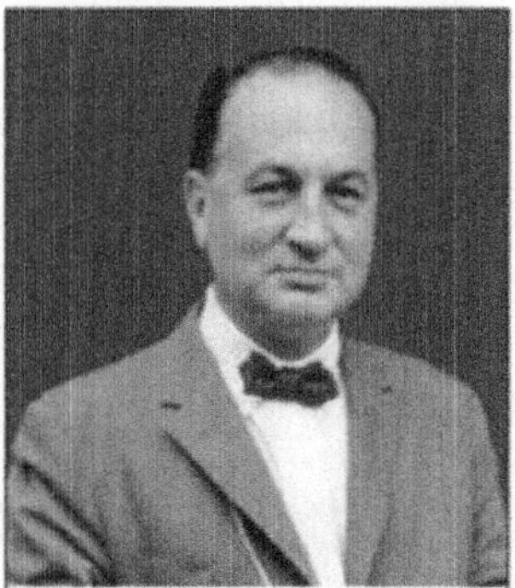

Robert E Gross MD
Chief, Cardio-Thoracic Service

During the seven months I spent on the Cardio-Thoracic Service, I enjoyed working with Dr. Gross. His surgical style was characterized by precision, distinction, joy, and beautiful gestures, which were the envy of most surgeons and something I aspired to emulate. He shared many personal qualities with my former British surgical mentor, Professor Robin Picher. He wielded a scalpel with graceful yet precise movements and executed his procedures with the speed and confidence of an experienced surgeon. After the Schuster fight, I scrubbed in with him on numerous intra-abdominal operations. In these, he also demonstrated the speed and élan of a surgeon well-acquainted with the intricate anatomy of a child's body.

He hardly spoke to me during this time. However, I drew out a smile from him when he saw me buying his "An Atlas of Children's Surgery" at the Co-op. I was thrilled to see his delight when I asked him to sign my copy. Even as he signed, he kept his comments to a minimum. I knew I would enjoy operating with him and his team because I valued a layer of silence to prevent any mistakes. Communicate to instruct. Avoid idle chatter.

My daily reading shifted from general surgery to "The Surgery of Infancy and Childhood, *Its Principles and Techniques*," initially published in the U.S. by W. B. Saunders Company in 1953. It was out of print, and secondhand copies were highly priced. I had to settle for the Asian edition published in Tokyo, as it was less expensive. I used the Atlas daily; it described general surgical, thoracic, and cardiac operations, illustrating each step of each operation in detail. The descriptions of the techniques honed my surgical knowledge and skills. Both books became my bibles, and I integrated the general education and operative skills I learned at the Children's Hospital into my surgical expertise.

Like most other service chiefs, Robert Gross graduated from Harvard Medical School with an M.D. in 1931. Between 1934 and 1936, he conducted research in pathology, focusing on the patent ductus arteriosus anomaly, a short vessel connecting the aorta and pulmonary artery that fails to close at birth. Most infants with this condition died from heart failure, though some lived as cardiac cripples into childhood. Through his research, Dr. Gross discovered a method to tie off the duct, thereby establishing normal surgical circulation. This allows for healthy growth into adulthood if successfully performed on a young child. He repeatedly practiced and perfected the technique on his pathological specimens, but it had yet to be applied to a living patient.

Dr. Elliot Cutler, the chief of surgery at Peter Bent Brigham Hospital from 1932 to 1947, was a renowned cardiac surgeon who performed the world's first successful mitral valvuloplasty in 1923, opening a scarred mitral valve in a patient with mitral stenosis.

Impressed by Robert Gross's ability to successfully ligate a patent ductus between the aorta and the pulmonary artery on a pathological specimen, he offered him a position as a surgical resident in his training program. Both agreed and predicted that ligating a patent ductus would be the world's first successful operation carried out by a surgeon on the large vessels of the heart, bringing fame and prestige. Perhaps Dr. Cutler dreamed of being that surgeon.

During pregnancy, the placenta develops in the uterus, supplying the growing baby with oxygenated blood and nutrients through the umbilical cord. The blood flows into the baby via the right ventricle, from which it is pumped into the pulmonary artery and directed toward the lungs. However, the fetus's lungs are filled with amniotic fluid, preventing the blood from entering them. As a result, blood is redirected away from the lungs through the open duct back to the aorta.

Typically, after birth, the ductus arteriosus closes as the baby brings breathing oxygen, transforming into a fibrous strand that connects the aorta and the pulmonary artery. In approximately 4,000 babies, the ductus arteriosus fails to close, allowing normal circulation to establish while the duct remains open. Consequently, oxygenated blood from the lungs flows through the low-pressure pulmonary artery into the left ventricle. From there, it is forcefully ejected into the high-pressure aorta. However, since the ductus arteriosus remains open, the blood flow short-circuits back into the pulmonary artery. It is recycled to the left ventricle, leading to increased workload and progressive heart failure, ultimately resulting in the child's death.

By 1938, when Dr. Gross was a senior resident, Dr. Cutler appointed him a visiting surgeon at Children's Hospital in Boston. Dr. Gross was consulted by a young pediatrician regarding a patient with patent ductus arteriosus. He examined the patient and recommended surgery to tie off the duct. Under anesthesia, he opened the chest of the seven-year-old girl. He performed the first-ever ligation of the ductus after obtaining permission from the acting chief of surgery at the hospital while Dr. Cutler was away.

However, Dr. Gross's status was that of a senior resident acting as the chief surgical resident, employing a new operative technique that had not yet received formal approval from the relevant authorities! The operation was successful. The girl was out of bed the next day and discharged ten days later. Dr. Gross became an instant pioneer in cardiac surgery. When Dr. Cutler returned, he heard the news. A livid, perhaps even jealous, Dr. Cutler was defeated in the race to be the first to perform this operation.

He fired young Robert Gross.

It's not the first time in medical history that an audacious surgical act has resulted in a firing. In 1929, at the age of 25, while undergoing surgical training in Berlin, Dr. Werner Forssmann inserted a ureteral catheter into his vein. He advanced it into the right atrium of his heart, thus becoming the first person to catheterize a heart. He was fired. In 1956, he won a Nobel Prize in Medicine. This anecdote reminded me of my hilarious and daring use of Dr. Fuller's non-crush clamp to perform circumcisions. It serves as a big hurrah for creative imagination that works. Still, it also serves as a strong reproach for the unethical practice of what is called "independent research on patients and oneself."

The ousted Dr. Gross returned to his home in Vermont and began constructing a barn. Legend has it that when he was lured back to the Children's Hospital as the Chief of Cardiovascular Surgery, he accepted but insisted on completing the barn first.

Dr. Gross successfully operated on ten other children by ligating the ductus. In the case of an eleventh child, the ligature separated two weeks after the procedure, resulting in the child's death from a massive hemorrhage. Following this death, the method was modified. The ductus would be clamped doubly, divided between the clamps, and each end would be sutured or sewn shut.

The high point of a senior or chief resident's experience on Dr. Gross's service was being guided through the division of the ductus by Dr. Gross—the pioneer teaching a disciple! This operation saved countless lives.

I watched with envy because I was only in my third year as a junior resident, destined by Dr. Moore never to have the opportunity to perform one of these procedures with the pioneer. After all, I wasn't going into the field of Thoracic Surgery. However, if a chief thoracic resident suddenly had to drop out for any reason, I could operate my nervousness and junior resident status. Such moments made me reflect on FDR's saying, 'The only thing we have to fear is fear itself.'

On a Monday morning, we operated on a seven-year-old child with a patent ductus arteriosus. She appeared small and vulnerable in her lonely anxiety, lying awake on a pediatric OR table, surrounded by a host of white-clad adults in masks and caps in a silent, white-tiled room where a mysterious formula of equations and numbers had been scrawled with a black Sharpie on the wall for all to see, and where nurses fussed about, attaching patches to her. Only those exchanging transactional messages spoke in low tones. This was the anesthesiologist's moment. We were secondary as surgeons. Dr. Gross's nurse stood beside the young girl, comfortingly touching her shoulder and murmuring words of reassurance that we couldn't hear.

As the patient was gently sedated, Dr. Gross, his chief resident, and I scrubbed in, put on our gowns, and gloved up. The cotton gowns covered our fronts and sides, leaving our backs exposed. We moved toward the table to begin the operation when we received the signal.

We watched the anesthesiologist showcase his artistry as he checked the position of the intra-tracheal anesthesia tube and the aeration of each lung before securely taping the tracheal tube to her upper lip. It was evident that the anesthesiologist and the surgeon were executing a well-rehearsed, choreographed procedure that had been performed to perfection many times before. Once the anesthesiologist was fully satisfied, he straightened up, switched from manually ventilating the patient to using the anesthesia machine, and nodded—at last, the sign!

At this point, the circulating nurse stepped forward. The circulator attached a board to the right side of the table, securing the child's arm and palm in an upward position. She moved a side table with two small cups containing sterile solutions to the side of the arm. Inserting her sponge on a clamp into the clear, sterile Hibiclens solution, she washed, dried, and draped the forearm, exposing the wrist. After this, the chief resident stepped forward and percutaneously inserted a tiny catheter into the patient's right radial artery to monitor blood oxygen levels throughout the operation continuously.

We observed him from the opposite side of the O.R. table. The catheter insertion was challenging; the artery of a seven-year-old girl was smaller than the radial arteries, into which I had repeatedly inserted catheters during my time in the Cardiac Service at Brigham.

Once the chief resident finished that task, he turned to the complex formula of numbers and equations that determined the amount of anticoagulant heparin to inject into the patient. He drew the solution from one of two open containers beside him and injected it into the artery.

We watched in horror as the hand progressively darkened and became jet black, looking like a mummy's petrified hand. He had drawn up and injected the wrong solution—Hibiclens instead of heparin—because the cups were not labeled. Dr. Gross rushed over to examine the little girl's hand, but the damage had been done. Copious amounts of saline, followed by heparin solution, were flushed and infused down the catheter to wash out the poison to save the child's right hand. The black hand gradually became gray like a corpse's, suggesting that a selected degree of tissue death had occurred, eventually leading to some functional loss. Only time would tell the degree of function of her hand.

The chief resident was also a victim of this accident, appearing ashen, pale, and trembling in disbelief over the unfortunate event he had caused. The scrub nurse offered him some orange juice and helped him remove his gown before he left the O.R., likely to pray at his small cemetery of regrets.

Dr. Gross and the team faced a more significant predicament. The child with the patent ductus had experienced a major adverse effect that could potentially result in the loss of her right hand. The dilemma was whether to close the ductus or abort the operation.

Dr. Gross, the anesthesiologist, the scrub nurse, and Elsie huddled around the patient. The group mumbled among themselves. Heads nodded. A consensus had been reached. They separated and returned to their action stations. Was the chief resident coming back? Was this my chance to step forward and do the operation?

The hand remained a dull gray, reminiscent of Fred's hand in medical school. Despite the gloom that enveloped the team like thick fog, the chief resident returned. We all washed, gowned, and gloved once more. Dr. Gross again left his unsterile back exposed. By now, the child's chest had been washed and draped, and everyone took their positions according to their seniority and role. The anesthesiologist was at the head of the table. As a second assistant, my place at the O.R. table was next to Dr. Gross, who faced the chief resident, ostensibly responsible for operating, at least the part involving the dissection of the ductus arteriosus and its division. I stood very close to Dr. Gross, observing the procedure with intense concentration, memorizing every step so that I could perform the entire operation if called upon as a substitute.

Dr. Gross made a curvilinear incision below the girl's left breast, entering the chest by cutting through the intercostal muscles and throughout the length of the third intercostal rib space. He divided the third and fourth costal cartilages. Like the adult operations I had assisted, an intercostal spreader was placed, providing a clear view of the left deflated lung and the large vessels: the aortic arch, the pulmonary vessels, and the heart. The pulmonary artery was as large as the aorta, each measuring approximately 7 mm in diameter, while the left ventricle was enlarged. Dr. Gross and the chief resident could feel a thrill in the surrounding structure while I, pressing closer to Dr. Gross, could hear it. The ductus was enormous and nearly as wide as the diameter of the aorta. I was awestruck to think that this shunt between the two major vessels was the cause of this child's failure to thrive for the past seven years. The resident dissected the ductus, freeing it from the surrounding tissues, while almost skeletonizing it. With each step, the resident looked up to see if Dr. Gross approved. The small space between the aorta and the pulmonary artery was visible.

To see what the resident had dissected, I pressed closer to Dr. Gross. The left half of my body was almost behind his right back as the chief resident placed a clamp on the aortic side of the ductus and another one on the pulmonary side. Once the clamps were in place, the resident accepted a long scalpel with a fresh blade offered to him by the scrub nurse so that he could cut across the ductus. This he did.

As this was happening in front of me, I could see in my peripheral vision that Elsie had placed a green sterile towel over Dr. Gross's back, covering the gap in his gown to prevent contaminating the front of my gown with his back. She attached the towel using two towel clips that had sharp, pointed tips. The first secured the towel to Dr. Gross's gown effortlessly. She placed the second one while the resident was transecting the ductus. The second towel clip pierced Dr. Gross's shirt and penetrated his skin. Without turning around, he sharply commanded, "Take it off." The resident glared at him as Dr. Gross forcefully repeated, "Take . . . the clamp . . . off!"

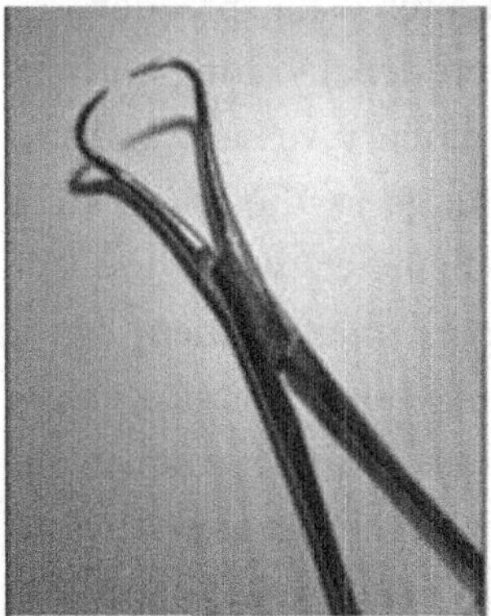

Surgical Towel Clamp

The resident removed the aortic clamp, unleashing a tidal wave of warm red blood that sprayed in all directions, drenching the anesthesia's drape and my glasses.

"Not you, you idiot!" he cried, flinging several surgical towels and sponges into the field to control blood loss, yelling, "The back ones." His immediate response stemmed the massive blood loss; however, the patient's blood pressure fell precipitously. Dr. Gross promptly reapplied the clamp to the aortic side of the ductus, stopping further hemorrhage.

The clamp in his back was removed.

That night, I reflected on the events of the day. The damaged hand was likely due to a rare anatomical anomaly in which, in 10% of patients, the ulnar artery in the hand is underdeveloped. In 90% of cases, the radial artery is the dominant one. This explains why we measured the pulse in the radial artery. The incorrect solution was injected, leading to an immediate adverse effect that frightened me. How many times had I taken medications prepared by nurses, trusting in good faith that what I was injecting into a patient was indeed the medication I had requested? In this instance, the medical error occurred because the two different solutions were not properly labeled. Looking underneath the dressing, I could see the patient's hand was pink and improving. I felt remorse for what I had witnessed and vowed that I would never make this mistake with one of my patients.

The incident lasted only a few blinks of the eye, yet it burned into my brain. I replayed it repeatedly, realizing how my enthusiasm for observing the division of the duct by pressing

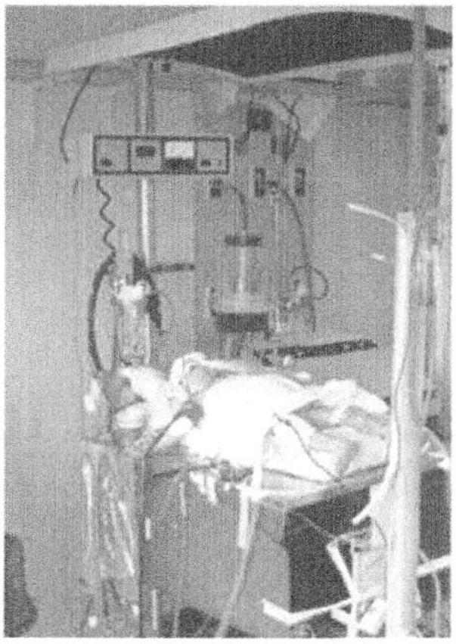

closely to Dr. Gross had inadvertently contributed to the error. Future gowns were designed to wrap around the entire body.

By the end of his career, Dr. Gross had done 1,610 operations with minimal mortality.

The year at the Children's Hospital solidified my ongoing interest in training in Boston. My knowledge and maturity in surgery greatly increased, not only in the operating room but also in my realization that to advance along an academic path, I needed to conduct research. Dr. Folkman made this clear to me. I forged friendships with Alberto and Alden, and I regret not getting to know Mort Kahan, as we never had the opportunity to work together again. I should have better balanced my home and professional life.

46

THE HOLDING UNIT

Wherever the art of medicine is loved,
There is also a love of humanity.
—Hippocrates

My next rotation involved returning to the Brigham Emergency Room. Unlike the Children's, orientation was unnecessary; the Brigham felt like home. One was expected to pick up where one had left off a year earlier.

Dr. Robert Osteen, the senior resident, informed my fellow resident, Howie, and me about the new on-call schedule. The 24-hour on-call hours were divided into 12-hour shifts. I will cover the E.R. from 8 a.m. to 8 p.m. and then go home. While I was in the E.R., Howie covered the Industrial Accident and Surgical Follow-up clinics before transitioning to the E.R. for the night shift and the next day's E.R. day shift, after which he would go home. This meant we were on constant duty for 36 hours and home for 12! We were tough Brigamites.

Nuala gave me a friendly, welcoming hug as I walked into the Emergency Room.

"See," she said, sticking forward her left leg, "it's fixed, thanks to you. I'm back to normal." Still in a playful mood, she said in a sexy voice, slightly lifting her skirt, "Do you want to see where it was done?"

"Oh yes. Show me," I replied, playing along with her. She stepped back and, in her good-humored voice, said, "Over there," pointing to The Pike where the O.R.s were. We burst into laughter, amused by her Irish sense of humor.

"I'm so glad you had it done. You look great. Some operations help patients 100%, and some help the surgeon," I hesitated for the punch line, "100%." Our playful banter attracted attention from those around us, including colleagues and patients, drawing curious looks their way.

"Are you back for a second round of E.R. work?"

"Yep. I genuinely missed the E.R., just interacting with patients and helping them."

"You haven't seen our newly built Holding or Purgatory Unit."

I laughed.

She guided me by the elbow toward an alcove in a spacious room. Eight beds lined the walls of this windowless, rectangular, white-walled ward, four on each side, although it could accommodate twelve beds. Dr. Osteen huddled with the residents from the Ward Service at the foot of a bed, discussing a patient.

During my years away, a much-needed Med-Surg Holding Unit was built next to the Emergency Ward. It addressed a critical need for managing in-house bed utilization at Brigham.

The purpose of this unit was to accommodate overnight patients who were ill but not sick enough to require admission. Bob Osteen held administrative responsibility for supervising surgical patients with ambiguous or poorly defined diagnoses, who were later admitted from the E.R. to the Holding Unit for further observation, examination, and testing. Each late afternoon, Dr. Osteen conducted rounds with either me or Howie on the surgical patients we were overseeing in the unit. The policy was that after three days, the patient had to be transferred to a medical or surgical ward or discharged.

Nuala asked me to see a college student. "You know, from one of our many schools. She lost her tampon. Would you see her, find it, and get her out of here? She's been waiting quite a while and is acutely embarrassed, poor kid."

Mary Lou greeted me shyly, then turned to face the wall, blushing with shame.

"How long ago did you lose it?' I asked.

"The string broke off five days ago," she muttered.

"Let's see what we can do to help you."

Nuala had already placed the young girl in stirrups and covered her with a sheet. I sat down on a stool and scooted between Mary-Lou's legs while Nuala adjusted the light to focus on my patient's perineum. The smell was overwhelming, almost nauseating. I backed off. Nuala gave me a face mask onto which she had squirted 2% Xylocaine, which left a yellow spot and smelled of banana to mask the putrid smell emanating from Mary-Lou's crotch. While Nuala steadied my patient's knees, I slowly inserted a vaginal speculum with flat duckbill blades into Mary-Lou's vagina. Nuala once more adjusted the light. With a pair of forceps, I fished about the apex of the vagina. The smell was overpowering, and the light wasn't optimal. Finally, I saw a crunched-up black object behind the underside of the cervix. I grasped it with forceps and gently withdrew it, placing it into a kidney-shaped dish. Despite the banana smell, the rotting odor from the decaying blood smelled like wet gangrene before an amputation.

"Breathe, honey, just pant. Yes, that's right—just pant. The doctor is finished," Nuala said reassuringly.

"Got it, Mary-Lou. These things sometimes happen," I said,

lying since this was the first time I'd fished something out of a vagina.

"I'm just going to irrigate this area, and you'll be right as rain." After irrigation and suction, I backed out while Nuala finished Mary-Lou's care, gently removing her legs from the stirrups. Turning to me, Nuala asked, "Should we send it to pathology? I mean, there isn't much to see."

Yes, I've already filled out the form. I suppose, for insurance purposes, pathology just has to identify and acknowledge what we removed.

"What a welcome back case!" she said with a wink. "We kept it just for you."

Not infrequently, I encountered surgical patients with atypical abdominal pain that didn't align with the usual pain pattern and wasn't associated with specific diseases. Upon examination, the abdomen wasn't significantly painful, and their physical signs, blood work, and X-rays didn't lead to a definitive diagnosis. Could the abdominal pain be caused by an underlying lung or cardiac issue, pancreatitis, or compromised blood flow to the small bowel? Perhaps it was a small diverticulum perforation in a patient with diverticulitis developing into an abscess, or even typhlitis, a suspected colon inflammation seen in patients with undiagnosed leukemia. The typical clinical features include fever, low white cell count, and vague abdominal pain in the right lower quadrant. Time was necessary to allow the illness to resolve or manifest further.

In the past, we kept them in an E.R. cubicle for 12 to 24 hours while we observed them. We would examine them frequently, repeat their blood work, and look for clues about what illness was developing in their belly. Depending on our findings, we would determine the patient's disposition. With our limited cubicles, this resulted in a backlog of patients who needed to be seen and a long wait in the E.R. to see a doctor.

In the past, we would send patients home and ask them to

return if their condition worsened. Often, we never saw the same patient again. If their symptoms deteriorated, they would seek care at another E.R. and be admitted or even operated on without our knowledge, which was unsatisfactory for us.

Now that we have a holding unit in place, we can admit them for observation. This represents a significant step forward in patient management and care.

Thirty-two-year-old Mary Haskell's primary complaint was a gradual "loss of appetite" accompanied by vague abdominal pain. Her temperature was normal, and neither a repeated abdominal examination, including a pelvic exam, nor her blood work, along with radiological and ultrasound studies of her pancreas and ovaries, provided a definitive clue leading to a diagnosis and treatment. There was too much intra-small bowel gas to visualize the appendix. I was mystified regarding the diagnosis but suspected it to be chronic typhlitis or even appendicitis. From experience, I knew that the vague complaint of "loss of appetite" indicated that not all was well, even if we couldn't identify the cause.

I followed her for three days in the Holding Unit. She gradually felt somewhat better when I asked her, "Are you hungry?" or "Would you like a juicy hamburger?" She repeatedly said no.

If I admitted her with suspected appendicitis, I would not be able to operate because I was in the E.R. and not on the Ward Service. Wanting to solve this mystery, I decided to examine her intra-abdominal organs, particularly her appendix. I consulted a gynecological colleague with whom I had assisted on numerous hysterectomies in the past while on the Ward Service. He came to the E.R. and saw her promptly. He, too, was not impressed by her physical findings.

"I think I'll admit her to my service, and we'll look into her abdomen. If it's appendicitis, you can do it."

I eagerly agreed.

Before the advent of CAT or MRI scans to visualize the

intra-abdominal organs, our only options were to admit her and operate with a presumptive diagnosis of appendicitis or to have the gynecologist insert a scope to examine her internal organs.

Mary Haskell agreed to be admitted.

In the O.R., my gynecological colleague inserted a scope through the umbilicus. The view of the organs left me awestruck. "Wow, this is awesome!" I nearly shouted in my excitement. I saw her uterus, fallopian tubes, and ovaries, all of which appeared normal. I was gazing into the future of laparoscopic surgery.

Standing beside him, I was eager to find out if my suspicion that we were dealing with the unusual condition of chronic appendicitis or typhlitis was accurate. I kept looking through his scope at the various organs. The cecum looked normal. We unraveled this surgical mystery by ruling out suspect organs that could become inflamed and diseased—one by one. At last, we scrutinized the final suspected culprit: a shaggy, thickened, chronically inflamed appendix.

Since laparoscopic surgery was not yet available, I made an incision at McBurney's point in the right lower abdominal quadrant with his assistance, removed a swollen and edematous appendix, and then closed the wound.

The patient was subsequently admitted to the ward service. A few days later, her appetite returned, and she was discharged once she could eat and drink a reasonable amount of food. Many eyebrows were raised at the unusual collaboration between a surgical resident and an attending physician in the gynecological service. When questioned, I explained that the GYN attending had the right tool, namely a laparoscope, and that I had the scalpel.

The case was discussed during M&M, and I had to explain myself to Dr. Moore. The discussion centered on sensitive turf issues: Should a gynecologist assist me in removing an appendix, as I had just done? Did this imply that a general surgeon could now remove an ovary?

A year later, I met Dr. Collins's nurse while walking on The Pike.

"I haven't seen you for some time," she said.

"I spent the last year at the Children's Hospital. I'm back now. How are you?"

"Well, thanks to you . . ."

"Me?"

"Yes, you! Dr. Collins sent me to attend a course in Human Sexuality in California."

"Hah!" I smiled.

There was a positive outcome to my telling Dr. Collins that he should address the frequent questions posed by his patients about when they could have sex after their heart operation. I waved to her as we went our separate ways. She was one of my favorite nurses—always smiling, friendly, and attentive to the needs of patients and residents. Now, with her knowledge of Human Sexuality, she would answer this question for Dr. Collins's patients.

The issue of sex arose with most of my patients during my career. To my chagrin, like Dr. Collins, I neglected to address the topic of human sexuality with many patients until the husband of a seventy-two-year-old woman asked me, "When can we resume sex?" I was taken aback by his frankness and embarrassed by my failure to address the matter. As a young surgical attendant, it didn't occur to me that elderly couples engaged in sexual activities. Boy, was I mistaken. "Whoever said money makes the world go round forgot about sex."

47

FOLLY OR PAYBACK?

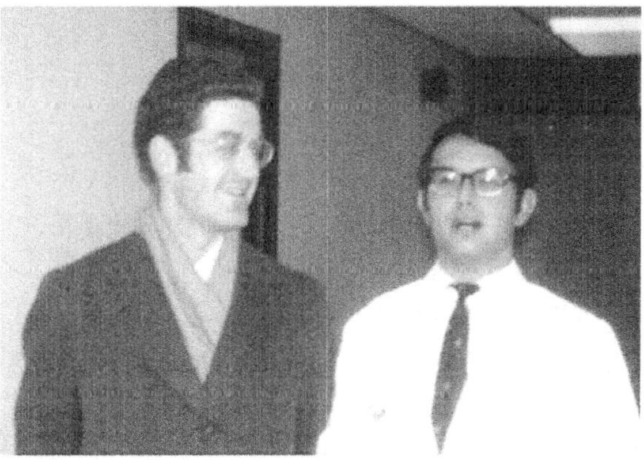

Drs. Howard McCormick III & Michael Meguid

To err is human. To forgive is against departmental policy.
—Anonymous

Since some patients who came to the E.R. didn't have a primary attending physician, we would follow up with them after their initial E.R. visit, usually to remove sutures, change dressings, adjust medications, or, if needed, order additional blood tests or follow-up X-rays.

When I saw patients in the Follow-up Clinic, I would end my note by writing 'RTC 1/12,' meaning 'returns to the clinic in one month,' just as I had done at the Children's and in England. The E.R. secretary interpreted this to mean that I wanted the patient to return on January 12th of the following year. This became apparent when she told me that on January 12th, I would have a bumper clinic, as many patients would be returning that day! We laughed heartily at the error caused by different cultural interpretations.

During the third week of December, Howie approached me. "Hey, Mike. What do you think if I take a week off and you cover both the E.R. and the clinic, which is pretty light work, and then when I come back, I'll cover both, and you have a week off?"

"You mean a break, like a holiday?"

"Yeah."

"And is that legal? I mean, permitted. You are a categorical resident and safe. You are part of the Harvard establishment. I'm only provisional and could be fired, so I'm at greater risk. Shouldn't we clear this with our chief resident, Bob Osteen, who is a congenial and pleasant colleague?"

"As long as both clinics are covered and the work gets done, no one will know, no one will care, and we'll both have an extra week of vacation during this festive season. I'll go down to Georgia to see my southern belle, and you can see your folks in England," he said confidently.

"Sounds too good to be true, Howie."

"It'll work. We'll be OK," he reassured me in his deep Southern voice.

"Let me check with my wife, and I'll get back to you."

Victoria and I discussed the issue from various perspectives. A one-week holiday just before Christmas with our family, whom we hadn't seen since leaving England, was appealing, primarily since Victoria could obtain two relatively inexpensive coach tickets on BOAC (British Overseas Airways Corporation), as British Airways was then called. She scheduled a week off and ensured that our passports had the necessary documents to allow us to return to Boston and continue our studies.

Howie and I agreed to execute our plan. I drew the short straw and chose to work from Monday night through the following Monday morning of the week before Victoria was free, during the third week of December, one week before Christmas. "Well then, I'll take the week before you go," Howie said with a smile.

Howie disappeared on Monday evening, along with his radio and favorite Howard Cosell. I covered his night call, which was busy until about 11 p.m. Then, sporadically, every few minutes or hours, the night nurse would open the door of the on-call room and yell, "You have a patient waiting."

On this occasion, it was an overweight man with an impressively large belly, coming off a late day shift, complaining of back pain in the lumbosacral area. I ordered a set of back X-rays, which took almost an hour to obtain—too short to lie down again and too long to wait in the E.R. When he was eventually wheeled back from X-ray with his films, they showed some degenerative disc disease and a significant degree of lumbar lordosis or extension, likely compressing a lumbar disc that impinged on a nerve. I showed him the films in the faint hope it might motivate him to moderate his food intake, lose weight, and relieve the pressure on the spinal nerve. I gave him some pain meds to take immediately and a prescription for the following days, then referred him to the orthopedic attending on-call for follow-up.

I returned to my bed in the E.R. on-call room. While drifting off to sleep again, I thought my hope that the patient might lose weight was silly. How many patients had I seen here and in England who expressed this desire to drop a few pounds? It seemed part of modern humanity's daydream, as even I sometimes worried about gaining a pound or so, despite being frantically busy.

An on-call pattern formed in my mind when the 24-hour E.R. traffic was slow, guiding me to potential windows of time when I could shower and shave in the morning, eat breakfast, change into fresh clothes, sneak off to lunch, or take a bathroom break; when I could squeeze in a cat nap for 10 or 20 minutes (with the cooperation of the E.R. nurses); and when I could have dinner. Initially, a couple of nurses asked me where Howie was, and I'd say we changed on-call schedules. I wasn't keen on having our arrangement known. Between E.R. cases, I attended to patients in the Resident's Follow-up Clinic and the Industrial Accident Clinic, working with Bob Osteen. Fortunately, he didn't ask questions about Howie, although he must have wondered why I showed up every day.

From day to day, I toiled like the Energizer Bunny, as the days flowed into nights filled with unpredictable amounts of rest and sleep, which merged into another full day of handling emergency cases, broken up by erratic meals and insufficient drinking water. The workload began to take its toll. I couldn't remember the day or the patients I had seen. One day morphed into another night, and the demand for my sleep became progressively greater. Was the nurse's call about a patient needing to be seen a dream or reality? Did I jump out of bed to respond to the nurse's call immediately, or had I fallen asleep again? Had the night nurse called me twice, or was that my imagination? Thus, seven days passed as I transformed from a mindful human surgeon into a sleep-deprived robotic zombie, healing and caring for patients on autopilot. I skipped breakfast, showering, and shaving to grab a few more minutes of sleep. I lived on coffee and the knowledge that when Howie returned Monday, I'd be free to rejoin the normally functioning human race.

Howie reappeared in high spirits, talking even faster than

usual about everything he had done. A haggard version of myself vanished and went home, where I declined the lunch my dear wife had packed for me, opting instead for a four-hour nap, a shower, a cup of tea, and some clean clothes. She drove us to the airport, arriving two hours early for our 8 p.m. flight to Gatwick Airport in England so we could secure two exit seats with more legroom for the overnight flight.

The clerk at the check-in desk, dressed in a BOAC uniform and resembling a stewardess, was astonished when she saw our tickets and said, "Goodness. Two Doctor Meguids."

While she fussed over checking our passports and tagging our two bags, I asked her, "Could we have two seats in the exit row?"

"I'm just looking," she replied. There was a pause as she tapped the keyboard. The pause grew longer as she made a phone call. Two more ground crew members appeared at the desk. They spoke while pointing to the seating plan. We began to wonder what the problem was; boarding passes were usually issued quickly.

"Is there a problem with our tickets?" I asked, fearing the worst.

"No, not really. Except we don't have seats for you," she revealed, shattering our expectations and leaving us in disbelief.

My heart sank. "How can that be? We booked some time ago," I stated as a more experienced ticket agent joined the others at the counter.

Together, they reviewed the seating plan in a huddled discussion.

"It reminds me of the problem we had with BOAC in Antigua after our honeymoon almost five years ago when we were trying to return to London," Victoria told me. I nodded, feeling more agitated and frustrated. My chronic sleep deprivation didn't help my anxious mood.

Turning to Victoria, I said quietly, "It's good we came early. It looks like they've overbooked the flight," I added. "I want to get a seat so I can sleep."

"We're so sorry about the delay in finding your seats; we have a huge party on board. We're working on seating you. In the meantime, can we invite you to wait in our private Executive Lounge until it's time to fly?" said the senior Stewardess, leading us down a corridor to a BOAC Private Lounge. Ushering us in, she pointed to the bar, "Do help yourself to a drink. It's complementary," she added. We were the only passengers in a large windowless room.

Victoria sat down with a copy of Vogue. I was parched and gravitated toward an expansive self-serve bar that impressively occupied an entire wall of the room. As I looked around for some water to quench my chronic thirst, a bottle of Jack Daniel's whiskey caught my eye. Instead of water, I decided to kill two birds with one stone. Make yourself a drink, I thought, to satisfy my thirst and unwind from an endless week.

I dissolved two sugar cubes by adding a little water to a whiskey glass, then added two dashes of Angostura bitters. After that, I filled the glass with small ice cubes, poured a generous amount of whiskey, and finally added a piece of orange peel. The aroma of my Old Fashioned was exquisite, and each sip was divine. The thought of John Rackey crossed my mind, along with his lessons on how to make this drink.

Not realizing how dehydrated and thirsty I was, I drank it instead of sipping it as I sat beside Victoria. "I nearly forgot to tell you that John Rackey telephoned me some time ago."

"What did he say? How are they, Margaret and their two girls?"

I couldn't talk to him. I was between cardiac cases, rushing along The Pike from the I.C.U. to the second case. I said I'd call him back. I meant to, but I was overwhelmed, and I forgot. When I called the following day, there was no answer or a message on the machine. I was beginning to feel fatigued. The ongoing stress of the past week was catching up with me, affecting my thought process.

Another passenger had joined us in the lounge; it was now 7:30 p.m.

Victoria didn't want a drink, so I made another Old Fashioned and sipped it more slowly. Turning to Victoria, I said, "He seemed agitated."

Looking up from her magazine, she said, "Who?"

"John Rackey, of course. Who do you think we were talking about? He seemed agitated, and his voice was urgent, as if he wanted to discuss something. I wish I had talked to him."

At first, she didn't respond and said, "You know those drinks are strong."

"Margaret did write to me," I said, sitting with my eyes closed.

"Margaret?"

"Yeah. John committed suicide."

"When?"

"It would be about a year ago now."

"And you didn't tell me?"

"Sorry, I forgot. I've been working nonstop for quite a while. And now I've got a tremendous headache. Remind me in England, and I'll tell you," I whispered.

The other passenger stood up and left the lounge; it was 20 minutes to eight. We chose to wait for the agent, so I poured myself another drink. It tasted delightful, and the sugar was invigorating since I hadn't eaten much all day.

We were growing increasingly worried. No BOAC personnel had entered this glamorous waiting room since we had been shunted in. It was nearly 7:50 p.m., and the flight was set to leave in ten minutes. Had they forgotten about us?

Just then, the door opened, and the supervisor walked in.

"We're terribly sorry you've had to wait so long." We stood

up, gathering our hand luggage, unsure of what would happen next. I drained my glass.

"We're ready to go. We found you two tickets in first class, and we'd like to apologize for the inconvenience," she announced, handing us the boarding passes. A wave of relief washed over us as we realized we were about to travel in comfort, away from the busy coach section.

Victoria and I exchanged glances, hardly believing our luck —residents traveling first class again, just like on our Mexico trip! It was a moment of sheer disbelief. Wow, being a doctor must be a very prestigious profession.

We thanked her, boarded the plane, and settled into our seats, the only empty ones in first class. It was a luxurious experience, featuring plush leather seats and ample legroom located in the third row from the bulkhead.

There was a movie screen in front of us. As we settled in, the purser (head steward) welcomed us aboard and handed us the menu. He then asked Victoria, seated by the window, "Can I get you a glass of Dom Pérignon 1968, madam?"

"Thank you. That would be lovely."

Turning to me in my aisle seat, I nodded yes before he had time to ask.

I studied the exquisite menu, which featured only the foods we could dream of enjoying one day when we became affluent. After being starved and barely eating for the past week, the promised evening meal made my mouth water.

Before I could study the breakfast menu, the steward returned with two glasses of Dom Pérignon. Victoria and I toasted to our health, well-deserved rest, and good fortune at being in First Class once again. I wasn't fond of Champagne, but feeling thirsty, I downed my bubbly.

Appetizers

Caviar

Presented with a traditional selection of finely chopped chives, grated egg, sour cream and lemon, served with melba toast and blinis.

Cream of mushroom soup

Topped with chives.

Salad

Seasonal leaves served with dressing.

Main Course

Pan-fried beef tenderloin

Served with jus lié, steamed snow peas, carrots and new potatoes with herbs.

London chicken

Chicken in a traditional British spice marinade, served on aromatic rice with fried onions and pistachios.

Pan-seared salmon trout

Served with mashed potatoes, sautéed kailan and beurre blanc with roasted almonds.

All our meals are served with freshly baked bread.

Dessert

Orange frangipane tart

Served with citrus compote.

Chocolate tart

Layered chocolate and orange mousse topped with dark chocolate ganache, served with citrus jellies.

Seasonal fruit

An assortment of fresh cut fruit

Cheese board

A carefully chosen assortment of fine boutique cheeses from around the world, served with crackers and accompaniments.

Chocolates

A voice came onto the PA system. “This is your captain. We have a problem with engine number two. We’ve ordered a replacement, which is coming from JFK in New York.”

“This will probably delay us by about two hours. I’ve given the purser and the ladies in coach the green light to proceed with the meal service, giving you more time to sleep. In the meantime, I’ll keep you updated as we change engines.”

Suddenly, I started to feel unwell. Fatigue washed over me like a giant tidal wave. I sank deeper into my seat, longing to lie flat. Only my seatbelt prevented me from slipping onto the cabin floor as the world around me gradually began to fade to black. First, my hearing blurred into the noise surrounding me, and then my eyelids became overwhelmingly heavy—heavier than lead. A buzz filled my head, dissolving any memory of time or place as I drifted into a state of disconnection from the moment. I wanted nothing more than to sleep. To be dead to the world.

The last thing I remember was the empty champagne glass falling to the cabin floor and Victoria's voice.

"Are you all right?"

"Unnhh?" No further answer.

That's all I remember. I was out, swimming in my mind in a continuous, dark, cold world, occasionally hearing the clink of cutlery.

A man knelt in the aisle, asking if I had any pain. I was unable to respond. I couldn't even open my eyes. It wasn't a dream. He took my pulse and blood pressure and listened to my heart while speaking into a phone, transmitting my biometrics to some distant place.

Victoria's voice, "He's a surgical resident at the Brigham and very tired . . . Was on duty for one whole week . . . Didn't get much sleep . . . Probably the alcohol . . . Yes, he's my husband . . . No, he has no medical history . . . He takes no meds . . . Just was awake most of last week . . . Now, too much to drink."

The male voice repeated everything over a static-filled radio. As quickly as he had appeared, I heard him groan as he rose from the aisle.

"He'll be OK."

I briefly managed to open my eyes as I became aware of the man who had leaned over me, watching him leave. The commotion around me faded. I could sleep, reeling in my world of unfamiliar alcohol intoxication.

I woke suddenly to the cabin's darkness, coldness, and the noise of the jet engines.

Refreshed.

Cold.

Shivering.

Starving.

The cabin was dark. Victoria was asleep, leaning against the window on a pillow. All the passengers around me were asleep except for the lady in 5A, who had her reading light on. I turned mine on as well and signaled to the purser. He arrived.

I smiled. "I'm starving. Could I please have the caviar and the beef tenderloin, followed by the orange frangipane tart?"

"Under the circumstances, sir, I think the best thing for you would be some tea and toast."

And that's what I received. I was too embarrassed to ask for chocolate. I found it frustrating that he judged me. I had worked hard to care for patients—older men like him—and all he offered me was tea and toast, which was a definite disappointment. It was a moment of great sorrow during which I felt disgraced and humiliated. However, the tea and toast were divine.

Shirley was pleased to see us. She was in a good mood and emotionally stable. She quizzed her daughter about our life in Boston while we enjoyed her wholesome cooking. Victoria and I have been able to sleep together in her house since getting married. I spent a lot of my time catching up on sleep. On two occasions, I jumped out of bed in the middle of the night yelling, "I'm coming, I'm coming . . . " believing the E.R. night nurse had called me to see a patient. Victoria jumped out of bed, crying, "It's O.K., it's O.K., you're at home, come back to bed." She grabbed me by my pajamas just in time, for I had reached the landing at the top of the staircase. She held me back from tumbling down.

For the next 30 years, we would go to the Isle of Wight for

each summer vacation because "it could be granny's last summer."

Upon returning and resuming my E.R. duties, Dr. Osteen asked, "Did you have a good time?" He noticed the surprise on my face. "We were looking for you. Howard," and I noted the formal use of his name, "got a sore throat and became sick on Tuesday. He couldn't function most of the week, so I did both his work and mine."

Howie, you wimp! How could you get sick? I couldn't process that he didn't have the guts to push through. Even if you're dying, keep your end of the bargain—you, the one who boasted of having gone to military school. Didn't they teach you honor? As a provisional resident, I am expendable and must appear as the clever conniver working the system. In contrast, feeble Howie, under the protective gown of a categorical resident, was the poor victim of my scheming. What a twerp!

I awaited the reprimand, the humiliating thunder and lightning, the mandatory smack on my bare backside as vindictively delivered by the head boy at the English School in Cairo, or the call to the grammar school headmaster's office in Manchester for a verbal reprimand. Worse, I anticipated a disciplinary, angry rant from Dr. Moore, which would lead to shame, embarrassment, and rejection, followed by a disciplinary letter and dismissal.

What would I do then? I spiraled into despair. I felt the intense insecurity of social anxiety, anger, and the loneliness of the situation I was in. I could not eat, sleep, focus, or confront Victoria, fearing a lecture instead of a sympathetic hug. I had probably burned my bridges by leaving London. I couldn't see the security advantage of having passed the Primary FRCS. I had squandered the opportunity for an interview with Professor Wilkinson and the job offer from Professor Clark. It was never a good time to be fired, especially now, considering that Victoria was in the middle of her pediatric residency and doing well. Where would I go? Who would console me? Who would give me another chance at residency?

After a while, reason told me I was merely a body, a clog in the system's wheel. The system needed me, so my firing wouldn't be abrupt. The system would extract its payback. Yet, my folly of trusting Howie to keep his bargain and failing to be present when needed—the infamous AWOL—would leave another stain on my record, counted against me when the two-year commitment was over.

One thing was for sure: I couldn't count on Howie in this highly competitive work environment. I had to push through on my own to avoid the stigma and shame of being unable to fulfill my commitments. Therefore, I was glad to move on to my next rotation and work with friends again.

Fifty years later, Howard called me at home in Marco Island. After some polite chatter, he apologized for letting me down. There is a difference between offering an apology and the other person accepting it. That's the grudge one carries if the apology isn't accepted. Upon hearing his offer, I accepted it. A few months later, he died.

48

SYMPHONY OF SORROWS

A physician is obligated to consider more than a diseased organ,
more even than the whole man.
He must view the man in his world.
—Harvey Cushing

Burbank Hospital was about fifty miles northwest of Boston, situated in Fitchburg, Middlesex County. This community hospital did not have living quarters, so I drove to and from the hospital daily. Each day, I could see the visible changes of the seasons outside my VW Bug window. I cherished the late winter drive as spring approached, filling me with hope for a better year ahead.

I collected my thoughts of the day while driving through the leafy darkness of still-sleepy Brookline. Turning onto Route 9 and heading west, I accelerated onto Route 128, staying within the speed limit. As I played Tchaikovsky's Symphony No. 6 on my tape deck, I was enveloped by its intense Allegro non troppo. The piece began with a solitary bassoon, foretelling a dark aura, which was lifted by a cascade of furious strings struggling against the blasting wind instruments, together creating a tempestuous and dramatic mood.

This exquisite orchestral music, aptly named the Pathétique —a Franco-Russian term meaning passionate or emotional— conveys a sense of existential torment that reflects my feelings about the residency. The music illustrates the intense clash between the orchestra's booming wind instruments, which rattled my windows and uplifted my spirits, and the pronounced, frantic struggle of the strings that resonated in my ears as I experienced the powerful and loud musical conflict descending into darkness.

The stark reality of being a provisional resident alternated with my fleeting hopes for acceptance and advancement to a categorical resident. The music resonated with my mood swings, which were soothed by the medicine of operating. This freed me from the constraints of the Brigham program, allowing me to exercise the full extent of my surgical craft and care for patients like those I'd operate on during this exciting rotation at a community hospital.

The music was like the cool morning air whizzing past me as I turned off Route 128 to take Route 2, heading Northwest toward Fitchburg. As I was about to go under the Route 128 bridge, I saw a tornado in the otherwise bluish-gray sky heading northward in front of me.

The wind funnel twisted in the distance, perhaps a mile away. The car began to buckle back and forth as I felt the pressure shift in my eardrums. I veered onto the road's shoulder, parked, got out, and ran a few feet ahead into the shadow of the overhead bridge before flinging myself into a ditch. The twisting wind, swirling with leaves and dust, whisked over me and moved away. When calm returned, I cautiously got up and approached my car. The traffic flow resumed, and I maneuvered into it, knowing I was about 15 minutes late. Were the Pathétique and the Twister omens of work to come at Burbank?

Arvin Phillipart was my senior resident. I had worked with him at the Children's Hospital, and he was one of my favorite Brigham seniors. He fully trusted me, which boosted my self-confidence and motivated me to give my all to this rotation.

Dr. Ross, the chief of surgery, reflected Dr. Moore in looks, speech, and mannerisms, but not in intellect or curiosity. Like most Brigham-trained alumni, he remained a friend of Dr. Moore. He was tall and lean, wearing horn-rimmed glasses with worn leather patches on the elbows of his herringbone jacket. A thoughtful man of few words, he operated in stillness, like the desert in Egypt, the silence of the afternoon heat that suspended thought in Cairo. Unlike Arvin, who was interested in thoracic surgery and handled those cases, Dr. Ross was a skilled general surgeon. Early on, I learned that he was awkward in the O.R., fussy, and tended to micromanage the nurses, who didn't show affection toward him because he was a cold fish. In my mind, after giants like Drs. Collins, Murray, Folkman, Peña, Gross, and even Filler, he lacked the self-assurance of a surgeon, which he concealed behind a screen of few words.

Burbank offered an excitingly steep clinical and surgical learning curve. I was like a joyful kid in a candy store, being taken through and assisting with a wide range of operations that spanned the spectrum of a community's surgical problems. My experience propelled me into almost vertical growth, like a rocket into the stratosphere of routine operations. I cut skin, dissected tissue, clamped off structures, divided them, tied off vessels, removed diseased organs or structures, and closed many abdomens to the tempo of the music that still filled my ears.

Similar to my earlier experience in the Ward Service, I was closely supervised throughout each operation, but was also given the autonomy to follow up on patients post-operatively. The daily notes and blood work I gathered after assisting a patient provided the private surgeons with a clear picture of my pre- and post-operative skills. I helped them save time for office work or an extra cup of coffee at home. The range of my surgical activities is best described in the letter I sent to Dr. Ross upon completing my rotation:

Dear Dr. Ross,
Per your request, I have enclosed my operating list. I performed 130 operations on 111 patients. The discrepancy arises because several patients underwent multiple procedures, such as a cholecystectomy, an appendectomy, and a tubal ligation in one case. All patients who had a tubal ligation also underwent an appendectomy when the organ was present. A few patients had their original colostomy sites revised. In contrast, some patients had a hernia repaired, along with varicose vein stripping in women or a vasectomy in men.

The most common operation I performed was a hernia repair—about twenty-four, mostly proper, indirect, inguinal hernias. The second most common procedure I assisted on with the attending surgeon was cholecystectomy, varicose vein ligation with stripping of the veins, and D&Cs in non-pregnant women. One of the most memorable operations was a transthoracic hiatal hernia repair in a patient with a lower esophageal

Schatzki's ring (an abnormal ring of tissue narrowing the esophagus at the stomach).

Among the most exciting operations was an exploratory laparotomy for the perplexing diagnosis of hematemesis [profuse bleeding via the rectum], accompanied by melena [black, tarry stools] and a hematocrit of 20. During an upper GI endoscopy, we finally identified a peptic ulcer. While we worked up this patient, we replaced his blood volume over 18 hours. Throughout this period, his hematocrit levels fluctuated between 18% and 25%. A gastrectomy was performed, which effectively stopped the bleeding.

By far, the most pleasing operations were four caesarian sections. The birth of a healthy, wanted, and loved baby remains one of the most emotionally gratifying experiences. From the perspective of a junior resident, the more fundamental to personal growth were the numerous new operating procedures I was introduced to for the first time. These included several hemorrhoidectomies with Dr. Rollo, a couple of simple mastectomies, numerous hysterectomies, a vena cava clipping for severe pelvic thromboembolism, and a suprapubic prostatectomy. In the latter case, the tip of the latex glove on my index finger was cut off. Using my naked finger, I then enucleated the prostate with the nail of my bare finger.

The aura of the operating room has attracted me ever since I was eleven years old, when I underwent an appendectomy in Cairo. As a second-year medical student, I've been holding retractors and observing countless operations. I read up on each and would dry-run them on paper. But here at Burbank, under the careful guidance of your staff, I was allowed to operate. The tremendous sense of satisfaction quelled the frustrations that had accrued since my early days as a medical student. My childhood dreams of becoming a surgeon are becoming a reality. Also, the nursing staff at Burbank Hospital do a tremendous job; they are courteous, knowledgeable, and helpful.

I wish to thank you for the opportunity and experience I had while working with you. I learned a great deal from you, and I believe I made a constructive contribution to Burbank Hospital's continued excellent reputation.

Sincerely yours,
Michael Meguid

```
PS: Thank you for giving me time off to
spend Christmas with my wife.
```

One concern I didn't mention was my apprehension about a nagging ethical question regarding the removal of a normal appendix alongside a primary diseased organ, such as in a cholecystectomy or tubal ligation. I understood that the private surgeon was accommodating the patient; however, given the very high frequency of adhesions that develop in the abdomen after an operation—up to 80% later in life, according to the American College of Surgeons—these can cause bowel obstruction, acute abdominal pain, and a diagnostic dilemma, which made me cautious about the automatic removal. Did the patient have appendicitis? Patients often did not remember that their appendix had been removed, and there was no scar to confirm this. But that was back when CTs and MRIs didn't exist.

As a second-year resident, I observed the reality of community surgical practice, free from the constraints of academia, and aimed to learn rather than question or critique. After all, I aspired to be like them—in the trenches of surgery—competent, average, practical surgeons, marginally constrained by questionable ethical operations.

49

THOSE PESKY HEMORRHOIDS

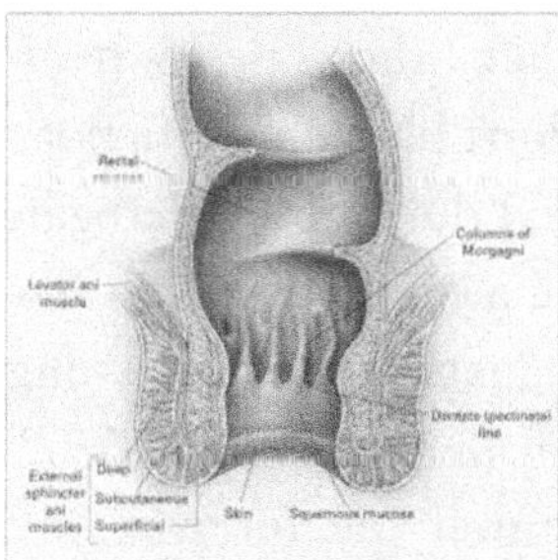

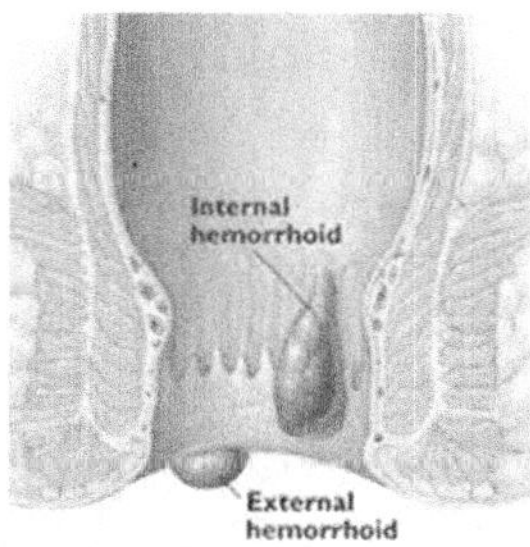

graphic credit: Mayo Clinic

Why do they call it an asteroid when it's outside the hemisphere,
But call it a hemorrhoid when it's in your ass?
—Ano Nymous

The eccentric lecturer, wearing a short white coat that signified he was a surgical registrar at the University College Hospital, insisted on pronouncing "canal" to rhyme with "anal"—A-nal KAYnal—eliciting loud chuckles from the medical students, predominantly men in the audience. Thus, an anatomy lecture on the anal canal began during medical school nearly seven years ago.

"While the A-nal KAYnal is only one and a half inches long,

it is a wondrous structure that terminates at the 30-foot-long GI tube. The GI tube starts at the stomach, includes the lengthy small intestine, the shorter large colon which contains the rectum, and the A-nal KAYnal, which ends at the anal verge," he said.

He enthusiastically lectured as we sat attentively in the amphitheater, taking notes. He began drawing the anal canal in 3D with various colors on the chalkboard. "It is as clever as your index finger," he proclaimed, turning his head over his right shoulder as he drew. "It can distinguish air from liquids and solids." Then, he recited a soliloquy he had written, intending to hold his students' attention.

My name is A-nal KAYnal. It's OK; you can snicker; for although you chuckle, you seldom think of me except when my cousin Royd and his twin brothers, those pesky hemorrhoids Frick and Frack, act up. Please don't blame me; it's not my fault. It's no use calling me an asshole; I don't find it derogatory. It's a compliment, a celebrated name, a noble name, invoked many times in the world, in lots of languages, numerous tongues, but most regally sounding in guttural German: 'Asch Loch!'

By that time, he had captured my interest. My female colleagues murmured in disapproval, while my classmates giggled with delight. We sat listening as he continued his monologue. I wondered if I should be taking notes.

He resumed, "I am bathed in blue blood. I am nobility. Show me a King or Queen, president, consort, or Nobel Laureate living without me or someone in Holy Orders who doesn't lust for me. I was with you when you won the Fulbright and Rhodes, the Grammy and Oscar, the Pushcart, Pulitzer, and Booker Prize."

He continued, "Adam and Eve showed a fascination for me and, in the process, discovered tomfoolery. I've traveled and lured travelers to find comfort and relief while in the remoteness of Bedouin caravans, in the privacy of deep-sea subs, and

while on the dark side of the moon. I was there when explorers discovered the Americas. I lived in Samaria, the Gobi, and Antarctica. I'm immortalized by gonorrhea, feared for HIV, honored by herpes, and flattered by flatulence. I'm the nexus, the tunnel, the conveyor of crap, the doyen of diarrhea, and the fashioner of farts, linking mouth to anus."

My fellow students and I stopped scribbling and listened intently to the lecturer—now comedian. He finished his 3D color drawing and recited the importance of the A-nal KAYnal.

We cheered.

He bowed gracefully.

In a twist of mannerism, his voice became serious as he reviewed the anatomy, pointing to the dentate line. "It divides the A-nal KAYnal into an upper one-third and a lower two-thirds." The upper zone is lined by simple columnar epithelial cells with long folds of mucosal lining that end in anal glands that secrete lymph." He paused and looked at the audience, riveted in their seats on the wooden benches. Then, as if sharing a surgical trade secret, he lowered his voice and said, "The upper part is supplied by the superior rectal artery, which I've drawn here," raising his voice, "but essentially, this segment of the A-nal KAYnal is also not sensitive to needles. A cancer growing in this area will metastasize or spread to the lymph gland in the abdomen." He sounded serious, and I took the appropriate notes.

The lower part is also divided into two sections by the white line of Hilton, which forms the boundary between the anus and the skin. For those interested in money," there were cheers in the audience, including me. "Above it, the mucosa isn't sensitive to needles. We listened below . . ." he stopped. He hesitated, "A needle prick will make your patient howl with pain because the mucosa is more sensitive than the skin. After all, its embryonic origin is skin.

Lowering his voice again, he whispered, "A patient in pain

means they'll be reluctant to pay. So, the sensible thing is to numb it with Lidocaine." I scribbled furiously. "But even more importantly, a cancer in this area drains to the lymph glands around the pubic bone—the famous inguinal lymph nodes." As he spoke, he drew an arrow to the superficial inguinal nodes beneath the skin of the groin.

We shuffled about in our seats. "The blood supply here is significant. It spells money," he said, pointing to his diagram. "Here is the inferior rectal artery and its accompanying rectal veins that bulge and bleed—the three pesky piles, or Royd, Frick, and Frack, that are internally causing painless bleeding, itchiness, and trouble sitting." We sat in anticipatory hush.

"The enlarging uterus during pregnancy increases intra-abdominal pressure, causing these veins to dilate, become tortuous, and bleed. Additionally, many trumpet players, weightlifters, or individuals with advanced liver disease have a higher risk of hemorrhoids, while cancers in this area spread directly to the liver." He paused again, viewing his diagram over his shoulder, then turned to us, saying, "Regarding money," he paused, "Ladies and gentlemen can easily survive without annoying, painful hemorrhoids. But surgeons can do so only with great difficulty unless they can operate on them."

The class cheered once more.

Reliving that lively anatomical lecture on the anal canal felt like a dream as I assisted Dr. Rollo with a hemorrhoid operation time and again, performing them under his supervision. He took the time to teach a very logical method for conducting this operation. I named the procedure "Dr. Rollo's Painless Internal Hemorrhoidectomy," and it has served me well throughout my years of operating. I have also enjoyed teaching it to generations of residents.

Once the patient has been anesthetized and intubated to ventilate the lungs, they are positioned in a lithotomy position by raising the table to the surgeon's eye level and tilting the head down. The circulating nurse secures the patient's legs in stirrups, similar to how it is done in gynecological procedures.

Dr. Rollo then dilated the anus by inserting first one well-lubricated, gloved finger. Then two fingers, gradually proceeding to dilate and relax the anal opening until there was space for his well-lubricated fist to fit into the opening of the anal verge—the five-finger dilatation. "After all," he told me, "a woman dilates much wider to let the baby's head and shoulders through her vagina."

When he finished, the circulating nurse cleaned and dried the perineum. Sterile leggings were draped over each limb, and sterile drapes were placed under the buttocks. A lithotomy drape covered the area except for a square window over the perineal region, providing visibility and access to the anus.

Dr. Rollo first inserted a hemorrhoidal retractor. After opening its duckbill, I, the assistant, held it in position to provide him with a perfect view of the anal canal and the upper part of the rectum. Standing to his left and peeking with my right eye, I could see what the master surgeon was doing more or less.

With the patient's back and nose facing upwards in the 12 o'clock position, the internal hemorrhoids are positioned at the 4, 7, and 11 o'clock locations. These anatomical sites remain relatively constant as they correspond to the arrangement of the hemorrhoidal veins descending from the gut's blood supply. Occasionally, an accompanying artery lies beneath the vein and is not easily visible. Dr. Rollo would then inject the base of each hemorrhoid with a premixed combination of 1% lidocaine and 1:50,000 epinephrine to cause the venous structures to constrict, limit their bleeding, and provide temporary numbness and paralysis to the rectal wall.

"When you do this," he said, "make sure you don't advance the needle tip of your syringe too far into the base of the hemorrhoids." He continued, "Remember Alcock's or pudendal canal?"

"Remind me."

He placed my finger against the back wall of the canal and pressed it down. I could feel a bony groove on either side of the pelvis.

"I feel the canal," I said, pleased to connect an anatomical fact from the past to its practical application.

"Well, the pudendal nerve lies within the canal. It runs toward you through the perineum muscles, accompanied by the perineal artery, and supplies not only sensation to the anal skin but also innervates the sphincters for the bladder and the rectum. If you advance your needle too far and hit the bone while injecting, then you'll paralyze the bladder muscle and prevent the bladder from contracting, so the patient won't be able to urinate for quite some time."

He paused, looked me in the eyes, and then made the cardinal pronouncement: "The numbness of the anal skin and the rectal muscles make this hemorrhoidectomy a relatively painless procedure."

"Brilliant." I was in reverence.

He then proceeded to suture ligate the base of each hemorrhoid, laying down three knots. He locked the last tie of the knot with a jerk of his hand to prevent the suture from slipping open when it swelled, leading to bleeding. Once the suture was tied, he cut out the internal hemorrhoid above the suture knots.

"To close the anal mucosa from around the dissected-out hemorrhoid, I use a 2-0 chromic suture that starts at the base where we have cut the hemorrhoid and then suture the edges of the mucosa toward the anal verge."

"I see that you left a gap between the mucosa and the skin at the verge," I said. He completed my thoughts, "To let any oozing blood out so it won't build up inside the anal canal."

I nodded.

I removed the hemorrhoidal duckbill retractor, and we observed how the anal sphincter slowly began to contract again, forming the recognizable anus.

"The last thing I do is to divide this band of superficial muscle underneath the skin that I've dissected out, but only in one place. It is the most superficial sphincter of the three bands that make up the external sphincter. I do not touch the internal sphincter."

"Wouldn't this make the patient incontinent?"

It relaxes the sensitive area around the anal verge, preventing pain as the anus begins to contract immediately after an operation and afterward.

Before Dr. Rollo trained me in his technique for performing a painless hemorrhoidectomy, I was taught various methods to prevent residual bleeding in the canal.

"You receive many referrals for this operation, right?" I asked.

He nodded. "Not only has this operation got my four kids through college, but I enjoy doing it because," his triumphant signature said, "The end is in sight from the very beginning!" We chuckled, clearly savoring this glorious moment.

50

THE BURBANK BLUNDER

I have learned that people will forget what you said and did but never forget how you made them feel.
—Maya Angelou

The Continuing Medical Education Program was under Dr. Ross's supervision. An upcoming evening speaker was unable to attend, and he asked me if I would be interested in speaking to the surgical community at the hospital—the surgeons I knew and interacted with daily, who were training me—on a topic of my choice.

I paused. I hesitated.

The mere thought terrified me; I was just a resident who, having arrived in America 18 months earlier, had devoted all my time and energy to learning the art of surgery. I had never needed to prepare a formal presentation. I didn't see myself as qualified to make such an educational leap. I deferred to Dr. Ross's suggestion.

He persisted. He needed a speaker, and my Queen's English accent seemed to command attention, no matter the topic.

To make me feel more comfortable, he said, "You know, you

can talk about your experiences with the British and American healthcare systems." It's just, you know, a chat among friends." As an incentive, he added, "There is a free dinner followed by only a 45-minute talk." I still hesitated primarily because I had never given a speech to an audience; I wasn't familiar with the topic, I wasn't a healthcare expert, and the thought of standing in front of an audience terrified me—I'd probably forget most of what I intended to say.

"You have two weeks to prepare for the talk, and in case I didn't tell you, there is a $250 bonus."

I viewed the invitation as a compliment and felt flattered. The remuneration was equivalent to five blood donations at the Children's Hospital, making it very appealing. I questioned whether two weeks would be enough time to thoroughly research a new topic and create a balanced presentation for an engaging talk, without the distraction of fancy slides. Additionally, there was no facility for me to make them.

The Fitchburg community epitomized quintessential Americana. This rotation provided my first experience with the primary American model of community surgical practice, in which a primary care doctor refers a patient to a surgeon of their choice, creating a competitive system within the community. Patients requiring surgery are admitted to a local hospital where the surgeon is authorized to operate. After the procedure, the patient is seen post-operatively in the surgeon's office before being discharged. The patient's insurance company receives the bill for the visit and the cost of the operation, activating a complex reimbursement system. This private practice competitive structure is euphemistically known as the "Kill to Eat" model: If you do not operate, you do not eat. It motivates surgeons to collaborate with internists and nurses, but primarily with primary care physicians in the community, who would make referrals to them.

In contrast, Brigham was a teaching hospital. Most professors were salaried by the university and compensated for teaching, conducting research, and performing administrative duties, a model known as the "Triple Threat." Until my Fitchburg rotation, I had primarily been exposed to the academic system at Brigham and Children's Hospital.

In the British model, like its American counterpart, the GP refers a patient with a surgical issue to a Surgical Consultant within the National Health Service. However, unlike the American model, British surgeons faced limitations due to specific hours or working sessions. New patients were placed on an ever-lengthening waiting list for openings in the surgeons' sessions. The delay resulted in dissatisfied patients and contributed to the British National Health Service's poor reputation. That was socialized medicine!

When comparing the tension surrounding earning a living between the British and American models, the liberal "Kill to Eat" model is clearly superior for a cutting surgeon and his bottom line. Burbank Hospital epitomized most community hospitals in America, where the "Kill to Eat" model quietly prevailed, and the practice of the "Triple Threat" model did not exist.

Dr. Ross invited Victoria and me to his home on a weekend when we were both off. Armed with a bottle of wine and Victoria carrying some flowers, we joined the Rosses at their warm and lovely home for an early Sunday dinner. Dr. Ross and his wife were very hospitable and kind. To my surprise, the librarian was also invited. I was astonished because such liaisons in hospital friendships always intrigued me. She was a middle-aged divorcee, while the Rosses could have easily been her parents.

I often spent a couple of hours each day between cases in the library reading about surgery—the etiology, pathology, types of operations, and their complications. Usually, I was the only one in the room. Each time I asked her for a book or whether she could photocopy a paper about a study concerning an operation, she would willingly oblige, handing me the work but then lingering, trying to initiate some conversation, which invariably veered towards my or her personal life. At first, I thought she was kind and eager to help me, but over time, I realized she was lonely and sought a closer friendship. I found her obsequiousness unwelcome and did not wish to encourage her intrusion on my study time between operative cases. I eventually used the library for only brief sit-downs, aiming to avoid developing a connection beyond the patron-librarian relationship. It was her library, her space, and it seemed I was the only regular patron.

From the start of dinner, she dominated the conversation and steered it away from surgery—a topic that two surgeons enjoyed discussing—heightening the tension in the room. Victoria didn't warm up to her, which made the lighthearted conversation feel awkward with the quiet Mrs. Ross.

After dinner, she suggested we play Charades. Since most people in the room were physicians, our identity was firmly rooted in reality, and miming seemed like too much work. She pranced before us, dancing around like Isadora Duncan, while our half-hearted guesses were mainly wrong. The whole performance felt painful. Yet Dr. Ross encouraged her to continue reluctantly while we remained her captors. The evening dragged on when it should have developed into some spontaneous, congenial conversation. It ended early since we had to drive a fair way to Newton Highlands.

I finally relented to Dr. Ross's persuasive arguments and agreed to give a talk. I decided partly because, at the Brigham, I had recently attended a couple of Grand Round lectures by two British physicians. The first was a visitor; the second was a non-operating surgeon, Dr. Andrews, who sat in a small office far removed from the department and conducted academic work, assisting in one of Dr. Moore's many projects.

After M&M, Dr. Andrews gave a talk on the British and American healthcare systems. He spoke eloquently, as if addressing a packed house in Parliament, and was warmly received by the faculty, residents, and medical students who filled the auditorium.

Despite the controversial topic that sparked many restless murmurs among the audience, Dr. Moore, a self-proclaimed Anglophile, led an impressive charge in an energetic, erudite, and learned discussion during the Q&A session—an intellectual dialogue. If the audience judged the content of Dr. Andrew's talk poorly or found it irrelevant to surgical practice in Boston, they skillfully kept their opinions to themselves.

The aging, ever-academic Dr. Andrews provided the audience with a reference list of medical papers on his topic, primarily published in the British Medical Journal (BMJ). Recognizing it as a valuable resource for my proposed talk, the obliging librarian at Burbank Hospital obtained most of the papers referenced in the BMJ for me. I prepared my presentation using this body of work, taking copious notes without a slide presentation.

The dreaded evening arrived: the buffet dinner with beef, corn on the cob, potatoes, and green beans, followed by ice cream. I ate very little, as I felt more nervous than hungry.

I noticed that the audience was greater than the sum of the hospital surgeons I knew. Others, too, had gathered. An influx of unrecognized community physicians from all medical disciplines outnumbered the usual friendly faces. A restless and curious tension replaced the gemütlich environment as the audience settled into their seats, and the room grew hot and stuffy.

It was a meeting of the Western North District Medical Society. On stage, flanking me to my left were the Secretary and Treasurer, and to my right was the Vice President—hardly a chatty environment of surgical friends, as had been suggested.

Dr. Ross introduced me after the Secretary and Treasurer delivered some society business. Rising center stage, I nervously stood before a larger gathering of physicians than I had imagined.

Unaccustomed to giving presentations, I read from my prepared notes. As I progressed, the subject matter caused disquiet and agitation among a few vocal audience members. The increasingly restless members interrupted me, seeking clarification on specific points. I wasn't familiar with the subject's nuances, so my answers raised more questions. This disrupted my presentation, as the atmosphere in the room became chaotic with several separate group discussions within the audience that I found unruly and that the Secretary could not control.

Unlike at the lofty Brigham, where this subject was discussed leisurely and scholarly in line with an intellectual dialogue, here at the down-to-earth Burbank Hospital, they wanted me to cut to the chase and give them the bottom line. In my nervousness, I awkwardly handled the Q&A session that followed. Unfortunately, it seemed to leave the audience with the overall belief that I had predicted: that with time, healthcare in the U.S. would become more controlled by others rather than physicians, which smacked of socialized medicine.

Some audience members conveniently overlooked the fact that forms of socialized medicine already existed in the United States. The U.S. Department of Veterans Affairs, the Indian Health Service, the U.S. Public Health Service, and Kaiser Permanente, among other smaller health services, thrived and operated alongside the "Kill to Eat" model.

I recognized my mistake. I had misjudged the audience. This wasn't "a chat among friends," as billed by Dr. Ross, nor was it an academic presentation among experts interested in civil debate; instead, it was a presentation to a specific audience that relied on the only reimbursement model that supported their families, paid for their children's college education, covered their mortgage, car or boat payments, and financed their annual vacations on Cape Cod. They couldn't envision a government-salaried position or a third-party regulating reimbursement and insurance, which would limit their ability to practice. They were not interested in hearing from a junior resident with no standing or qualifications in this field on such a sensitive topic. They interpreted my talk as lauding the National Health Service in a Queen's English accent. The meeting ended in disarray.

I expected the audience to appreciate the talk. Instead, I was left with the clear impression that more people came for the free meal than for the topic or content of my talk.

I was upset.

Dr. Ross was disappointed. A cognitive dissonance came between us, and retrospectively, my talk may have embarrassed him.

The ripples of my induced disquiet even reached the friendly, middle-aged librarian who, despite not having attended the meeting, felt obliged, based on rumors, to behave indifferently toward me. Gone was her pleasant attitude. The library had been my refuge, and now there was nowhere to hide. Such was my discomfort at Burbank.

What could I do about it? I was passing through their community and nearing the end of my rotation. No matter how much I tried to explain that the thesis of my talk was merely a comparison between two systems, not a judgment of one as better, I learned that explanations weren't the way to dig out of a hole. A gloomy cloud of disappointment hung over my head and followed me around the wards and O.R. There must have been some negative feedback to Dr. Ross, too, which eventually found its way to Dr. Moore. I held my breath, wondering what fury would befall me.

In this now cool and somewhat unfriendly atmosphere, I

assisted Dr. Rollo, whose positive outlook on life lifted my spirits. As a general surgeon, he had a tendency toward anal diseases, a five-star Michelin reputation for treating hemorrhoids, skill in successfully operating on them, a strong standing in the community, and indifference to the murky waters of hospital politics, intrigue, and the swirls of toxic rumors. What a gentleman, a surgeon, and a tonic for me.

On the dark Friday, December 24, 1971, Christmas Eve, as I drove under heavy clouds and a gray sky to Burbank Hospital for early morning rounds before heading to the operating room, my disposition had changed. Once, I relished the anticipation of greeting my patients with joy and a positive attitude, knowing I had the support of the attending surgeons. On this post-blunder day, I drove in with apprehension and self-doubt. I felt that I was no longer regarded as a trustworthy member of the surgical team and that I was seeing their patients, not mine, during rounds. The surgeons viewed me differently from the initial impression they had of me. My disposition verged on the depressive. Listening to the emotionally laden Tchaikovsky Symphony No. 6, the Pathétique, playing from my tape deck, my mood mirrored the enraged and melancholic motif of Tchaikovsky's music, winding down to its concluding finale, which represents death.

The weather was near freezing.

It rained.

The roads were slick.

I turned off my music to concentrate more fully on the traffic and the elements. My windshield wiper blades smudged the glass more than they cleared the persistent precipitation. As I drove slowly, navigating traffic and peering through the relatively clear areas of my windscreen, I made a mental note to replace them.

While working with patients during my ward rounds, I glanced out of the hospital's large windows and noticed it had started snowing. As the snow began accumulating on the parked cars, the usual traffic sounds in the parking lot grew muffled. The thought of being stuck in the hospital, now in what felt like an indifferent environment, struck me. I was eager to drive home before the roads became impassable due to the accumulating snow and shifting drifts, akin to a sandstorm. Dr. Ross suggested I spend Christmas Eve with Victoria. The staff would cover for me in my absence, and I truly appreciated this friendly gesture. Shortly after 11 a.m., the snowfall eased, and the sound of snowplows scraping asphalt became audible.

I bolted.

I drove home through the snow and the occasional flurry. The roads to our home were plowed, sanded, and treated with salt. As I arrived, suddenly, bright midday sunshine followed the snow squall.

As I entered our small flat, I was enveloped by the scents of roasting beef, parsnips, and carrots from her cooking, and overwhelmed by the Christmas songs performed by King's College Choir, Cambridge. I felt homesick for England.

Victoria had prepared an excellent meal. I loved coming home and embracing her, regardless of my mood. The comfort of her hug, her face next to mine, the kisses we exchanged, and the imprint of her body against mine reinforced the memory of our love.

I changed into some festive clothes, and we celebrated Christmas Eve with a fine beef roast, Yorkshire pudding, and baked vegetables, which I shared in silent contemplation, attempting to put behind me the bitter failure. I didn't have the gumption to tell Victoria the story of what I considered my Burbank blunder. My personality is such that I could not share the pain and disappointment with her. Maybe I should have, but I had previously experienced a less-than-consoling response to my mental aches and pains, and I didn't want to spoil the excellent festive environment she had created in our little home.

After our customary Christmas calls to Victoria's mother, Shirley, and our mother in England, we enjoyed Christmas pudding set afire with brandy and exchanged gifts. The best gift was snuggling together and finding comfort in her embrace.

51

THE REPLY

The best time to respond to a friend's letters is when you receive them. The warmth of friendship and the intelligence gained then cooperate most effectively.
—Seneca the Younger

I hadn't expected a reply from Dr. Ross after our cognitive dissonance—a psychological state of discomfort that occurs when a person has conflicting beliefs, values, or attitudes. In our case, it pertained to my presentation and how the whole issue was initially presented to me. I took his request, on parting, to send him a letter enumerating all the operations I had done to remind myself that he was still the boss. No other Attending was ever curious enough to know what I had done.

Somehow, our cognitive dissonance became widely known. The German language has a phrase that aptly describes the atmosphere in a room when people who were once friendly toward one another suddenly avoid each other out of discomfort or deliberately refrain from talking to one another due to an awkward interpersonal situation. It is "Dicke Luft," meaning thick or heavy air.

Our uncomfortable feelings arose because we had fundamentally conflicting feelings, assessments, and mindsets concerning my talk. In my case, I hadn't delivered a satisfactory message to the "Kill to Eat" audience. I hadn't reinforced their belief system, not that I was set to change minds, but to present what I believed were different—the US and the British mainstream systems. In Dr. Ross's opinion, I hadn't given a "Team player's talk."

He didn't control the end of the meeting. He didn't stand up, address the audience, or quell discussions; nor did he give a two-sentence summary of the talk with a positive angle to leave the audience in a more constructive frame of mind. Not doing this meant he didn't have Dr. Moore's leadership qualities. Essentially, he abandoned his speaker—a lesson I took to heart. I never applied to be a resident or an invited lecturer in the 25 years I ran my institution's invited speakers' program. Was his lack of action perhaps because he realized I had learned he had misled me about the nature of the audience, which added to his self-discomfort?

We both felt awkward the following month when I was still working at Burbank. I no longer enjoyed going there. We could have clarified the situation by mutually discussing it and achieving a more significant agreement to reduce the dissonance by the time of my departure at the end of January 1972, approximately 30 days after I had given the talk. This would have clarified the situation immediately. Years later, a casual comment by my senior resident, Arvin Phillipart, rang a bell: "Watch out for Dr. Ross." I didn't know what he meant by that.

I shouldn't have dismissed the comments, unaware of what would come when I returned to the Brigham. He signed his letter like Dr. Moore did, who was referred to by his initials, "F.D.M." So, by signing his note to me with "F.P.R.," which no one used at Fitchburg, was he trying to assume Dr. Moore's mantle of fame and authority?

I left with an unresolved situation and the knowledge that, in this case, he wasn't being entirely truthful with me. The librarian's frosty and dismissive attitude toward my presence after my talk should have told me he was a gossip and that he probably would bias any communication with Dr. Moore. I had worked with many first-class chiefs on numerous services. I wish that Dr. Ross had matched their mettle.

With the maturity and hindsight of age, now at 81, I should have gone to Dr. Ross's office and spoken to him. However, I believed that humans tend to think that when things go wrong, "it is my mistake," which regrettably colored my self-opinion for the rest of my clinical time at Brigham.

FREDERICK P. ROSS, M. D.
BURBANK PROFESSIONAL BUILDING
FITCHBURG, MASSACHUSETTS 01420

TELEPHONE: (617) 342-4521

7 March 1972

Michael Meguid, M.D.
Children's Hospital
300 Longwood Avenue
Boston, Massachusetts

Dear Mike:

Thank you for your operative list and your letter. I am glad that the Burbank experience seemed so worthwhile to you. I was particularly interested in your comment about Caesarean sections, this is an operation that I have never done and is almost certain that I never will!

Please give my best to Victoria. Do I gather from your comments that you are expecting a baby? Please keep in touch.

Best regards,

F.P.R.

Frederick P. Ross, M.D.

52

VISA VULNERABILITY

In the middle of our journey, I came to myself in a dark wood where the straight path was lost.
—Dante Alighieri

Returning to the Brigham after my rotation in Burbank, I felt unsettled because Ross had damaged my moral compass. Homecoming meant I was nearing the end of my PG-2/PG-3 year, a time marked by a sense of sadness and sentimentality. Of the two models of surgical life I had encountered, the "Kill to eat"—operate to eat, and the "Triple threat"—operating, teaching, and researching! I preferred the latter.

I still had several weeks of clinical work before starting my one-year term as a research fellow in Dr. Moore's lab. I was assigned to the intensely busy ER service, where I devoted myself to the wounded while feeling hurt myself. I wandered around, feeling lost and disconnected from the Brigham, just as I had once. I yearned to be part of a tight-knit resident team, as I had been with Mort, Howard, and other categorical residents —a sense of belonging.

My pilgrimage through paradise—the department of surgery—had turned into an odyssey through personal hell. I bumped into the administrative resident, Nick O'Connor, on The Pike. I inquired about changing my upcoming rotation from the West Roxbury VA to the Ward Service. I imagined that such a switch, where I would work within the mainstream hospital—the Brigham—rather than the VA, which was far removed from the Brigham in South Boston, would settle me.

Nick O'Connor, a tall Canadian, had completed five years of surgery and was looking to enter a residency in plastic surgery. He was antagonistic, if not unsympathetic, to my request. Such a switch wasn't possible because he had created the yearly schedule for each resident. There was a lack of conviction regarding Nick O'Connor's motives for not trying to change the schedule. He knew I was a provisional resident and didn't care enough to help me. He didn't say, "Well, let's see, or why not ask a fellow resident if he wanted to switch?" Nothing of the sort. He just continued on his way with a haughty attitude. Not helpful.

I worked in the ER for three months, followed by my final clinical rotation at the West Roxbury VA, which is considered one of the least desirable rotations because residents viewed the general surgical program as weak, and the chief at the VA primarily performed cardiac cases.

One of the main shortcomings of the training program was the lack of feedback after each rotation, whether positive or negative. Through my tactful inquiries among the surgeons I had worked with, who had been friendly towards me, consistently received the reply was that I was doing well and that Dr. Moore thought highly of me; however, the decision to advance to a senior or chief resident position was left solely to Dr. Moore.

During our residencies, Victoria and I emotionally transitioned from being ambivalent visitors to Boston to the apprehensive certainty of wanting to stay in the United States. After such a long absence, the idea of a professional life in London had become a vague illusion.

I wanted to hear Dr. Moore inform me that I had been selected to complete my surgical training at Brigham after my research year in his lab. After all, the decision to convert the program into a pyramidal structure by accepting only three residents seemed arbitrary. Why not take four? What was stopping the acceptance of a fourth resident? If that happened, I would graduate with a brand on my forehead: "Trained by FDM," a highly coveted and prestigious recognition that would open doors to elite jobs. As the Chief of Surgery, Dr. Moore decided on advancement to the higher resident levels and the path to success. In essence, he held our future in his hands.

The lack of certainty was very unsettling for someone on a non-immigrant visa. The implications of continuing at Brigham were far reaching. Harvard would convert our visa to a Permanent Resident Card (Green Card) due to a shortage of physicians or a maldistribution of physicians within the United States, thereby opening the path to citizenship and allowing us to live, work, and become citizens in the United States.

Dr. Moore's numerous letters conveyed an ambiguous message: you are a desirable resident, and there may be an opening. As I entered the lab, my mind remained suspended between two contradictory propositions: would my surgical training at the Brigham end after my time in the lab, or would a PG-4 position become available for me? I despised this ambiguity. I would have probably become a psychiatrist if I could tolerate such uncertainty.

No.

My personality was similar to that of a surgeon. In terms of my residency, issues were black or white, yes or no, and involved the question of whether to cut. Certainty underpinned my character. I would have accepted a definitive NO! Without such an invitation to continue my upward mobility, I could plan our life, as the decision also impacted Victoria. However, I'd enter the lab with uncertainty—a feeling of doubt, accompanied by negative emotions like fear, anxiety, and worry. The lack of control over our lives and the inability to plan or predict future outcomes were particularly distressing.

Would Dr. Moore offer me a future gateway?

That is not what happened.

Ironically, that is exactly what happened. Surprisingly, it did not unfold as either he or I expected—the opportunity arose in a whispered verbal offer from Dr. Moore to me when I was completing my two-year research in his lab, a couple of weeks before I was about to leave the Brigham. The outcome surprised us both.

53

PEAK PERFORMANCE

Even miracles take a little time.
—Anonymous

While I was intensely preoccupied with the last few months of my clinical work and lost in my thoughts, Victoria reminded me that I had filial duties at home.

In the late spring of 1973, Victoria was approaching the end of her residency and planned to get pregnant. The pill was stopped, and sex, once a romantic event, became a duty. Husband duty was like being a stud. It became a labor of love.

Once, making love was the fundamental language—an inseparable expression of the human soul, our spirituality, and sexuality—the common vernacular of the need to love, to be accepted, and to receive love as human beings. In return, we want to be touched at our mortal core and receive reassurance.

Now, instead, it became yet another task. There was no escaping the 1-2-degree Fahrenheit temperature spikes that remained steady for three days or more, which were associated with ovulation. I was clawed back from escaping through the front door: "You can't leave now; my temperature is up . . ." With a rising body temperature, Victoria didn't want to take a chance on a missed opportunity. I was no longer on clinical duty; I was now on sex duty. It didn't feel good—no sense of pleasure.

On the domestic front, the accusation was that I was escaping my "filial duties."

What the fuck.

Not again.

I'm drained!

It must have been crowded in those poor Fallopian tubes as thousands of travel-tired front-line competitors seeking the ovum fell back to rest. At the same time, millions more sperm arrived daily, if not hourly, each stepping up to the plate or jostling to be the first in line in some convoluted Fallopian race that made the Boston Marathon appear like a cakewalk—wave upon wave of sperm hustling to be the first to meet and greet the ovum—making the D-Day landings look like child's play. This was serious stuff with no end in sight.

Once I got home, it went on and on. Staying late in the E.R. was becoming increasingly attractive. I'm sure my brain's dopamine and endorphin levels—the body's feel-good hormones—were depleted and utterly spent. This paternal duty felt like a chronic emergency chore. How long will this last?

There was no escaping my dick's duty. My poor penis—that worn-out limp phallus—needs a rest, a 4th of July, a vacation, even a sabbatical.

Would the yearning or the simple pleasure of desire, longing, and lust ever enter her mind again? Would the simple joy of feeling a fine, stiff erection, just for its own sake, like a man would feel a fat, long cigar, ever be re-experienced?

And then . . . finally, she proclaimed, "I think I'm pregnant.

"Think? Please say you *are* pregnant."

"Yes."

"Thank goodness. Sometime in March or April, as the transition from cold, dark winter to bright, warm spring occurred, a new life sprang up within my wife.

I declared my variation of a Churchillian proclamation: Never was so much owed to so few, like Victoria and me, to so many!

54

VAUGHN AVENUE

The magic thing about home is that it feels good to leave.
And it feels even better to come back.
—Anonymous

We calculated that the magic date could have fallen sometime in October 1973, when our family was set to expand. Those were the days when ultrasounds weren't used to predict a baby's sex. However, the ultrasound revealed that the tadpole swimming around appeared healthy. We were grateful that our child would be okay and that our nuclear family would grow. We couldn't imagine a couple being unable to conceive; how very tragic that would be. Our child was a product of love and hard work, and we were happy. Our baby would be born after Victoria had completed her residency while I was in the lab. We needed a larger home, and since I had no idea where to look for it, I left this task to Victoria.

It had been an incredibly exhausting weekend on call. From the moment I walked into the hospital for the 7 a.m. shift, I was occupied with Saturday morning rounds until I finally went home on Monday after the evening 6 p.m. round—36 hours later. During the 7 a.m. rounds, I gathered a long list of scut tasks left unfinished by the residents I was replacing, along with two critically ill patients in the E.R. waiting for emergency operations. The days and evenings were long and challenging. Essential bodily functions like eating, urinating, defecating, pausing to catch my breath, and trying to get some sleep became distant secondary concerns compared to the care my fellow residents and I provided to our sick patients. As time went on and the tasks seemed endless and piled high, we were consumed by routine jobs and one operation after another. The lack of sleep made me anxious that I had forgotten something important that needed to be done, but since I hadn't written it down, I couldn't recall it. Irritability set in among my fellow residents during rounds throughout the day, and prolonged operations led to fuzzy thinking and impaired concentration.

The nurses were my shepherds, guiding me to ensure I meant what I said during rounds. The elderly, motherly nurses recognized the signs of sleep deprivation, noting how I schlepped around the ward in my O.R. blues, unshaven and probably not smelling great. Sleep was the most prominent thought in my mind. Sneaking away to lie down for a few hours of shut-eye filled me with guilt, given the long to-do list waiting for me. Once lying down with my shoes kicked off, I became aware of my throbbing legs and aching feet—appendages that supported me during operations and carried me across the ward on endless rounds. When the phone or my pager roused me from sleep, I felt groggy, disoriented, fatigued, sluggish, and irritable, struggling to concentrate—the state often referred to as "sleep inertia," "sleep desynchronization," or "sleep-psychosis"—a mental disorder where thought and emotions are so impaired that contact is lost with external reality, characterizing a temporary period of diminished cognitive function and reduced alertness that follows waking up from sleep, especially after inadequate rest.

Monday evening rounds couldn't come soon enough. After that, I drove to our two-room home, making sure that in my zombie state I didn't veer down Longwood Ave around Coolidge Corner and into Marion Street before parking behind our apartment.

"Darling, how are you? How was your weekend? I've made dinner for you, as you must be starving."

I'm fatigued, washed out—you know, in a zombie-like state. I could barely keep my eyes open driving home. All I want is a shower and to crash on my bed.

"I saw a perfect house for us! A typical New England Colonial-style house.

"Sounds nice."

"It's just the right size for us. It features a central entrance leading to a large sitting room with a fireplace, a children's room adjacent to a dining room, and a fully equipped kitchen. Upstairs, in addition to our master bedroom, there are two more bedrooms that we can convert into a children's bedroom and a bathroom. Victoria prattled on and on and on. I had long stopped absorbing the details as I stripped on my way to a long, hot shower. Her enthusiasm barely matched my impaired alertness and sense of dehumanization from sleep deprivation. Could she not see that I was a zombie?

"It sounds fantastic. I'm free next weekend," I said, hoping to end the conversation. However, I failed, as she kept talking.

"Oh no! We must see it tonight. The realtor says it's a very desirable house in a leafy, quiet district of Newton Highlands. The schools are among the best. There are other families with little children. "It's a safe district for children to play," she went on.

"Darling, I'm so tired. Can we discuss this tomorrow morning when I've had a chance to catch up on my sleep? Why don't you tell me all this over breakfast? I'm going to have a shower now."

She trailed me into the bathroom. "The realtor says it's well priced, and if we don't see it tonight, we'll lose it. Someone else will buy it."

I turned on the shower, and the mist quickly filled the small room. Victoria's voice reached me through the fog as the hot water cascaded down my neck, back, buttocks, and legs. It felt wonderfully relaxing, enhancing my soporific mood. If I closed my eyes, I might have fallen asleep standing in the shower.

". . . so, we need to see it tonight and make an offer." her voice reached me.

"I can't. I'm too tired to drive. And we have nothing to offer." I hope this last statement gives her pause and makes her drop the subject.

I'll drive, darling. You have to see it, and I can handle the paperwork for an offer. It doesn't need to involve you.

I could see that this was a no-win situation.

She drove west of Boston proper, along Route 9, turned onto the leafy street top, and stopped at Vaughn Avenue. The street was empty at 9 p.m., but halfway down, the third house on the left looked like a "Christmas Tree"—all lit up in the night's darkness. It was painted white, had an attractive red front door, a manicured lawn, and oak trees lining the sidewalks; it appeared like a dream. We sat in silence, admiring the view.

"It's enormous. We'll rattle in it."

"The washer and dryer in the basement are new, and the other half is finished, making it a perfect playroom or even an office for you," she said in a whisper.

I repeated, "Just look at it. It's too large.

It covers 2500 square feet and features a separate garage for your car. Additionally, it is within walking distance of the T, which I can use to commute to the hospital or work.

"How much are they asking for this palace?"

"About $43,000. The realtor says that if we make a down payment of $5,000, we can secure a mortgage for the remaining amount at 5.49%. She states that as two doctors, we'll have no problem getting the bank to give us a 30-year mortgage."

Turning to Victoria, I asked, "Are the three of us planning on staying in America, in Boston, for 30 years?"

"Who knows, but for the 30-year fixed interest rate, the best mortgage rate is 5.49%."

"We only have $2,000 in our account. How do we obtain the additional $3,000?"

As I fell asleep, I agreed with my wife to purchase the house. Being pregnant and envisioning herself graduating as a pediatrician changed her outlook on life. I was too tired to argue with her any further. There seemed to be no other way to increase our wealth than by investing in a house. As I was dropping off to sleep, I experienced a deja vu moment: Burley!

Dear Burley came to mind. "Ask Dr. Moore."

I wrote Dr. Moore a letter. He responded promptly. Dr. Ross, at Fitchburg, was the Treasurer of the "Friends of the Brigham" account.

I wasn't sure Dr. Ross would approve my request after my blunder. He did.

This led me to reevaluate the events that occurred at Fitchburg. My assessment on two fronts is wrong. Dr. Ross viewed my so-called blunder as a youthful mistake, which he contributed to by not informing me beforehand that my talk was intended for a wider audience, including members of the Western North District Medical Society.

What difference would that have made?

Frankly, some.

I would have transmitted the same information with a more appealing spin for the audience. However, that is my assessment at 80 as I write this.

45 Marion Street
Brookline
Mass. 02146

May 3, 1973

Dear Dr. Moore:

I wish to enquire whether it would be possible to borrow $3000 from the Surgical fund for a limited period of time in order to shore up our financial situation. We are in the process of buying a house and the money would go towards lawyer's fees, certain house-hold utilities, e.g. a stove and dishwasher, and for minor adjustments to the house.

As I mentioned to you, we are expecting a child in October and although Victoria is taking her Boards this summer, her work situation has, as yet, not been clarified.

I would appreciate discussing this matter with you further.

Yours sincerely,

Michael Hegeman

The second person I need to re-evaluate is Dr. Moore. I admired him as a leader and assumed he would care for his residents as well. However, that assumption was naïve. Why would he develop a fondness for me? My mistake was seeing him as the father figure I lost at age eleven. I felt flattered to be accepted as a resident in his program, but his apparent absence overshadowed this; he didn't have a surgical service, didn't operate, and, therefore, I lacked the close affiliation that comes from struggling through operations together or receiving direct guidance from him regarding surgical knowledge, skill, and patient care. This lack of surgical intimacy transformed him into a distant hero figure who intimidated me, and I longed for his love and approval. Of course, these were unrealistic psychological constructs.

In my mind, a surgeon operates alongside their trainee in the trenches, standing at the same O.R. table as Burley at the Brigham, Alberto at the Children's, and various surgeons at Burbank Hospital in Fitchburg. There is a certain magic when our gloved hands share the same blood, worry, and care for the patient. When our shared perspective on the human body becomes a source of wonder and beauty, it enhances the complex nature of the work. Isn't that what defines a surgeon? Unfortunately, that was not the case with Dr. Moore, and I had difficulty accepting that he was not a surgeon but the chief administrator and decision-maker.

We moved into 53 Vaughn Avenue, Newton Highlands. After a free weekend and catching up on my sleep, one of my first tasks was to assemble a crib. This came in a kit we bought at Lechmere's retail store. My second task was to prepare a vegetable bed in the backyard.

"How big?"

"Oh, about 3 x 5 feet."

"OK." I toiled with a hand trowel for hours, our only gardening tool. Just beneath the grassy soil lay piles of rocks, forming an endless array that I carted away. Topsoil was spread over the prepared patch, and Victoria began planting rows of seeds, including radishes, parsley, lettuce, and spring onions.

By the end of May, the surrounding trees had begun to bud and leaf, creating a canopy of shade that enveloped our vegetable garden—yet nothing flourished.

A surprise letter from Dr. Gilliland arrived, announcing his upcoming visit to Boston. I was delighted to meet and greet my first mentor from my first job—my medical internship at Bethnal Green Hospital—a professor of endocrinology at the prestigious Royal Postgraduate Medical School at Hammersmith Hospital in London. With his piercing green eyes and welcoming smile, Dr. Gilliland was a quiet, unassuming man gifted with immense personal charm. He had served as a medic with the commandos during World War II in Palestine and retained his vigor and military bearing.

Victoria roasted a leg of New Zealand lamb, served with potatoes, vegetables, and all the trimmings, and even prepared a Trifle Pudding for our guests. I bought some Scotch, which he enjoyed drinking before dinner. We were ready for his visit.

When he arrived, instead of the vigorous man I had known five years ago, we met a frail man who had lost the vigor of youth and a significant amount of weight. In his mid-fifties, he had been diagnosed and treated for esophageal cancer, undergoing radiation therapy and chemotherapy. We sat at the dinner table—one bulging Victoria, a lamentably tired me, and a weak and ailing former boss who nibbled at his meal, having refused a Scotch with ice. The topic of Professor Lord Rosenheim arose again, and how he had shunned me during a job interview at University College Hospital. "Well, dear boy, you were well qualified, but you're not one of his kind," he chuckled as his green eyes looked into mine across the table. I understood. Rosenheim hated Arabs.

He told us he was in Boston to see a surgeon at Mass General for a second opinion. It pained me immensely that my once-hero was sick, that I was helpless to reverse his cancer and weight loss, that he was wasting away before my eyes—I felt powerless. He wanted our help procuring a remote control for his TV in London so that he wouldn't need to get out of bed each time he tried to change the station. We only had a small black-and-white TV with rabbit ears at the time.

Victoria took him to a TV shop the following day, where they discovered he also needed a compatible TV set to use the remote device. She informed me of his visible disappointment. Witnessing this vigorous and intelligent man reflect on his existential situation filled me with overwhelming sorrow. I regretted not being able to shop with him. Instead, I returned to the ER at Brigham, once again depriving myself of the chance to say goodbye to a teacher who had become a friend. He had looked out for me by alerting Mr. Kingdom at University College Hospital about my services to him and even notifying Drs. Wilkinson and Nixon at Great Ormond Street Sick Children's Hospital to consider me for a surgical house job, which I wanted to pursue if the opportunity in Boston didn't work out. I have missed his presence in my life so much. When I returned to London, I would have visited him and his wife, who had once invited Victoria and me to their home in Swiss Cottage, Finchley. Now, I only hold onto his memory, which is positive, unlike my unresolved contention with my father.

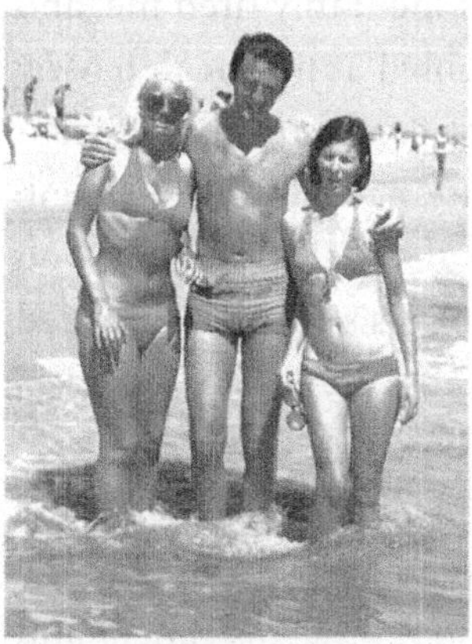

Once we had a house in Boston, and visitors came from England and Egypt. Over the summer, Victoria's medical school friend, Gillian, and her husband, Peter, visited us. We took them to Cape Cod. We established a routine of showing our guests all the tourist sites and restaurants in Boston. One of my favorite aunts was Tante Mustakima. Her son, Ali Moharram, in his early twenties, came to visit and stayed with us for six weeks. With summer over and the stream of guests gone, we looked forward to the arrival of our offspring—this joyful event.

55

THE STUDY THAT CONSUMED HIM

Commitment is what transforms a promise into a reality.
—Anonymous

Dr. Moore was engrossed in a national study from 1970 to 1975. Called "The Study on Surgical Services for the United States," known as SOSSUS, it was a comprehensive examination of surgical care in the United States, which consumed his time for five years at the expense of his other commitments. This study consumed him. It took away his time and dedication from the rounds with residents on the Ward Service and his commitment to me and other research fellows he had accepted into his lab, with whom he was to work closely on advancing his metabolic projects and his research legacy. But SOSSUS kept him preoccupied and often required him to travel to distant communities throughout the United States to gather data from various local surgical committees, exacerbating his absence from the Brigham, his lab, and his trainees. The study involved collecting information on the number of surgeons, the size of the community, whether the surgeons were too busy, how long it took for new patient appointments to be seen, the equipment wealth of the local hospital, the society and local politics that allowed for competitive surgical practice, and more, resulting in his absence.

When I entered the lab from 1972 to 1974, unaware of his total time commitment to the SOSSUS project, I often thought he and I would work together on his metabolic problems and legacy.

I was wrong.

I was a one-man team because he was unavailable when I had questions about my research project or how to present my data. As time progressed and the research became more sophisticated, Dr. Moore was perceived as an absent landlord in his lab. I wanted him to mentor me. Would Dr. Judah Folkman have betrayed his time to his research fellows?

Dr. Moore was focused on the SOSSUS study, which assessed the number of surgeons being trained and their subspecialties. Who was training them in each community across the U.S.? It also evaluated the current and future needs of surgeons in each discipline.

SOSSUS emerged at a critical time, marked by cuts in federal and third-party funding, a significant rise in the number of foreign medical graduates like Victoria and me, and increasing enrollments in medical schools. At the same time, fewer surgeons were filling budgeted surgical faculty roles in teaching hospitals, where the income was considerably lower than that of private practice.

Dr. Moore served as the vice-chair of the project sponsored by the American College of Surgeons and the American Surgical Association. Hundreds of community surgeons participated in a five-year effort to understand and improve surgical care delivery. The study collected and analyzed data on the number of practicing board-certified surgeons, their geographical distribution, workload, and the interactions of surgery with other medical specialties, the community, and the legal system.

The study highlighted the importance of maintaining clinical competence and providing adequate training for future surgeons. Published in three volumes in 1975, it offered recommendations on the training and number of surgeons required in each subspecialty to inform future healthcare planning.

He'd return with the facts to Boston and add them to his database. As he passed through the lab from his office to the door on the far side leading to The Pike, he'd occasionally walk by my desk and linger. "Imagine," he said, "Surgeons operate only on hernias for five hours twice a week and play golf on Wednesday . . ." Walking away from me down the lab toward the west door, he'd add, "Their surgical workloads are too low, and yet they make a living . . ." Since I didn't fully understand the context of his remarks about SOSSUS, his statements left me baffled. What did this have to do with my research problems?

Based on such information, the end product of the five-year commitment, among other suggestions, was to recommend that fewer general surgeons be trained, as it was projected that they'd have even less work to do. Fifty years later, it is evident that the inadequate supply of surgeons, including specialty surgeons in the United States, is partly due to the three-volume SOSSUS report published in 1975.

56

THE SOSSUS CONFLICT

Conflict is inevitable, but combat is optional.
—Max Lucado

Remembering that Dr. Moore wanted his residents to publish, I transformed my notes comparing the British and American healthcare systems into a manuscript after conducting in-depth research, dedicating my evenings to it after grueling hours in the emergency room. Writing, rewriting, and polishing the various drafts took nearly three weeks. I submitted it to Dr. Andrews for review, and he provided suggestions that strengthened the comparison between the two systems. The manuscript did not favor one type of arrangement over the other; however, like all stories, its conclusion remained ambiguous, allowing the reader to interpret its message.

Dr. Andrews declined my invitation to be a co-author because I conducted the research and wrote the manuscript. His scientific stance against being an "honorary author"—essentially meaning he was being given credit for work he did not do—was correct, as this practice is deemed unethical in academic circles.

Once I finished, I sent a copy to Dr. Moore for feedback. A week later, he returned the manuscript with some minor changes, but he did not include a cover note or request a discussion. Two weeks later, I completed my writing and continued to refine the manuscript during my free evenings. Out of respect for both men, I acknowledged Dr. Moore and Dr. Andrews for their contributions. Relieved and pleased with my work, I submitted the final draft to The New England Journal of Medicine. The manuscript took about eight weeks from my initial notes to submission. As was my practice, I sent both men a copy of the final manuscript, sensing that The Journal would either reject it outright since it was a single-author paper and I wasn't a healthcare expert, or review it before dismissing it. Frankly, I wasn't interested in the topic, but having an accepted paper in The Journal would enhance my curriculum vitae as a young surgeon trying to establish my reputation.

My focus was now on finishing my work in the E.R., where Nuala organized a small farewell party for me at the end of my shift before I started working at West Roxbury, Virginia.

The turbulence of the past few months has subsided, and the end of my clinical commitment to Dr. Moore's residency is clearly in view—three months to go.

West Roxbury, VA, here I come.

Emotionally, I rebalanced after the Burbank blunder. All was quiet, and my feelings aligned with the environment that required residents to submit two papers each year to ensure their upward mobility.

On the way home from the VA, I listened to Tchaikovsky's Pathétique Symphony No. 6, first in my car and then on my record at home on my Fischer stereo. Gradually, the music swells, reflecting my gloomy mood and representing the mourning of my clinical service in the E.R.—melding into the gently played, harmonious Adagio. It soon shifts to faster, more nervous, anxious, and uneasy intertwining notes from the full blast of trumpets, French horns, trombones, and tubas blaring, interweaving, and struggling against the violins, violas, cellos, and double bass, all filled with intense urges until it reaches a thundering climax underscored by the bass drum and cymbals . . . leading to a pause—a moment of complete, deadly peace before . . . And in that precious moment of quiet, the telephone rang.

It was Dr. Moore who called me at home in the evening. Imagine being at home, trying to unwind while listening to the marvelous Pathétique! I still remember the ringing—the invasion of my peace. I recall, fifty years later, as if it had happened last night, when Tchaikovsky's movement returned to the divine, lamentoso theme.

In a furiously agitated tone, he bellowed into the phone. He demanded that I withdraw the manuscript. "You aren't a Healthcare Policy Expert. The manuscript smacks of anti-American!"

My blood froze in my arteries as my heart stopped. My body tensed as if crushed in the vice of Dante's hellish making. Breathing ceased. My grip on the receiver tightened, fingers blanched, as our benefactor lashed me furiously while my guts twisted so tightly that I was going to crap on the spot. Unable to breathe or even to respond to the ceaseless vituperous assault on my senses, I took the verbal strikes, the body blows, and the crippling venomous flow coming through the phone. In my mode of paralytical fear, he continued to admonish me for attempting to talk, or did he mean to write about this topic and express what he considered my un-American views, etc., etc., etc. I heard the existential tones of Tchaikovsky's dying tones.

He could have told me, "You're an ungrateful resident for everything I've done for you." Instead, I heard him roar angrily, "I doubt that we have an opening here for you for promotion into a solid senior resident." He added, "You should continue your residency in Baton Rouge."

Did he say Baton Rouge? Baton Rouge?

Yes. Baton Rouge, during the tumultuous 1973 race riots in the South, felt to me like banishment to the intellectual desert of Siberia, far from the hallowed halls of Harvard.

He abruptly hung up.

I felt faint.

"What was that all about?" asked Victoria. I couldn't speak because my mouth was parched.

I sat down, nearly vomiting. My world had ended. My paper was misrepresented, leading to a downward spiral into Dante's last level of hell. I had dragged Victoria down with me, as she, too, was on a non-immigrant visa. Dr. Moore had thrown us into an existential crisis because he controlled our visa status.

I was devastated.

I was petrified.

Was I going to be fired?

I never expressed anti-American sentiments or thoughts, neither verbally nor on paper, because we had no anti-American feelings. America had become our home. So why would I feel that way? Anti-American? It made no sense. He did not provide an example of where an anti-American statement, sentence, or word appeared in the manuscript. Had he not read the manuscript? By now, the furor over the Burbank blunder should have passed. What had ignited those embers? What was the reason? What had triggered this outburst?

I was on my final clinical rotation a few months before joining his laboratory. I envisioned working with him because he no longer had a surgical service and didn't perform surgeries.

Dr. Moore wields power. Such was his control over our lives; such was our vulnerability. If he terminated our visa, he would force Victoria and me to return to London, both half-trained.

Given this crisis, neglecting past academic and professional contacts in London exacerbated the situation.

I sat down and, in a trembling voice, tried to explain to Victoria that I believed this phone call concerned the recent events in Burbank. The fallout seemed endless. Something or someone had precipitated this calamity. Dr. Moore had read the manuscript a week ago, and everything was fine. His anger didn't make sense, as it was disproportionate to the situation. Nightmares haunted me.

But the damage was done. From that moment, I felt the unease of a persona non grata, much like the feelings I experienced when my mother abandoned me at the age of 4. I recognized that my emotions were part of the symptoms associated with complex PTSD—the effects of anxiety and uncertainty. There was no calling his office for a dressing down with an explanation. No. Just vagueness, uncertainty, and no valid reason. "Anti-American" was an emotion; for a scientist, the description wasn't in keeping with an analytical mind.

Profoundly humiliated and feeling uncertain, I repented and withdrew the manuscript. Now I felt like Dante; except instead of his nine circles of Hell, I sat in a tub of doo-doo in my tenth circle of Hell!

Wherever I looked or walked around the hospital, I imagined people gazing at me strangely, knowingly, with disdain or pity. The feeling of drifting helplessly was paralyzing. I felt cast off.

For a brief moment, I wondered if his sudden decision was related to steroids, which are known to increase irritability, anxiety, aggression, and mood swings. When he experienced severe asthma exacerbations, the Chief Resident on the Ward Service had to rush to his home to administer a steroid injection to help with his breathing. Yet, in my vulnerability, I failed to consider whether he might be acting due to aggravating factors in his life that had nothing to do with me. I had no idea.

I was working in isolation. But now, with the vigor of life in my eighth decade, I look back with greater objectivity and clarity. I assess that he was so engrossed in the SOSSUS that my message comparing two different cultural healthcare systems was an irritation to the likely message of his major report.

Ironically, my last rotation during the two clinical years was at the West Roxbury Veterans Administration Hospital, where U.S. Veterans received free healthcare through America's most extensive socialized medical program. Driving to the Veterans Hospital in Jamaica Plain, I listened to Tchaikovsky's 6th Symphony, which was dramatic and haunting, matching my mood. At the VA, I was out of Dr. Moore's sight. I kept my head down, convinced the whole world could see my sense of shame.

My fellow resident at the VA was Hillel Laks, originally from South Africa, while the chief, Dr. Ernest Barsamian, was an Egyptian Armenian. They remained silent if they knew of my disfavor.

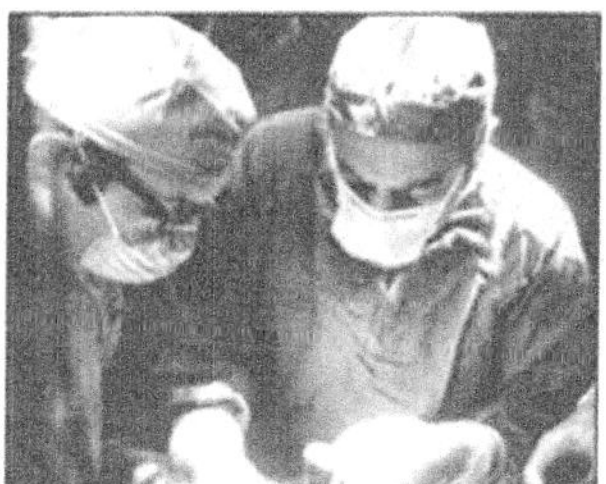

Drs. Meguid & Barsamian

Dr. Laks, who was interested in thoracic surgery, and I assisted Dr. Barsamian in performing cardiac operations almost daily. These procedures weren't as well-coordinated as at Brigham. Several minor problems—little "hiccups"—occurred in the choreography among the surgical, pump, and anesthesia teams. The operations didn't flow smoothly.

This irritated me and frustrated Dr. Barsamian, who seemed to struggle constantly. The veterans were not preselected, nor were the patients at the Brigham. They were elderly and less well-nourished than those at the Brigham. Most had smoked, had poor lung reserves, and some were alcoholics developing delirium tremors after alcohol withdrawal, prone to ripping out chest tubes, Foley urinary catheters, and dressings. Additionally, they had more advanced and established cardiac disease. The outcome wasn't as gratifying as Dr. Barsamian had hoped. Likewise, my time at the VA wasn't fulfilling, as I felt miserable most days due to the scarcity of general surgical cases and my persistent unease about my future.

My unhappiness intensified, and my stress skyrocketed when I received a letter from Dr. Moore dated March 23, 1972, ten days after I had received Dr. Ross's phony "Thank you note." The sight of that dreaded envelope filled me with discomfort in the pit of my stomach, even more than receiving a letter from the I.R.S.

After the telephone call and my withdrawal of the manuscript, I thought we had settled the matter.

Not so!

> I doubt that we have an opening here for you for promotion into solid senior residency work. I believe that you should plan elsewhere or, if you wish, into one of the surgical specialties here.
>
> Very truly yours,
>
> FDM: imh
>
> Francis D. Moore, M.D.

His letter was a two-page zinger about the manuscript—like a bullet crashing through me, reigniting an adrenaline rush. My eyes fell on the last paragraph—the verdict in his dictated letter. Its bluntness was inconsistent with the man of charm. Yet, in its decisiveness, it is stated unequivocally and unambiguously in the last paragraph—"**You are not wanted here.**" My gut reaction matched the news I had once heard, ". . . your mother wanted to abort you . . ."

The feelings that awoke in me were those defined by Complex-PTSD. This mental health state develops after an infant is raised with as few attachments and excessive tenderness is provided as occurs when a young child is abandoned by a parent and experiences prolonged emotional deprivation, which includes feelings of shame, guilt, worthlessness, and heightened emotional responses.

He had effectively shut the door to my clinical career at Brigham. I'd only a few weeks left before completing my VA rotation, after which I'd have to work alongside Dr. Moore in the lab on his projects for the next 12 months. With all the poison he was spewing, shaming me, and grossly inhibiting my sense of well-being, how could a creative, collaborative relationship work?

After his secretary had typed the letter, and possibly a day or two later, when he came to sign it, Dr. Moore added a handwritten postscript. This would be visible only on my copy, not the archived carbon, which he subsequently claimed would be locked up together with his personal papers for 100 years.

Did the handwritten note indicate a softening of attitude? Perhaps a pang of regret or guilt, since this retort didn't align with what he had observed over the previous one and a half pages. Did he fear that his letter, lacking the postscript, would lead to my quitting his program by the end of June instead of honoring my commitment to work in his laboratory? He wrote it because a truly powerful person wouldn't need to display his power to his subordinates. Instead, he possessed the omnipotence to be magnanimous.

Why wasn't I there now if I had been "highly desirable for that position" in September 1971? What had changed? Could it be that he decided it would be wise to hang onto me until it was crystal clear that he had enough categorical residents or others to fill the ranks of the last two senior years? If so, I was a mere cog in his residency wheel—an insignificant individual. He was no longer stringing me along for effectively he had fired me.

Whatever my private anxieties and uncertainty, the effect of his postscript was to soften my landing. Furthermore, he had bought himself 365 days to "must talk together some before you make solid plans." Did the "must" mean he cared? I was confused.

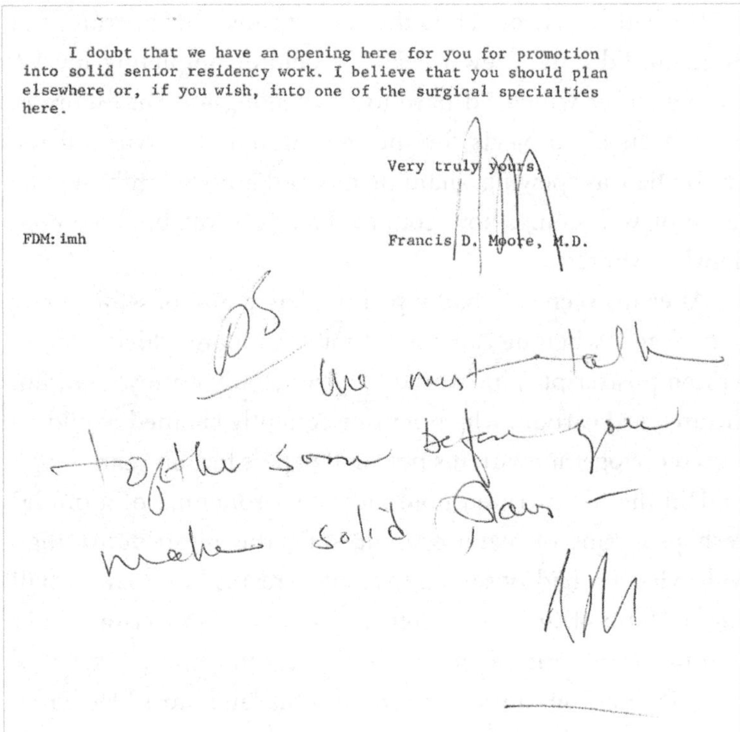

I doubt that we have an opening here for you for promotion into solid senior residency work. I believe that you should plan elsewhere or, if you wish, into one of the surgical specialties here.

Very truly yours,

FDM: imh

Francis D. Moore, M.D.

PS We must talk together some before you make solid plans —

Twelve months passed during the following academic year, from July 1972 to June 1973, when I was in the lab, and no such plans "to talk" were made. To me, a year felt like an incredibly long period of uncertainty. Since we didn't meet to discuss my future, my situation and uncertainty couldn't have been that urgent for him.

Dr. Moore's letter occupied my thoughts throughout the next day as I held a retractor, lost in contemplation, during one of Dr. Barsamian's lengthy cardiac cases.

I needed a Plan B.

I had to find another general surgery training program in Boston since Victoria had one more year at Children's to complete her training. We had made our domestic plans and wanted to stay in Boston, closer to England than elsewhere.

Despite being happy at the Children's Hospital, I was too embarrassed by my discomfort to ask Dr. Folkman for help finding a job. In my distress, I failed to recognize that he might have connections to the surgical world beyond those of Dr. Moore.

But Dr. Barsamian did. "Call Lester Williams at Boston City Hospital. He's looking for a resident," was all he said.

That evening, I drove home slowly from the West Roxbury VA Hospital, contemplating my conflicting interpretations of Dr. Moore's intentions while soaking in the stunning array of emotions boldly expressed in the loud and revolutionary slow tempo of the grand Finale—the Adagio Lamentoso of Tchaikovsky's 6th symphony. Like Tchaikovsky, I too tried to resolve my anguish. Listening to the Finale now became my tortured closing notes. The magnificent composition felt like a parallel to my life, as the slow music's downward slide from its high point, my vigorous surgical life at the Brigham and Children's Hospital, faded in tone and led to death's darkness, much like my Burbank Blunder, in parallel with Tchaikovsky's notes ending silently. I, too, fell deep into darkness.

I learned that I can't control the pain I experienced, nor the crap that gets put in my head from my own doing or that of others. However, I was learning that I could control how I responded.

"We must talk together before you make some solid plan" was clear to me. However, he was never available whenever I tried to set up an appointment with him. Months passed. Finally, after the pain of disappointment had faded and the "we must talk together . . ." had been scheduled, six months after his letter and three months into my time in the lab, I applied to Dr. Lester F. Williams at Boston City Hospital.

Dr. Williams invited me for an interview. I drove two miles across Boston from Brigham to Boston City Hospital, where I met Dr. Williams, Dr. Hirsch, Chief of Trauma, and Dr. Mannick, Surgeon-in-Chief of the Boston University Program.

During the interview, I gingerly mentioned the likelihood of staying in the lab at the Brigham for two years until June 1974 to complete my research. All the interviewees unanimously agreed that I could continue my surgical study and start my residency as of July 1, 1974.

Before I left the medical center, an unscheduled interview with Dr. Egdahl was arranged, as we shared mutual research interests. Dr. Egdahl interviewed me in his corner office suite at the top of the University Hospital. After reviewing my curriculum vitae, which included 18 published research papers, our interview became informal, resembling a conversation about our parallel research pursuits. The controversy at the time centered around whether the impetus for the response to the trauma event was transmitted to the brain via nerves, as he had demonstrated, or through blood messengers, as Dr. Moore believed.

As we chatted, I finally picked up a clue that had previously eluded me. Drs. Moore and Egdahl were rivals in research, and as it turned out, also in the struggle to become president of the prestigious New England Surgical Society, thereby becoming the influencer of the New England surgical world.

Although I fell in love with research in Dr. Moore's laboratory, I knew deep in my bones that I was always destined to be a cutting-edge surgeon. On my drive back to the Brigham, I felt the interview had gone well. I sensed that my future in completing the surgical residency was assured, as was Victoria's future. With these thoughts came a phrase from Nietzsche, "No one can build you the bridge on which you, and only you, must cross the river of life."

My vibes were confirmed when I received a letter from Dr. Lester Williams dated July 10, 1973. Clutching that lifeline letter, I slept peacefully that night in Victoria's arms, free from the tyranny of anxiety and worry. Our future in Boston was secured, as I had verbally accepted Dr. Lester Williams's offer.

Invictus
by William Ernest Henley

Out of the night that covers me.
Black as the pit from pole to pole,
I thank whatever gods may be
For my unconquerable soul.
In the fell clutch of circumstance,
I have not winced nor cried aloud
Under the bludgeonings of chance
My head is bloody, but unbowed.
Beyond this place of wrath and tears
Looms but the Horror of the shade,
And yet the menace of the years
Finds and shall find me unafraid.
It matters not how strait the gate,
How charged with punishments the scroll,
I am the master of my fate.
I am the captain of my soul.

EPILOGUE

Great is the art of beginning, but greater is the art of ending.
—Henry Wadsworth Longfellow

After completing his many administrative tasks, including the lengthy SOSSUS project, Dr. Moore retired and relocated to the Countway Library, where he began writing his memoir.

I had the chance to visit him on Friday mornings at the Countway starting in 1978, when I was an Associate Professor of Surgery at the City of Hope in Duarte, California, and also a graduate student in the Department of Nutrition and Food Science at the Massachusetts Institute of Technology in Cambridge, MA. I often took the red eye to Boston, arriving at 6 a.m. After showering at MIT, I would visit Dr. Moore by 8 a.m. Usually, the Thesis Committee met by 11 a.m., when I delivered my research progress reports.

During my visits, he perceived me differently due to the shift in power between us, which allowed him to speak openly about the past. Gradually, he revealed himself not as a giant of the academic surgical world, the revered Chief of Surgery, but as an ordinary, flawed man with the full range of feelings that come with being human—compassion, contradictions, regrets, slights, grudges, and the deep pain of disappointments. Now, in my eightieth year, I recognize some of the characteristics in myself. Nevertheless, he was a tantalizing and provocative person who would always remain my Chief of Chiefs.

Several years later, I would attend Dr. Moore's Memorial Service.

REFERENCES

Chapter 3. Brigham Façade and directory map: Courtesy of Catherine Pate, Brigham and Women's Hospital Archivist, Harvard Medical School, Center for the History of Medicine, Countway Library, Boston, Mass. With Permission.

Chapter 7. Illustrations of amputation from "Procedures in Vascular Surgeries," Published in 1960 by Little Brown and Co, Boston, MA, with Permission.

"Attitude," Charles R. Swindoll. Permission requested. Reply pending.

"You Mustn't Quit": By Edgar Albert Guest (1881-1959)—Public Domain.

"The Anesthetist" by Karin Cotterman. With permission, Canadian Medical Association Journal courtesy of Canadian Medical Association.

Chapter 11. Photograph of Dr. William Osler: By Elliott and Fry

(~1910) from the Welcome Collection 13318i. Johns Hopkins Octagonal Ward. Published on Wikipedia.com. Public Domain.

Chapter 12. Left Normal Large Bowel (L) and Diseased Sections of Bowel (R): With Permission National Institute of Diabetes and Digestive and Kidney Diseases, National Institute of Health

Chapter 13. Patient with Breast Tumor and Radical Mastectomy. Courtesy of Meredith Publishing Company, 1964 / Appleton-Century-Crofts Inc., 1958.Chapter 14. Side view of Breast: Illustration used with permission from geekymedics.com.

Chapter 15. Abdominal Walls and Common Incisions. Interior Gastrointestinal Section. Illustration used with permission from geekymedics.com.

Chapter 16. Liver, Spleen, Gall Bladder, Stomach Diagram, and Abdominal Hernia. Wikipedia.com. Public Domain.

Chapter 19. Powell K. Grocery shopping with my mother. Soft Skull Press. New York. NY. ISBN 9781593767

Chapter 20. General Hospital USA. Credit given to American Lore.
Chapter 26. Normal Coronary Artery and Narrowed Coronary Artery – Society of Thoracic Surgery. Wikipedia.com. Public Domain.

"Around the Corner" by Charles Hanson Towne. Public Domain.

Chapter 33. Habal MB, Meguid MM, and Murray JE: The long-scarf syndrome - a potentially fatal and preventable hazard. J Am. Med Assoc 1972; 221:1269-1270.

Chapter 39. Imperforated Anus. Modified from Monologues of a Pediatric Surgeon, 2011. Courtesy of Alberto Pena, Editor James P. Cunningham III. By Trent Muller, Esq.

Chapter 40. No Nose Baby: Photo from Reddit.com. Posted on Reddit.com.
Pharynx: Courtesy of the Canadian Cancer Society.

Chapter 42. "Annabel Lee" by Edgar Allen Poe, Public Domain.

Chapter 43. Dudrick et al. Long-Term Total Parenteral Nutrition and Growth, Development, and Positive Nitrogen Balance. With permission, Surgery 1968. 64, 134-142.

Chapter 49. External/Internal hemorrhoids. From King J E. In: Mayo Clinic on Digestive Health. *How to prevent and treat common stomach and gut problems*, 2nd ed. Rochester, MN; Mayo Clinic Press, 2004, page 47; With permission of Mayo Foundation for Medical Education and Research, all rights reserved.

Chapter 56. "Invictus" by William Ernest Henley, P.D. Public Domain.

Medical Illustrations, Chapters 10, 13,15, 25, 35, 39, 40, 44. Trent Muller, at trentmuller68@icloud.com, Marco Island, Florida.

SELECTED BIBLIOGRAPHY FOR GREAT JOYS, GREAT SORROWS

Alivizatos, P.A. *Mission ... at a Price*. A Transplant Odyssey. Ingram 2020.

Gawande, A. *Complications*. Metropolitan Books, 2002.

Gross, R.E., W.B. *An Atlas of Children's Surgery*. Saunders Company, 1970.

Holinger, D.P. 2020. *The Anatomy of Grief*. Yale University Press. New Haven & London. ISBN: 978-0-300-22623-2.

Kratzner, A. Harsh Nazi Parenting Guidelines May Still affect German children of today. *Scientific American*. January 4, 2019. https://www.scientificamerican.com/article/harsh-nazi-parenting-guidelines-may-still-affect-german-children-of-today1/

Larrey, D. J. *Memoirs of Military Surgery*. Part I. Cox and Son, St. Thomas's Street.

Lown, B. 1996. *The Lost Art of Healing*. Houghton Mifflin Co., New York. ISBN: 0-395-82525-3.

Moore, F. D. 1995. *A Miracle & a Privilege*. Joseph Henry Press, Washington, D.C. ISBN: 0-309-05188-6.

Pena, A. 2011. *Monologues of a Pediatric Surgeon*. ISBN-10: 0-9846432-0-6

Schein, M. Ed. *A Companion to Aphorisms & Quotations for the Surgeon*. Tmf Publishing Ltd, Shrewsbury, UK. ISBN 978 1 903378 6 8.

Selzer, R. 1976. *Mortal Lessons: Notes on the Art of Surgery*. Harvest Book, Harcourt Brace & Co., New York. ISBN: 0-15-600400-3

Warren, R. 1960. *Procedures in Vascular Surgery*. With permission. Little, Brown and Co.

ACKNOWLEDGMENTS

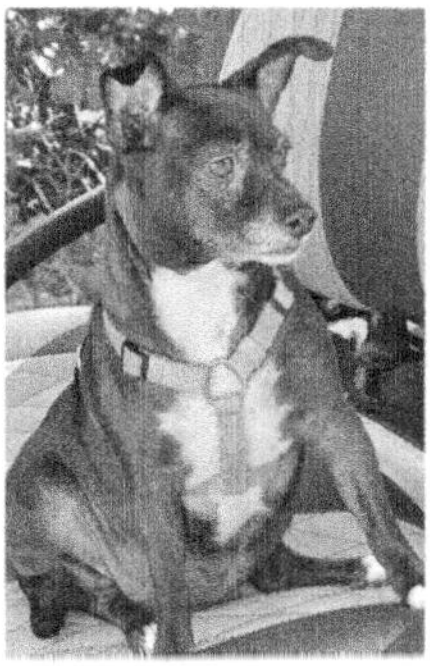

Writing can be a solitary task, but it was made less so by everyone who helped me tell this story. Family and friends generously assisted by reading, editing, making suggestions, and encouraging me to complete this work.

Among them is my dear Jo-Ann Sanborn, and friends Lori Stone, Joan Gerberding, Adrian Rubin, M.D., Mike Welsh, and my good friend Richard Lynn, M.D. Trent Muller kindly created some of the surgical anatomy diagrams that enhanced the book.

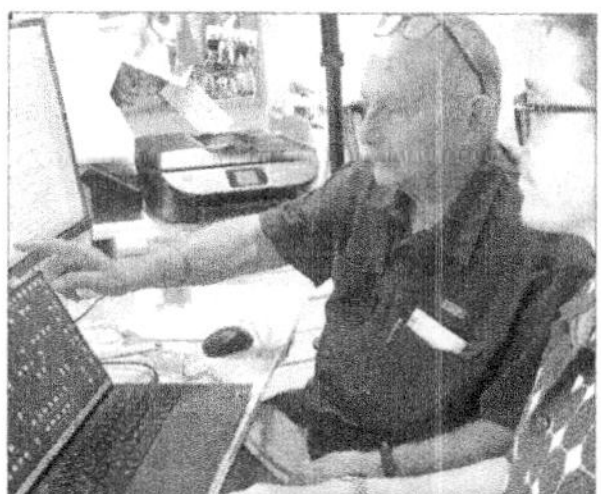

As always, I sincerely appreciate the magic of Carolyn Ring, who once again transformed a manuscript filled with numerous photos, letters, poems, and anatomical diagrams into *Great Joys, Great Sorrows.* Not to be forgotten is my rescue dog Sophie, who filled the void in my heart after Lucy passed away.

Great Joys, Great Sorrows,

A Surgeon's Odyssey Through Surgical Residency

Volume IV of a *Surgeon's Tale*

is available on Amazon, Kindle, and Audible.

Coming Soon:

Volume V--*The Enemy of Good is ... Better*

If you enjoyed the book, join other dear readers and

write a review on Amazon and Audible.

★★★★★

ABOUT THE AUTHOR

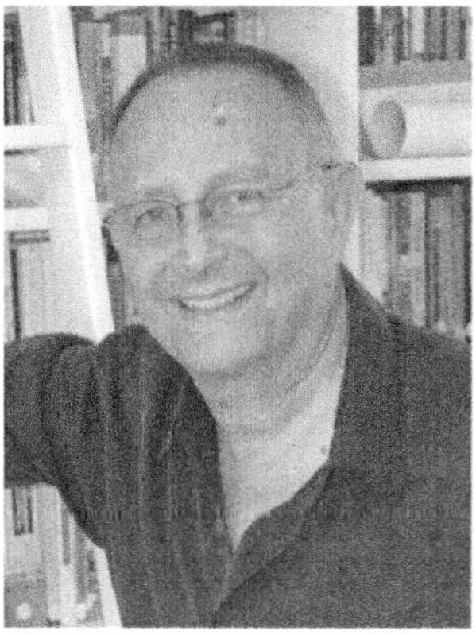

Born in Cairo into an Egyptian German culture, Dr. Meguid attended University College Hospital Medical School, London. He trained at the Peter Bent Brigham Hospital, Harvard, under the surgical pioneer Dr. Francis D. Moore and at Boston University under Dr. John A Mannick. He simultaneously studied with the renowned Vernon Young Ph.D., Hamish Monro Ph.D., and Nevin Scrimshaw M.D. Ph.D., at MIT in nutritional metabolism to develop and deliver lifesaving nutrition to his starving cancer patients. He is a Professor Emeritus of Surgery, Nutrition, and Neuroscience in Syracuse, New York, and Creator and Editor-in-Chief Emeritus of *Nutrition: The International Journal of Applied and Basic Nutritional Sciences*. Known by his peers as the velvet fist, he dished out exacting tough love to his residents because they were going to be our future surgeons, while being compassionate and patient-oriented.